ON CALL

D0922334

SURGERY

Be *on call* with confidence!

Successfully managing on-call situations requires a masterful combination of speed, skill and knowledge. Rise to the occasion **with W.B. SAUNDERS COMPANY'S On Call Series!** These pocket-size resources provide you with immediate access to the vital, step-by-step information you need to succeed!

Other titles in the On Call series

ON CALL
SURGERY

GREGG A. ADAMS, MD

Resident and Walter V. and Idun Y. Berry Fellow
Department of Surgery
Stanford University Medical Center
Stanford, California

STEPHEN D. BRESNICK, MD, DDS

Clinical Instructor
Division of Plastic and Reconstructive Surgery
University of Southern California, School of Medicine
Childrens Hospital, Los Angeles
Los Angeles, California

W.B. SAUNDERS COMPANY
A Division of Harcourt Brace & Company
Philadelphia London Toronto Montreal Sydney Tokyo

W.B. SAUNDERS COMPANY
A Division of Harcourt Brace & Company

The Curtis Center
Independence Square West
Philadelphia, Pennsylvania 19106

Library of Congress Cataloging-in-Publication Data

On call surgery / Gregg A. Adams, Stephen D. Bresnick.—1st ed.

p.   cm.

Includes index.

ISBN 0–7216–6432–6

1. Surgical emergencies—Handbooks, manual, etc.   2. Surgery—
Complications—Handbooks, manuals, etc.   I. Bresnick, Stephen D. II. Title.
[DNLM: 1. Emergencies—handbooks.   2. Surgery, Operative—handbooks.
WO 39 A213o 1997]

RD93.A32 1997   617'.026—dc21

DNLM/DLC   96–29954

Cover illustration is *OPUS 1972,* enamel on steel, by Virgil Cantini, PhD, from the private collection of the artist.

On Call Surgery   ISBN 0–7216–6432–6

Copyright © 1997 by W.B. Saunders Company.

All rights reserved.   No part of this publication may be reproduced or transmitted in any form or by any means, electronic or mechanical, including photocopy, recording, or any information storage and retrieval system, without permission in writing from the publisher.

Printed in the United States of America.

Last digit is the print number: 9   8   7   6   5   4   3   2   1

To our families

PREFACE

Many of the educational situations encountered during medical training occur during nights spent "on call." Although this is a time of learning, it is also a time of stress owing to fatigue, heavy workloads, and decreased availability of staff support. In addition, the on-call team may have responsibility for patients about whom limited information is available. *On Call Surgery* is designed to guide medical students, surgical house officers, and young practicing physicians through some of the more common clinical problems in a well-organized, concise, and informative manner.

Most medical didactic education starts with a disease process, then explains the resulting clinical findings. The training at the bedside, however, starts with a physical complaint or a finding, and the disease is revealed through careful listening, observation, and deduction. In order to facilitate this transition, the structure of *On Call Surgery* starts with the initial phone call describing a patient problem. A list of likely diagnoses is generated and a plan for assessment and management of the patient is outlined. Particular emphasis is placed on the special needs of the postoperative patient and on potential life-threatening situations.

The structure and content of *On Call Surgery* will be helpful as points of reference and guides to the management of many of the typical problems encountered while caring for surgical patients. We believe that the reader will find *On Call Surgery* to be one of the most valuable resources available.

Gregg A. Adams

Stephen D. Bresnick

NOTICE

Surgery is an ever-changing field. Standard safety precautions must be followed, but as new research and clinical experience broaden our knowledge, changes in treatment and drug therapy become necessary or appropriate. The editors of this work have carefully checked the generic and trade drug names and verified drug dosages to ensure that the dosage information in this work is accurate and in accord with the standards accepted at the time of publication. Readers are advised, however, to check the product information currently provided by the manufacturer of each drug to be administered to be certain that changes have not been made in the recommended dose or in the contraindications for administration. This is of particular importance in regard to new or infrequently used drugs. It is the responsibility of the treating physician, relying on experience and knowledge of the patient, to determine dosages and the best treatment for the patient. The editors cannot be responsible for misuse or misapplication of the material in this work.

THE PUBLISHER

ACKNOWLEDGMENTS

We acknowledge all of our teachers, including our parents, instructors, fellow residents and students, and especially our patients.

Specifically, we would like to thank William Schmitt, Lori Irvine, and the W.B. Saunders staff for their guidance and patience.

Thank you also to those who tolerated many late nights of typing and those many others who contributed, directly and indirectly, to this work.

COMMONLY USED ABBREVIATIONS

Abd	abdomen
ABG	arterial blood gas
ACE	angiotensin-converting enzyme
ACTH	adrenocorticotropic hormone
ADH	antidiuretic hormone
AF	atrial fibrillation
AIDS	acquired immunodeficiency syndrome
ALT	alanine aminotransferase (SGPT)
AP	anterior-to-posterior direction (as in path of x-rays)
ARDS	adult respiratory distress syndrome
ASA	acetylsalicylic acid, aspirin
ASD	atrioseptal defect
AST	aspartate aminotransferase (SGOT)
ATN	acute tubular necrosis
AV	atrioventricular
β-hCG	beta-human chorionic gonadotropin
BP	blood pressure*
BPH	benign prostatic hypertrophy
beats/min	beats per minute
BUN	blood urea nitrogen
°C	degrees centigrade
Ca^{2+}	calcium ion
CAD	coronary artery disease
CBC	complete blood count
CCU	cardiac care unit
CHF	congestive heart failure
CI	cardiac index*

*Denotes that a formula is listed in Appendix C

cm	centimeter
cm H_2O	centimeters of water*
CMV	cytomegalovirus
CN	cranial nerve
CNS	central nervous system
CO	cardiac output*
CO_2	carbon dioxide
COPD	chronic obstructive pulmonary disease
CPB	cardiopulmonary bypass
CPK	creatine phosphokinase
CPR	cardiopulmonary resuscitation
CPT	chest physical therapy
Cr	creatinine
CrCl	creatinine clearance
CT	computed tomography
CVA	costovertebral angle
CVP	central venous pressure
CVS	cardiovascular system
CXR	chest x-ray
D5NS	5% dextrose in normal saline
D5W	5% dextrose in water
D10W	10% dextrose in water
D20W	20% dextrose in water
D50W	50% dextrose in water
DBP	diastolic blood pressure
DDAVP	1-desamino-(8-D-arginine)-vasopressin
DI	diabetes insipidus
DIC	disseminated intravascular coagulation
dl	deciliter
DT	delirium tremens
Dx	diagnosis

*Denotes that a formula is listed in Appendix C

ECF	extracellular fluid
EDTA	disodium edetate
ECG	electrocardiogram
EMD	electromechanical dissociation
ERCP	endoscopic retrograde cholangiopancreatoscopy
ET	endotracheal
Extrem	extremity examination
°F	degrees Fahrenheit
FHx	family history
F$_{IO_2}$	fraction of oxygen in inspired air
GI	gastrointestinal system
g	gram
GN	glomerulonephritis
gran	polymorphonucleocyte, granulocyte
GU	genitourinary
H$_2$	histamine receptor (type 2)
H & P	history and physical examination
HAV	hepatitis A virus
Hb	hemoglobin
HBV	hepatitis B virus
HCl	hydrochloride, hydrochloric acid
HCO$_3^-$	bicarbonate ion*
Hct	hematocrit
HCTZ	hydrochlorothiazide
HCV	hepatitis C virus
HDV	hepatitis D virus
HEENT	head, eyes, ears, nose, and throat
HEV	hepatitis E virus
HIV	human immunodeficiency (AIDS) virus
HR	heart rate
HTN	hypertension

---

*Denotes that a formula is listed in Appendix C

Hx	history
ICF	intracellular fluid
ICP	intracranial pressure
ICU	intensive care unit
IJ	inferior jugular
IM	intramuscular
inf	inferior
INR	International Normalizing Ratio
I/O	intake and output measurements
IP	intraperitoneal
IV	intravenous
IVC	inferior vena cava
IVF	intravenous fluids
J	joule
JVD	jugular venous distention
K⁺	potassium ion
kg	kilogram
KUB	"kidney, ureter, bladder," a flat-plate radiograph of the abdomen
L	liter
LDH	lactate dehydrogenase
LFT	liver function test
LLL	left lower lobe (of lung)
LLQ	left lower quadrant (of abdomen)
LP	lumbar puncture
LR	lactated Ringer's solution
LUL	left upper lobe (of lung)
LUQ	left upper quadrant (of abdomen)
lymph	lymphocyte
MAO	monoamine oxidase
MAP	mean arterial pressure*

---

*Denotes that a formula is listed in Appendix C

mEq	milliequivalent
mg	milligram
μg	microgram
Mg²⁺	magnesium ion
MI	myocardial infarction
ml	milliliter
mm	millimeter
mm³	cubic millimeter
mm Hg	millimeters of mercury*
mmol	millimolar concentration
MOFS	multiple organ failure syndrome
mOsm	milliosmolar concentration
MRI	magnetic resonance imaging
MS	mental status
MSO₄	morphine sulfate
MSS	musculoskeletal system examination
MVP	mitral valve prolapse
N₂	nitrogen*
Na⁺	sodium ion*
Neuro	neurologic
NG	nasogastric
NPO	"nil per os," nothing by mouth
NS	normal saline
NSAID	nonsteroidal anti-inflammatory drug
O⁻	O type, Rh-negative blood
O₂	oxygen
O & P	ova and parasite examination of the stool
OR	operating room
OT	occupational therapy
P	pulse rate
PA	posterior-to-anterior direction (as in path of x-rays)

*Denotes that a formula is listed in Appendix C

PAC	premature atrial contraction
PA_{O_2}	alveolar partial pressure of oxygen*
Pa_{O_2}	arterial partial pressure of oxygen
$P[A\text{-}a]_{O_2}$	alveolar-arterial oxygen gradient*
PAR	"procedure, alternatives and risks," used with surgical consents
P_{CO_2}	partial pressure of carbon dioxide
PCWP	pulmonary capillary wedge pressure
PE	physical examination
PFT	pulmonary function test
pH	$(-)$ log of hydrogen ion concentration
PID	pelvic inflammatory disease
plt	platelet
PMHx	past medical history
PMN	polymorphonucleocyte, granulocyte
PND	paroxysmal nocturnal dyspnea
PO	"per os," by mouth
POD	postoperative day
post	posterior
PPN	peripheral parenteral nutrition
PRBC	packed red blood cells
PRN	"pro re nata," as necessary
PT	prothrombin time
PTT	partial thromboplastin time
PUD	peptic ulcer disease
PVC	premature ventricular contraction
PVR	pulmonary vascular resistance
R	right side
RAD	reactive airway disease
RBC	red blood cell, erythrocyte
resp	respiratory system

*Denotes that a formula is listed in Appendix C

RLL	right lower lobe (of lung)
RLQ	right lower quadrant (of abdomen)
RN	registered nurse
RR	respiratory rate
RUL	right upper lobe (of lung)
RUQ	right upper quadrant (of abdomen)
Rx	prescription
Sao$_2$	oxygen saturation of arterial blood
SBE	subacute bacterial endocarditis
SBP	systolic blood pressure
SC	subcutaneous
SG	specific gravity
SGOT	serum glutamic-oxaloacetic transaminase (AST)
SGPT	serum glutamic-pyruvic transaminase (ALT)
SIADH	syndrome of inappropriate ADH secretion
SL	sublingual
SOB	short of breath, shortness of breath
sp	species
S/P	status post (following)
SSS	sick sinus syndrome
SV	stroke volume*
SVC	superior vena cava
SVR	systemic vascular resistance*
SVT	supraventricular tachycardia
Sx	symptom
TFT	thyroid function test
TIA	transient ischemic attack
TID	"ter in die," three times a day
TKO	to keep open
TMP/SFX	trimethoprim/sulfamethoxazole
TOD	target organ damage

---

*Denotes that a formula is listed in Appendix C

t-PA	tissue plasminogen activator
TPN	total parenteral nutrition
TURBT	transurethral resection of bladder tumor
TURP	transurethral resection of prostate
Tx	treatment
UA	urinalysis
UO	urine output
URI	upper respiratory infection
UTI	urinary tract infection
VC	vena cava
VMA	vanillylmandelic acid
VP	ventriculoperitoneal
VS	vital signs
WBC	white blood cell, leukocyte
WPW	Wolff-Parkinson-White syndrome
wt	weight

CONTENTS

APPENDICES

INTRODUCTION

APPROACH TO ON-CALL SURGICAL PROBLEMS

Why write a book on surgical on-call problems? All surgical training programs require time spent "on call." This is the time overnight during which a physician is responsible for the care of hospitalized patients. These are times of extraordinary educational value as well as stress. While on call, the physician is typically among the first to encounter significant changes in the condition of a patient and variances in recovery patterns. Hence, it is a unique time to hone clinical skills. However, under current training practices, on-call physicians are also early in their education and may not have encountered a wide range of clinical situations. Being on call often requires many late hours and prioritizing of numerous tasks. In addition, being on call may also require "cross coverage," or responsibility for patients for whom the on-call physician may have little familiarity or information. Often life-threatening changes in a patient's condition may be hidden under seemingly innocuous symptoms. Knowledge and anticipation of these problems may make a great difference in the patient's outcome. It is useful, therefore, to have a scheme to evaluate and administer care to patients in a rapid but thorough and organized fashion.

This book provides an outline for the organization and implementation of care plans in response to many on-call surgical situations. It is written for the intern and junior resident, but we hope that the information will be useful for persons at all levels of training. Obviously, not all on-call situations could be covered, but emphasis has been placed on the more common and the more life-threatening problems.

The structure of this book follows closely the flow of information as it reaches the individual on call. Most chapters are divided into six major headings, as follows:

- Phone call
- Elevator thoughts
- Major threat to life
- Bedside
- Management
- Special surgical considerations

■ PHONE CALL

The first notification of a change in the status of a patient is often a phone call from the bedside caregiver. During that phone call the status of the patient and the urgency of the response must be assessed immediately. It is also important to determine whether the patient is pre- or postoperative. If necessary, orders for immediate action are given and initial laboratory studies are ordered. The bedside care provider should also be given an estimate of when to expect the physician's arrival at the bedside. Occasionally, the problem may be handled entirely over the phone, but much more often, a bedside evaluation is required to fully assess the situation. If there is any question, always err toward a bedside evaluation.

■ ELEVATOR THOUGHTS

The travel time to the bedside is wisely spent in consideration of the differential diagnosis of the presenting symptom. These are called "elevator thoughts." This term was coined by Shane A. Marshall, MD, and John Ruedy, MD, in the first edition of *On Call: Principles and Protocols,* and it refers to the long distances through the hospital that often have to be covered while on call. Elevator thoughts may also be used to organize a plan of action once at the bedside. The differential diagnoses given in this text are not meant to be complete; attention is given to those most common and to those that could be life threatening. Always bear in mind that there are many uncommon causes of symptoms, which can be diagnosed or treated with simple measures, and these must also be entertained. Know what the preliminary plan of attack will be before arriving at the bedside.

■ MAJOR THREAT TO LIFE

In any clinical situation there is a potential risk to life. Although this is thankfully uncommon, it is the anticipation of these complications or the treatments to avoid them that may lead to the hospitalization of patients in the first place. This section will focus on those observations and tests that will best ensure the safety of the patient. The major threat to life is rarely the most common option on the differential diagnosis list.

In clinical practice it is a reasonable educational tool to imagine what the major threat is to each patient each day, pre- and postoperatively, and to outline the plan of action. Although these threats may not become a reality, the anticipation of a bad outcome leads to appropriate vigilance and avoidance tactics and to suitable preparation in the face of an unfortunate event.

■ BEDSIDE
Quick Look Test

Once at the bedside, the first look at the patient is often the best assessment of the severity of the complaint. This begins as you enter the patient's room and involves a rapid scan of the patient's general condition. A patient who is calm and conversant, with stable vital signs, may require less speed of action than one who is acutely distressed or unstable. Patients may be divided into the following three broad groups:

1. Comfortable. At ease, with stable or normal vital signs.
2. Sick. Requiring attention; recent changes or abnormalities in signs or symptoms with an indication of patient discomfort.
3. Critical. Moribund or very unstable; about to die.

This "first look" should be practiced with every patient contact, such as on rounds in the morning or in the clinic, so that it becomes second nature.

Vital Signs

The next evaluation of any patient is a quick assessment of the patient's breathing, vital signs, and fluid status. Special note is made of any recent changes or instability. Breathing or circulatory difficulties are dealt with immediately as life-threatening conditions.

Selective History, Chart Review, and Physical Examination

Next is a limited and directed history and physical examination, which is generally problem directed. This departs from the standard 30- to 60-minute interview practiced in medical school or the unhurried evaluation of a new patient. The motivation is different when the physician is on call. A specific complaint is to be addressed, and although that often expands into an assessment of several systems, other aspects of the patient's care, unrelated to the current complaint, do not need to be evaluated at this time. Sources of pertinent information are obtained from the bedside caregiver, from the patient, and from the chart. Remember that much information has already been obtained and is organized in the bedside chart, but be careful not to rely completely on this information. Circumstances may dictate further questioning and examination not already documented.

■ MANAGEMENT

Emergency measures and initial laboratory studies are described in an Initial Management section.

Further management issues, based on findings in the history and physical examination, are then discussed in Definitive Management.

SPECIAL CONSIDERATIONS FOR SURGICAL PATIENTS

Surgical patients are different from other patients in the hospital. Physiologic changes in their condition that become apparent on call may be due to the disease process that prompted their admission or may be due to the surgical procedure that was used to treat them. Often the same symptom will require different considerations in a preoperative patient than in a postoperative patient. Also important are the time elapsed since the day of the operation and the type of procedure performed. This section will be devoted to considerations that are specific to the surgical patient. Problems and considerations specific to individual surgical specialties will also be addressed.

■ PREOPERATIVE CONSIDERATIONS

Preoperative patients are broadly divided into the following three categories: elective, urgent, and emergent.

The elective patient may not be acutely ill but may require a surgical procedure. A good example is the patient admitted for bowel preparation before abdominal surgery or the patient admitted for diagnostic procedures. Perturbations in their health, such as fever or chest pain, may be enough to cancel an elective procedure, pending further evaluation of the problem.

The urgent patient may be more ill, and the disease state that was the reason for admission may cause changes in the patient's condition. Knowledge of the pathophysiology of the disease will often make it easier to anticipate and circumvent these problems, but occasionally a patient's condition will deteriorate to the point that urgency becomes emergency.

The emergent patient requires the most immediate attention and thought. Any patient, including an elective patient, can become an emergent patient at any time. In the assessment of the emergent patient, always consider whether it is appropriate to move the patient to an intensive care unit or to the operating room. Also ask yourself whether you need assistance in assessing or dealing with the problem, and call in extra help as needed. Being on call is a learning experience, and there is no reason to avoid consulting with others.

Preoperative patients soon will be in the operating room, where their condition may drastically change. Therefore, preparation of the patient for surgery should be considered when conditions allow. Postoperative patients will do best when they have had adequate preoperative hydration, nutrition, and pharmacologic preparation. Specific considerations including preoperative antibiotic therapy and bowel preparation will be addressed in subsequent chapters.

■ POSTOPERATIVE CONSIDERATIONS

The delivery of anesthetic agents and the performance of major surgical procedures may have profound physiologic effects on a patient. Fluid shifts are common, and the patient may require hemodynamic monitoring, fluid resuscitation, and electrolyte measurement. Specific organ physiology may be permanently altered, as with the transplantation of a kidney or with extensive bowel resection. Various surgical results may need to be protected, such as the integrity of a new anastomosis or the blood flow to a free-flap graft. Many postoperative considerations are specific to the procedure performed and will be addressed in the appropriate chapters.

Hypothermia is a common postoperative finding. Although found mostly after extensive surgical procedures, it is of general interest because it may occur in a variety of patients, regardless of the procedure performed.

A core temperature of <36°C persisting 1 to 2 hours postoperatively is a significant complication. It is frequent after extensive intra-abdominal procedures and in septic, seriously injured, and very ill patients. Common etiologies include long periods of time with the patient's skin or abdominal contents exposed to subphysiologic temperatures, or massive rehydration with cool replacement fluids.

Expect patients with hypothermia to have vasoconstriction with an associated increase in systemic vascular resistance (SVR). Hypothermia may contribute to tachycardia and to hyperventilation, especially in the setting of shivering. In addition, as the patient is rewarmed, cooler peripheral beds are reperfused, which may slow further rewarming and contribute to postoperative acidosis.

The treatment includes awareness of the potential for hypothermia in the operating room, rapid operative procedures, warm intravenous (IV) solutions, warmed humidified gases in ventilated patients, and warming blankets.

Hypothermia alters mental state and prolongs the half-lives of many medications. It is also possible to overcorrect in the treatment of hypothermia, and the result should not be confused with postoperative fever (see Chapter 11).

DOCUMENTATION OF ON-CALL PROBLEMS

An important aspect of management of on-call problems is the appropriate documentation of events. This is essential for the continued efficient care of the patient. In addition, the medical chart is a medicolegal document, and it should be as accurate and complete as possible. Documentation is required for every patient evaluated. This may be just a short note for a simple problem, or it may require a complete rendering of a complex intervention.

An example of an on-call note is as follows:

Resident On-Call Note   *(Date and Time)*

Called by RN to evaluate patient because of fever.

The patient is a 65-year-old man who is 2 days status post exploratory laparotomy for presumed bowel obstruction; 20 cm of questionably necrotic small bowel was removed, and a primary anastomosis was performed without complication. His postoperative course has been complicated by initial shortness of breath associated with a mild fever (38.0°C) and an oxygen requirement on postoperative day 1, which resolved with diuretics and ambulation. His course since has been uncomplicated. He has been ambulatory without difficulty but has not yet been ready for oral feedings. His current therapies include IV hydration with 5% dextrose in one-half normal saline (D5½ NS) at 75 ml/hr, nasogastric suction, parenteral antibiotic therapy, ambulation, and incentive spirometry.

(List current medications.)

The physical examination is directed toward the evaluation of the problem described.

Vital signs (VS):	Temperature: 38.6°C
	Pulse: 107 beats/min
	Respiration: 20/min
	Blood pressure: 136 mm Hg/ 85 mm Hg
Head, eyes, ears, nose, and throat (HEENT):	Nasogastric tube in place, normally functioning. Output over the last 24 hours: 1550 ml (75 ml in the last

	hour. Green, nonbloody fluid). No sinus tenderness.
Cardiovascular system (CVS):	Regular rate and rhythm, mild tachycardia. No murmur.
Respiration:	Basilar rales with poor aeration. Incentive spirometer hidden in bottom drawer of personal items. No documented use since last shift.
Abdomen:	Wound clean without discharge. No erythema. Abdomen is soft, with mild incisional tenderness. No peritoneal signs. No organomegaly.
Urinary:	No urinary catheter. Urine output is >800 ml/shift. No dysuria complaints. No tenderness over bladder or flanks.
IV sites:	No erythema. Day 2 of current site (left dorsal hand).
Legs:	No calf tenderness.

Laboratory analysis, as follows, is dictated by the history and physical examination:

Complete blood count (CBC):	
White blood cell (WBC):	6700/μl
Hemoglobin (Hb):	12 g/dl
Hematocrit (Hct):	42%
Platelet (Plt):	267,000/μl
Urinalysis:	No WBC, 3 to 5 red blood cells, occasional epithelial cells. Negative for leukocyte esterase, specific gravity: 1.125.
Chest x-ray:	Bibasilar atelectasis without specific infiltrate.

The diagnosis and treatment should be clear; list any further studies that might be useful. Also list who might have been contacted.

Assessment:	Probable atelectasis; must also consider pulmonary infection or reaction to antibiotic therapy.

Treatment:

Postoperative day 2.
Day 2 antibiotic therapy *(list agents used)*.
1. Incentive spirometry every hour, the importance of which was reiterated to the patient and his family.
2. Continue antibiotic therapy.
3. Repeat chest x-ray and CBC in A.M.
4. Consider sputum analysis.
5. Plan discussed with RN and chief resident *(time)*.

■ COMMUNICATION

Complete medical care is a team approach, and adequate communication is vital for consistent and appropriate treatment of patients. It is important to document the chart in a complete and *legible* fashion. Do not forget that many practitioners and others read and rely on the information written in the medical record, e.g., the primary care team, the nurses directly involved in the patient's care, the consulting teams, and often the patient or family. Any of these individuals may contribute significantly to the care of the patient.

Often, medical approaches to treating patients on call represent differences in treatment philosophies, and these may be educational. Remember as well that communication should occur in all directions along the hierarchy of caregivers, to interns and to medical students, and to family, bedside caregivers, chief residents, and attending physicians.

4

ON-CALL HAZARDS

The practice of medicine has inherent risks. The exposure to blood- and secretion-borne disease is significant and should always be considered. Specifically, the transmission of human immunodeficiency virus (HIV) to a health care provider from an infected patient, although infrequent, is always a risk. Hepatitis B and hepatitis C are other blood-borne pathogens. Hepatitis B is particularly worrisome because only a small viral inoculum can result in disease transmission. Precautions must *always* be taken, especially in those patients about whom you have no firsthand knowledge (Table 4–1).

Table 4–1 □ UNIVERSAL PRECAUTIONS TO PREVENT TRANSMISSION OF HIV

Universal Precautions

Because a medical history and physical examination cannot reliably identify all patients infected with HIV or other blood-borne pathogens, blood and body fluid precautions should be consistently used for all patients, especially those in emergency care settings in which the risk of blood exposure is increased and the infection status of the patient is usually not known.

1. Use appropriate barrier protection to prevent skin and mucous membrane exposure when exposure to blood, body fluids containing blood, or other body fluids to which universal precautions apply (see below) is anticipated. Wear gloves when touching blood or body fluids, mucous membranes, or nonintact skin of all patients, when handling items or surfaces soiled with blood or body fluids, and when performing venipuncture and other vascular access procedures. Change gloves after contact with each patient; do not wash or disinfect gloves for reuse. Wear masks and protective eyewear or face shields during procedures that are likely to generate droplets of blood or other body fluids to prevent exposure of mucous membranes of the mouth, nose, and eyes. Wear gowns or aprons during procedures that are likely to generate splashes of blood or other body fluids.
2. Wash hands and other skin surfaces immediately and thoroughly following contamination with blood, body fluids containing blood, or other body fluids to which universal precautions apply. Wash hands immediately after gloves are removed.
3. Take care to prevent injuries when using needles, scalpels, and other sharp instruments or devices, when handling sharp instruments after procedures, when cleaning used instruments, and

Table continued on following page

when disposing of used needles. Do not recap needles by hand; do not remove used needles from disposable syringes by hand; and do not bend, break, or otherwise manipulate used needles by hand. Place used disposable syringes and needles, scalpel blades, and other sharp items in puncture-resistant disposal containers, which should be located as close to the use area as is practical.

4. Although saliva has not been implicated in HIV transmission, the need for emergency mouth-to-mouth resuscitation should be minimized by making mouthpieces, resuscitation bags, or other ventilation devices available for use in areas in which the need for resuscitation is predictable.

5. Health care workers with exudative lesions or weeping dermatitis should refrain from all direct patient care and from handling patient care equipment until the condition resolves.

Universal precautions are intended to supplement rather than replace recommendations for routine infection control, such as hand washing and use of gloves to prevent gross microbial contamination of hands. In addition, implementation of universal precautions does not eliminate the need for other category- or disease-specific isolation precautions, such as enteric precautions for infectious diarrhea or isolation for pulmonary tuberculosis. Universal precautions are not intended to change waste management programs undertaken in accordance with state and local regulations.

Body Fluids to Which Universal Precautions Apply

Universal precautions apply to blood and other body fluids containing visible blood. Blood is the single most important source of HIV, hepatitis B virus, and other blood-borne pathogens in the occupational setting. Universal precautions also apply to tissues, semen, vaginal secretions, and the following fluids: cerebrospinal, synovial, pleural, peritoneal, and amniotic.

Universal precautions do not apply to feces, nasal secretions, sputum, sweat, tears, urine, and vomitus unless they contain visible blood. Universal precautions also do not apply to human breast milk, although gloves may be worn by health care workers in situations in which exposure to breast milk might be frequent. In addition, universal precautions do not apply to saliva. Gloves need not be worn when feeding patients or wiping saliva from skin, although special precautions are recommended for dentistry, in which contamination of saliva with blood is predictable. The risk of transmission of HIV, as well as hepatitis B virus, from these fluids and materials is extremely low or nonexistent.

Use of Gloves for Phlebotomy

Gloves should be effective in reducing the incidence of blood contamination of hands during phlebotomy (drawing of blood samples), but they cannot prevent penetrating injuries caused by needles or other sharp instruments. In universal precautions, all blood is assumed to be potentially infectious for blood-borne pathogens. Some institutions have relaxed recommendations for the use of gloves for phelobotomy by skilled health care workers in settings in which the prevalence of blood-borne pathogens is known to be very low (e.g., volunteer blood donation centers). Institutions that judge that routine use of gloves for all phlebotomies is not necessary should periodically reevaluate their policy.

Gloves should always be available for those who wish to use them for phlebotomy. In addition, the following general guidelines apply:

1. Use gloves for performing phlebotomy if cuts, scratches, or other breaks in the skin are present.
2. Use gloves in situtations in which contamination with blood may occur—for example, when performing phlebotomy on an uncooperative patient.
3. Use gloves for performing finger or heel sticks on infants and children.
4. Use gloves when training persons to do phlebotomies.

From Rubin RH: Acquired immunodeficiency syndrome. Scientific American Medicine, Dale DC, Federman DD, Eds. Section 7, Subsection XI. © 1996 Scientific American, Inc. All rights reserved.

Before blood contact occurs, find out what the hospital policies are regarding treatment of significant blood-borne exposures. Know where to seek first aid as required. And make sure that your tetanus and hepatitis B vaccinations are up to date (Table 4–2).

Table 4–2 □ FIRST AID AFTER BLOOD OR BODY FLUID EXPOSURE (DO NOT DELAY!)

1. Immediately clean the exposed site. For skin sites, wash with detergent and water or a 1:10 bleach solution. For eyes and other mucous membranes, use saline or water. Wash for 5 minutes.
2. Save the instrument in a sharps container for testing later.
3. Seek out a supervisor for instructions. A specific protocol may be in place for your institution.
4. Serum probably will be drawn from you and the patient from whom the fluid originated.
5. Make sure tetanus and hepatitis B vaccinations are up to date.
6. Some institutions recommend zidovudine (AZT) prophylaxis.

PATIENT-RELATED PROBLEMS: THE COMMON CALLS

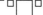

ABDOMINAL PAIN

One of the most common calls, abdominal pain, is also one of the most difficult to evaluate. Whole textbooks have been written on the approach to abdominal pain in surgical patients. This chapter is not meant to replace those books, but it will cover many of the common calls in the hospital. The first major decision to be made is whether the patient needs an operation immediately (acute abdomen). Once that is decided satisfactorily, the remainder of the evaluation may be performed.

■ PHONE CALL

Questions

1. **How severe is the pain?**
2. **Is the pain localized or generalized?**
3. **Are there any changes in vital signs, such as fever, hypotension, or tachycardia?**
4. **Is the patient taking pain medications or steroids?**
   Both of these may mask or alter pain perception.
5. **Has the patient undergone a surgical procedure? If so, how long ago?**
   Incision pain is common immediately following an abdominal procedure. Also be mindful that adhesion formation following an abdominal procedure may cause bowel obstruction many years later.
6. **Is a nasogastric (NG) tube in place? Is it functioning normally? Have there been changes in the trends of volume output and fluid characteristics?**
7. **Are there any other symptoms, such as vomiting, dysuria, diarrhea, or bloating?**

Orders

If an NG tube is in place for luminal decompression and it is not functioning, it may be flushed with 20 to 30 ml of normal saline (NS). Do this yourself if the patient has had a luminal perforation or an anastomosis in the proximal GI tract.

Degree of Urgency

If there is a significant change in vital signs or symptoms, or if the pain is a new symptom, the patient must be evaluated immediately. Recurrent and minor pain may be evaluated in 1 to 2 hours.

■ ELEVATOR THOUGHTS

- Localized abdominal pain
    This is best organized by the location of the pain (Fig. 5–1).
- Generalized abdominal pain
    Many etiologies of abdominal pain have aspects of both localized and generalized pain (Fig. 5–2), often with progression from one to the other over time.

■ MAJOR THREAT TO LIFE

- Luminal perforation
- Infarction
- Sepsis after intra-abdominal abscess
- Ruptured aortic aneurysm with exsanguinating hemorrhage

■ BEDSIDE

Quick Look Test

Mild abdominal pain is associated with only minor discomfort. The more severe the pain, the more uncomfortable the patient will appear. If the patient has an acute abdomen, impending hypovolemic shock may be present and the patient may be lethargic or even moribund. Patients receiving narcotic medication or steroids may be deceptively comfortable despite serious pathology. Pain and inflammatory responses (including fever) may be blunted. Patients with peritonitis (acute abdomen) will be still, because any movement of their abdominal wall will cause pain. Patients with renal or biliary colic will be agitated and will often have "caged cat" restlessness as they try to find a comfortable position.

Airway and Vital Signs

Tachycardia and hypovolemia are associated with shock. Fever is an indication of infection or inflammatory etiology, although it need not be present to make such a diagnosis. Tachypnea may be present due to a lower lobe pneumonia, or it may indicate progressive acidemia from necrosis of the bowel, which is more serious.

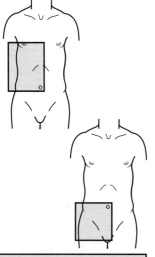

RIGHT UPPER QUADRANT PAIN
Gallbladder and biliary tract
Hepatitis
Hepatic abscess
Hepatomegaly due to
    congestive heart failure
Peptic ulcer
Pancreatitis
Retrocecal appendicitis
Renal pain
Myocardial ischemia
Pericarditis
Pneumonia
Empyema

LEFT UPPER QUADRANT PAIN
Gastritis
Pancreatitis
Splenic enlargement, rupture,
    infarction, aneurysm
Renal pain
Myocardial ischemia
Pneumonia
Empyema

RIGHT LOWER QUADRANT PAIN
Appendicitis
Intestinal obstruction
Regional enteritis
Diverticulitis
Cholecystitis
Perforated ulcer
Leaking aneurysm
Abdominal wall hematoma
Ectopic pregnancy
Ovarian cyst or torsion
Salpingitis
Endometriosis
Ureteral calculi
Renal pain
Seminal vesiculitis
Psoas abscess

LEFT LOWER QUADRANT PAIN
Diverticulitis
Intestinal obstruction
Appendicitis
Leaking aneurysm
Abdominal wall hematoma
Ectopic pregnancy
Ovarian cyst or torsion
Salpingitis
Endometriosis
Ureteral calculi
Renal pain
Seminal vesiculitis
Psoas abscess

Figure 5–1 □ Common etiologies of localized abdominal pain by quadrant. (Modified from Schwartz SI, Shires GT, Spencer FC: Principles of Surgery, 5th ed. New York, McGraw-Hill Book Co., 1989. Reproduced with permission of The McGraw-Hill Companies.)

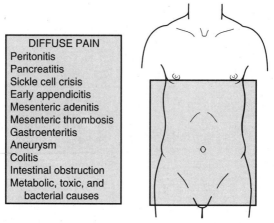

DIFFUSE PAIN
Peritonitis
Pancreatitis
Sickle cell crisis
Early appendicitis
Mesenteric adenitis
Mesenteric thrombosis
Gastroenteritis
Aneurysm
Colitis
Intestinal obstruction
Metabolic, toxic, and
   bacterial causes

Figure 5–2 □ Common etiologies of generalized abdominal pain. (Modified from Schwartz SI, Shires GT, Spencer FC: Principles of Surgery, 5th ed. New York, McGraw-Hill Book Co., 1989. Reproduced with permission of The McGraw-Hill Companies.)

Initial Assessment

A preliminary assessment helps in making the final diagnosis and deciding if the patient needs surgery immediately.
1. Assess for an acute abdomen.
   A rapid examination of the ill-appearing patient is a prudent start. Questions may be asked of the patient while the examination is being performed. The presence of an acute abdomen is a surgical emergency, and exploratory laparotomy is indicated for diagnosis and potential repair of the problem. It is not an easy diagnosis, but some specific clues are helpful. The presence or absence of these symptoms individually does not make the diagnosis, but in combination, and taken in context with the history, a decision may be made. It is not unusual to have to make a rapid decision without having many pieces of the puzzle.
   ■ Abdominal distention
     May be present with acute obstruction or progressive ascites.
   ■ Quiet abdomen
     The lack of bowel sounds indicates a functional ileus or peritonitis. As a diagnostic symptom it is not very sensitive, because bowel sounds are rarely completely absent; it may merely take several minutes to note them. High-pitched, rushing, or "tinkling" bowel sounds indicate possible obstruction.

- Peritonitis

    Severe pain to palpation or rigid abdominal musculature (involuntary guarding) is evidence of peritoneal irritation. This may be focal as in appendicitis, or it may be generalized as with rupture of the viscus. It may be apparent from gentle shaking of the bed or the patient, or by percussion or palpation of the abdomen. Rebound tenderness may be present but is a less specific finding.

- Hypotension

    A precipitous decrease in blood pressure associated with abdominal pain is a surgical emergency. You do not need to know the exact diagnosis before an exploratory laparotomy in a gravely ill patient.

2. Treat hypotension with aggressive fluid resuscitation, as necessary.

    Do a complete fluid assessment (see Chapter 12). Orthostatic blood pressure and pulse measurements will aid in diagnosing intravascular volume deficits. If surgical treatment is required, the patient should receive aggressive fluid resuscitation as described in Chapter 17 while preparations for transfer to the operating room (OR) are being made.

3. If the patient does not have an acute abdomen, then the remainder of the history and physical examination may be performed.

Selective History and Chart Review

- Gather a complete history of the pain.

    Important features include the following:

    1. Time of onset

        Many pain syndromes change over time. A classic example is the progression of appendicitis from periumbilical pain to right lower quadrant (RLQ) pain. The duration of the pain may suggest the location of the symptoms. Was the onset sudden or gradual? Did the pain awaken the patient?

    2. Location

        Review Figures 5–1 and 5–2. Note whether pain is epigastric, umbilical, prepubic, right or left, and upper or lower; changes in location are important. Pain may also be difficult to localize specifically; this is common in very old or very young patients. Most children will point at their belly buttons when asked to locate the pain.

    3. Radiation

        Pain can radiate to the back, groin, chest, and so on (Fig. 5–3). Radiation of pain occurs when the pain fibers from the affected organ are supplied by nerve roots

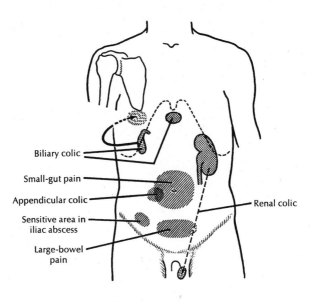

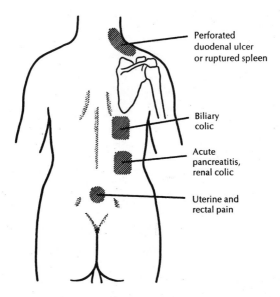

Figure 5–3 □ Common cutaneous sites of referred pain by etiology. (From Cope Z: Cope's Early Diagnosis of the Acute Abdomen, Revised by William Silen, 16th ed. Oxford, Oxford University Press, 1983, pp 11, 141 by permission of Oxford University Press.)

that also have a cutaneous sensory distribution. Pain in the diaphragm from a left lower lobe pneumonia or perisplenic abscess is radiated to the left shoulder because of mutual innervation by the C-3, C-4, and C-5 nerve roots.

4. Quality of the pain

    Pain can be stabbing, aching, cramping, burning, and so on.

5. Fluctuations in the pain

    Pain can be constant, colicky, intermittent (at what intervals?), increasing, and so on.

6. Factors that lessen the pain

    These can include position, meals, defecation, and time.

7. Factors that make the pain worse

8. Changes in the frequency or character of the stool

    Changes can include diarrhea, constipation, or change in color or caliber.

9. Associated symptoms

    Symptoms can include fever, nausea, vomiting, dizziness, dysuria, and cough.

10. Character of the vomitus, if the patient is vomiting

    Clear fluid indicates obstruction proximal to the sphincter of Oddi; bilious vomitus indicates a more distal obstruction. Feculent material indicates a distal colonic obstruction. Does the vomiting relate temporally to the pain?

11. Character of the stool, if the patient has diarrhea

    Bloody stools or those containing mucus indicate an invasive enteritis or inflammatory bowel disease. Clear liquid may indicate a viral etiology. Diarrhea is sometimes associated with a high-grade obstruction, because fluid materials are the only types that may pass. Does the diarrhea relate temporally to the pain?

12. Time of the patient's last meal

    Is the patient anorexic?

13. Whether the patient is passing gas

    Passed gas is largely swallowed air and indicates complete bowel continuity. A lack of flatus may indicate ileus or obstruction.

14. Prior abdominal procedures

    How long ago were procedures performed? Were any organs resected? Adhesions formed following an abdominal procedure are the major cause of mechanical bowel obstruction.

15. Family history of abdominal pain syndromes

    These can include familial Mediterranean fever and sickle cell anemia.

- Note if the patient is taking steroids, pain medications, or nonsteroidal anti-inflammatory drugs (NSAIDs).
- Does the patient have a past medical history of abdominal pain (see Figs. 5–1 and 5–2)?

    The most common recurrent abdominal pain syndromes include

    1. Peptic ulcer disease

        Does the patient use histamine H_2 blockers or other antacids routinely?
    2. Alcoholic pancreatitis

        Any prior admission for ascites or abdominal pain?
    3. Gastritis

        This is common after steroid or NSAID administration.
    4. Nephrolithiasis
    5. Cholelithiasis or cholecystitis
- Is there a history of peripheral or cardiovascular disease?

    Atherosclerotic plaque formation may be present in the mesenteric vessels as well, resulting in mesenteric ischemia.

Selective Physical Examination

VS: Repeat now.

MS: Lethargy (hypotension and narcotic pain medication).

HEENT: Icteric sclerae (hepatitis, cholangitis, and cholelithiasis).

Flat neck veins (hypotension).

CVS: New murmur or S_3 (myocardial infarction).

Resp: Decreased breath sounds, dullness to percussion, rales (pneumonia or pleural effusion).

GU: Dysuria (urinary tract infection [UTI]).

Skin: Edema, jaundice, spider angiomata, caput medusae (liver failure).

Wound: Discharge or erythema (wound infection).

Tubes: NG tube in place. Functioning well?

Abd: The aspects of a focused abdominal examination are as follows:

1. Observe: Look at the comfort of the patient. Look for distention. Often the large colon may be seen in outline in cases of distal obstruction. Ascites may be evident by bulging flanks. Peristalsis or outlines of bowel loops may be visible. Look at the position of the patient. An agitated, moving patient probably has biliary or renal colic. The still, quiet patient may have peritonitis. Look at the skin. Look for retroperitoneal bleeding and blood that ex-

travasates along tissue planes, which may present as bruising along the back, flanks, or abdomen.

Grey Turner's sign: Ecchymosis noted in the groin or flanks.

Cullen's sign: Ecchymosis noted in the peri-umbilical region.

2. Position: The patient should be supine with the knees bent slightly to relax the abdominal muscula-ture. Some examiners prefer to approach an abdominal examination from the same side of the bed each time.

3. Locate: Ask the patient to point to the location of the greatest pain. This is not always possible if the pain is generalized. If a point of maximal pain is identified, do not start the palpation at that spot or the patient will not trust you enough to relax for the remainder of the ex-amination.

4. Auscul-tate: Listen for bowel sounds in all four quadrants. Note high-pitched or rushing sounds, which may indicate obstruction.

5. Percuss: This may elicit tenderness in peritonitis; if so, resort to light palpation. Determine the liver size and the tympanic quality of the abdo-men. Distal obstruction may produce large gas pockets if the ileocecal valve is compe-tent. Is there localizable percussion tender-ness? (RLQ suggests appendicitis, prepubic suggests UTI.) Percuss for fluid waves and shifting dullness (ascites).

6. Palpate: Palpate gently at first, with gradual increase in pressure. Note tender areas and areas of referred pain. Note masses and regions of pulsation (as an artery). An acute abdomen may be rigid with "board-like stiffness," or tenderness may be more localized.

7. Re-bound: Rebound tenderness is an insensitive finding associated with peritonitis. *Direct rebound* is tenderness over a region when palpation pressure is quickly released. *Indirect rebound* is pain referred elsewhere with the same movement. Appendicitis may have direct re-bound over McBurney's point and may have indirect rebound to McBurney's point when pressure is released from elsewhere in the abdomen. Rebound itself does not make the

diagnosis of peritonitis. An apprehensive patient usually has some element of rebound.

8. Guarding:
Peritonitis is marked by guarding. *Voluntary guarding* is more insensitive and relates to the voluntary contraction of abdominal musculature to limit the pain anticipated by the patient (such as during an abdominal examination). Like rebound tenderness, this is present in many apprehensive patients in the absence of peritonitis. *Involuntary guarding* results in a rigid abdomen and is an ominous sign of acute peritonitis that requires immediate exploratory laparotomy. Guarding may be present only as unequal muscle tone in one region of the abdomen compared with another.

9. Hernias:
Examine the abdomen and the groin for evidence of hernias.

10. Rectal examination:
Rectal examination is absolutely necessary in the evaluation of abdominal pain. Evaluate for prostatic pain (prostatitis) and palpable, tender masses (appendicitis, tumor, or abscess). Guaiac-positive stool may be present with peptic ulcer disease, Meckel's diverticulum, inflammatory bowel disease, or intussusception.

11. Pelvic examination:
Pelvic examination is absolutely necessary in the evaluation of lower abdominal pain in a woman. Discharge indicates vaginitis or cervicitis. Cervical motion tenderness is present in cervicitis and pelvic inflammatory disease (PID). Adnexal masses may be palpable and tender.

12. Special examinations:
Murphy's sign: Have the patient inhale while firm pressure is held under the costal margin on the right. A positive sign is pain and abrupt cessation of respirations with palpation of a tender gallbladder.

Psoas sign: With the patient prone or on the side, extend the leg at the hip. A positive sign is painful extension, as with psoas abscess or retrocecal appendicitis.

Obturator sign: With the patient supine, bend one knee creating 90° angles at the hip and knee, and rotate the foot outward (internal rotation at the hip). A positive sign is abdominal pain with this maneuver, as with retrocecal appendicitis.

13. Additional tests:

- Laboratory examination
  1. Complete blood count (CBC) with differential

     An elevated white blood cell (WBC) count supports an infectious or inflammatory etiology.
  2. Urinalysis (UA)

     WBCs with or without red blood cells (RBCs) are associated with UTI; occasionally, a retrocecal appendicitis that lies in contact with the ureter may cause minor pyuria. RBCs indicate nephrolithiasis.
  3. Serum amylase

     Elevated levels suggest pancreatitis.
  4. Liver function tests (LFTs)

     Useful in evaluating patients with suspected hepatitis and biliary tract disease.
  5. Beta-human chorionic gonadotropin (β-hCG)

     Always rule out ectopic pregnancy in women.
  6. Stool studies

     If the patient has diarrhea, especially with evidence of invasion (bloody stools, leukocytosis, and fever), send stools for fecal leukocytes, culture and sensitivities of all pathogens, and analysis for ova and parasites (O&P). Send stool for *Clostridium difficile* toxin titer if the patient has had recent antibiotic treatment.
  7. Other tests as symptoms dictate
- Three-way abdominal films

  This includes a posteroanterior (PA) chest x-ray, and kidney, ureter, bladder (KUB) films done in the supine and upright positions. The important features to note are as follows:
  1. Free air under the diaphragm

     This is most likely seen under the right diaphragm on the CXR, as this is the higher side. This indicates a rupture in a viscus such as perforated ulcer or diverticulum. Free air is normally noted on x-ray after an abdominal procedure and may be seen for up to 7 days postoperatively. Air may also be noted in the biliary tree. A lateral abdominal x-ray may also demonstrate intraperitoneal air.
  2. Dilation of loops of bowel

     This may be in the small or large intestine. The dilation occurs proximal to an obstruction. The obstruction need not be complete to cause dilation.
  3. Air/fluid level

     This may occur throughout the intestinal tract and denotes stasis or ileus. It may be functional or secondary to obstruction.
  4. Gas pattern

     Is the gas equally distributed all the way to the rectum? Rapid transit of luminal contents, such as in diarrhea, will leave little gas in the bowel.

5. Inflammation of the bowel wall

This is most easily seen where two loops of bowel are side by side.

6. Air in the bowel wall

Also called pneumatosis intestinalis, it is a characteristic of necrotizing enterocolitis.

7. Stones

Nephrolithiasis and occasionally cholelithiasis may be diagnosed on plain films.

8. Loss of the psoas shadow

This may indicate a retroperitoneal process.

9. Thumb printing

This is evidence of edema or thickening of the bowel wall.

- Ultrasonography

This is used to evaluate specific complaints where indicated, such as in cases of suspected pancreatitis, cholecystitis, nephrolithiasis, appendicitis, or ovarian pathology. Liver and spleen may also be readily visualized in cases of trauma.

- Computed tomographic (CT) scan with contrast

This is useful to evaluate mass lesions in the abdomen and to assess the patency and continuity of the intestines. A noncontrast abdominal CT may be used to diagnose appendicitis.

- Angiography

Where indicated, selective vessel angiography can aid in the evaluation of aneurysms, arterial obstructions, or ruptures.

■ MANAGEMENT

Definitive management of the patient is dictated by the suspected diagnosis.

Gastritis or Peptic Ulcer Disease

Mucosal injuries in the stomach and duodenum have a spectrum of severity ranging from gastritis to acute or chronic peptic ulcer disease. The hallmark is GI bleeding.

- Clues to diagnosis:
  - History: Common in men in their 30s and 40s. History of stress, NSAID use, steroid use, or tobacco or alcohol abuse. Dyspepsia is a common symptom.

- Pain: Sudden onset. Constant. Burning or stabbing. Relieved with food.
- Location: Epigastrium, occasionally radiating to the back.
- Exam: Epigastric tenderness. Stool may be guaiac positive.
- Studies: Evaluation for *Helicobacter pylori.* Upper endoscopy in the stable patient is diagnostic >90% of the time.
- Acuity: Routine to urgent.
- Treatment: Bland diet.

  Medications (Table 5–1).

  Evaluation for coagulopathy and hyperacidity states.

  Do not administer antacids before endoscopy, as this will obscure the examination.

  Surgical therapy is reserved for treatment of chronic or severe symptoms or of bleeding that continues for 6 to 8 units over 48 hours.
- Notes: If hematemesis is the prominent symptom, an urgent upper endoscopy is required to rule out esophageal varices.

Perforated Peptic Ulcer

Perforated peptic ulcer disease occurs more frequently in the duodenum than in the stomach.

- Clues to diagnosis:
  - History: Common in men in their 30s and 40s. History of peptic ulcer disease. Use of NSAIDs, steroids, or sympathomimetic drugs. Tobacco or alcohol abuse. Stress.
  - Pain: Sudden onset. Severe burning or stabbing.
  - Location: Localized to epigastrium but generalizes over time. Often radiates to the back or shoulder.
  - Exam: Peritonitis is common with severe epigastric tenderness caused by the chemical burn of gastric acids on the peritoneum. Stool may be guaiac positive. Impending shock and hypovolemia are the norm. Intestinal fluids may travel down to the RLQ, and symptoms may mimic acute appendicitis. Abdominal distention.
  - Studies: Elevated WBCs. Free air under diaphragm on chest x-ray in 75% of cases.
  - Differential diagnosis: Acute appendicitis with perforation. Acute cholecystitis.

Table 5–1 ◻ COMMON MEDICATIONS USED TO TREAT GASTRITIS

Secretion Blockade

Medication*	Receptor Blockade	Dose†
Cimetidine (Tagamet)	H_2	300 mg IV every 6–8 hr, or 400 mg PO every 6 hr, may be given 800 mg PO twice per day
Ranitidine (Zantac)	H_2	50 mg IV every 8 hr or 150 mg PO twice per day
Famotidine (Pepcid)	H_2	20–40 mg PO or IV every day, IV form divided twice per day
Nizatidine (Axid)	H_2	300 mg PO every day (or may be divided twice per day)
Omeprazole (Prilosec)	H^+K^+-ATPase	20 mg PO every day

Acid Neutralization‡

Magnesium Containing	Aluminum Containing	Combination Agents
Milk of magnesia	ALternaGEL	Alka-Seltzer
Mag-Ox 400	Alumina	Maalox
Uro-Mag	Alu-Cap or Alu-Tab	Mylanta
	Amphojel	Bicitra

Protective Coating

Medication	Dose
Sulcralfate (Carafate)	1 g PO 4 times per day
Bismuth subsalicylate (Pepto-Bismol§)	2 tbsp or tablets PO every 0.5–1 hr as needed. Do not exceed 8 doses/ 24 hr

*Higher doses of secretion blockade medications may be required to treat hypersecretion states such as Zollinger-Ellison syndrome. Check gastric pH frequently to monitor therapy; aim for pH>5.0.

†All H_2-receptor antagonist doses must be reduced in patients with renal failure.

‡These may be administered in doses of 1–2 tbsp PO every 2–4 hours with "holds" for side effects, such as for diarrhea with magnesium-containing antacids and for constipation with aluminum-containing antacids.

§In patients with guaiac-positive stools, avoid the use of Pepto-Bismol, as the bismuth will turn the stool black and may be confused with melena. Note also that Pepto-Bismol contains salicylates.

IV = intravenously; PO = by mouth.

Acute pancreatitis.
Intestinal obstruction.
Perforated diverticulitis.

- Acuity: **Emergency.**
- Treatment: Nothing by mouth (NPO).
Fluid resuscitation as necessary.
Emergency exploratory laparotomy with repair.

Ascending Cholangitis

Results from bacterial infection of the bile in settings of stasis or biliary obstruction.
- Clues to diagnosis:
  - History: Often history of surgery on the biliary tract or adjacent structures. History of biliary colic.
  - Pain: Sharp, colicky.
  - Location: Right upper quadrant (RUQ) with radiation to the back.
  - Other signs and symptoms: Nausea, vomiting, jaundice, fever, and chills. *Charcot's triad* of fever with chills, RUQ pain, and jaundice is variably present and should not be relied on.
  - Exam: Hypoactive bowel tones. Often signs of peritonitis. RUQ tenderness with a positive Murphy's sign.
  - Studies: Elevated WBCs and bilirubin. Blood cultures may demonstrate growth of the causative microbe. Ultrasonography may reveal dilation of the gallbladder or the biliary tree with or without stones. Endoscopic retrograde cholangiopancreatography (ERCP) may demonstrate dilated and ectatic bile ducts but may not visualize beyond the obstruction. Transhepatic cholangiography is diagnostic, and a T-tube may be left in place for external drainage.
- Acuity: **Emergency.** Sepsis is likely.
- Treatment: NPO.
Fluid resuscitation as necessary.
Appropriate antibiotic therapy.
T-tube drainage.
Emergency surgical management is reserved for rupture or gangrene of the gallbladder, signified by evidence of sepsis.

Acute Cholecystitis

The spectrum of gallbladder disease includes biliary colic, chronic cholecystitis, and acute cholecystitis. Biliary colic describes intermittent pain in the RUQ after ingestion of fatty foods. This starts as discomfort, then crescendos into severe pain, which resolves in a short time. It is caused by incomplete obstruction of the duct with a stone. It is treated with fluids and pain relief measures. Chronic cholecystitis is the result of multiple inflammatory attacks on the gallbladder resulting in scar tissue and impaired function. Acute cholecystitis is a current inflammatory attack on the gallbladder. It is associated with complete occlusion of the duct by stones in 90% of the cases.

- Clues to diagnosis:
  - History: Common in women in their 30s to 60s. Often a known history of biliary tract disease or symptoms of biliary colic. Pain tends to increase 1 to 2 hours after fat intake. 75% of patients have had gallbladder symptoms in the past. The common mnemonic aid used to identify patients at risk is the "5 Fs:" fair, female, fat, forty, and fertile. Pain often wakes patient.
  - Pain: Dull to colicky, may be constant. Onset may be sudden.
  - Location: RUQ with radiation to the right subscapular region. Often the pain begins in the midline, then resolves and recurs in 6 to 8 hours in the RUQ. May generalize with gallbladder rupture or severe infection.
  - Other signs and symptoms: Nausea, vomiting, fever, and jaundice if significant obstruction exists. In chronic obstruction, urine may be tea colored and the stool may be clay colored.
  - Exam: Hypoactive bowel tones. Often signs of peritonitis, but some patients present with colicky pain. Right rectus muscle spasm may be present. RUQ tenderness with a positive *Murphy's sign.*
  - Studies: Elevated WBCs, bilirubin, and LFTs. Stones are uncommonly seen on plain films (<15%). Ultrasonography is the scanning method of choice and may reveal thickening of the gallbladder wall, pericholecystic fluid, stones in the gallbladder or the bile ducts, and dilation of the gallbladder or the biliary tree. Nonurgent gallbladder function tests include techne-

tium Tc-99m radionuclide scanning. Liver is visualized within 5 to 10 minutes, followed by visualization of the gallbladder and the bile ducts. Failure or delay of gallbladder filling is abnormal. 95% of patients with nonvisualization of the gallbladder who are symptomatic have acute cholecystitis. A nonfilling gallbladder noted in a patient whose symptoms have resolved indicates chronic cholecystitis.

- Differential diagnosis:
Acute appendicitis.
Coronary artery disease.
Fitz-Hugh-Curtis disease.
Hepatitis.
Obstructive jaundice due to cancer.
Pancreatitis.
Peptic ulcer disease.
Pyelonephritis.
Renal colic.
Pneumonia.

- Acuity: Urgent.
- Treatment: NPO. Fluid resuscitation as necessary.
Appropriate antibiotic therapy.
Pain relief.
If ducts are dilated, transhepatic cholangiography with placement of a T-tube may be palliative.
Likewise, ERCP with sphincterotomy may allow passage of an obstructing stone.
Emergency surgical management is reserved for rupture or gangrene of the gallbladder, indicated by impending sepsis.

- Notes: Most acute cholecystitis is "cooled off" with antibiotic treatment until the WBC count normalizes prior to attempting cholecystectomy.

Pancreatitis

Pancreatitis may be acute, chronic, or relapsing.
- Clues to diagnosis:
  - History: Patients in their 20s to 50s with prior pancreatitis or alcohol abuse or a history of cholelithiasis.
  - Pain: Rapid onset; severe, deep, constant, and progressive. May be colicky.
  - Location: Epigastric with radiation to the back and both costal margins.

- Other signs and symptoms:

  Nausea, vomiting, and anorexia.

- Exam:

  Hypoactive to absent bowel tones. Epigastric tenderness. Hemorrhagic pancreatitis may be associated with retroperitoneal bleeding and blood that extravasates along tissue planes (*Grey Turner's sign* or *Cullen's sign*).

- Studies:

  Elevated WBCs and serum amylase are diagnostic. P-amylase is specific to the pancreas, and isoenzymes are useful in differentiating from salivary amylase. Serum lipase is also a highly specific test. Plain films may reveal calcification of the pancreas, pleural effusion, or a "sentinel loop" of bowel. CT or ultrasonographic scanning may be useful in assessing complications such as pseudocyst.

- Differential diagnosis:

  Acute appendicitis.
  Acute cholecystitis.
  Acute renal failure.
  Choledocholithiasis.
  Peptic ulcer disease.
  Mesenteric ischemia or thrombosis.
  Myocardial infarction.
  Small-bowel obstruction.

- Acuity:

  Urgent. **Emergent** if shock is apparent.

- Treatment:

  NPO.
  NG suction.
  Fluid resuscitation.
  Pain management. **Meperidine (Demerol) 50 to 150 mg intramuscularly (IM) every 3 to 4 hours, as necessary,** is thought to be more appropriate than MSO_4, because it causes less spasm of the sphincter of Oddi.
  Support respirations.
  Surgery is rarely required except for complications such as phlegmon, hemorrhagic pancreatitis, or pseudocyst.

- Notes:

  Patients with fever should be assessed with a CT scan to rule out pancreatic abscess. The severity of acute pancreatitis may be predicted by *Ranson's criteria,* which are summarized in Table 5–2. The larger the number of positive signs, the more severe the case. Patients demonstrating >4 positive

Table 5–2 □ RANSON'S CRITERIA FOR PREDICTING THE SEVERITY OF ACUTE PANCREATITIS

Initial	Over the First 48 Hours
Age >55 yr	Hct drop >10%
WBC >16,000/mm³	BUN rise >5 mg/dl
Blood glucose >200 mg/dl	Serum calcium <8 mg/dl
Serum LDH >350 IU/L	Bicarbonate deficit >4 mEq/L
Serum SGOT >250 Sigma	PaO₂ <60 mm Hg
Frankel U/dl	Fluid gain >6 L

WBC = white blood cell (count); LDH = lactate dehydrogenase; SGOT = serum glutamic-oxaloacetic transaminase; Hct = hematocrit; BUN = blood urea nitrogen; PaO₂ = arterial partial pressure of oxygen.

signs are at greater risk of developing hemorrhagic pancreatitis.

Hepatitis

Hepatitis may be acute, chronic, or relapsing. Etiologies include viral infection and alcohol or other toxin ingestion.
- Clues to diagnosis:
  - History: Exposure to known infectious agent or toxin.
  - Pain: Gradual onset of severe, achy pain.
  - Location: RUQ with radiation to the back and right costal margin.
  - Other signs and symptoms: Nausea, vomiting, anorexia, jaundice, and fever.
  - Exam: Normal to hypoactive bowel tones. Epigastric and RUQ tenderness. Note that the entire liver will be tender, including the lateral aspect. Palpate the low lateral intercostal spaces; this will be useful in differentiating hepatitis from acute cholecystitis.
  - Studies: Elevated WBCs and LFTs are suggestive in viral etiologies. Serologies are available to diagnose the specific causative agent.
- Acuity: Routine to urgent.
- Treatment: Fluid resuscitation and pain management. Enteric or blood precautions as necessary. Acyclovir may have a role in chronic hepatitis B (HBV) infection. Surgery is rarely required.

■ Notes:

Five distinct viruses cause hepatitis: hepatitis A (HAV, formerly infectious hepatitis), HBV (formerly serum hepatitis), hepatitis C (HCV, formerly a subset of non-A, non-B hepatitis), hepatitis D (HDV, also known as delta-associated hepatitis, which requires concomitant HBV infection for replication), and hepatitis E (HEV, viral cause of non-A, non-B hepatitis). HAV and HEV are transmitted in a fecal or oral manner, and the remainder of the viruses are transmitted parenterally.

Hepatic reserve is estimated by the *Child's classification* (Table 5–3), which estimates risk based on biochemical and physical examination findings.

Acute Appendicitis

■ Clues to diagnosis:

■ History:	Characteristic pattern of pain progression.
■ Pain:	Initially a generalized ache, which progresses within 6 to 8 hours to localized severe ache.
■ Location:	Epigastric, then periumbilical, then RLQ (McBurney's point). As the appendix is variable in its location, the origin of the localized pain may vary.
■ Other signs and symptoms:	Anorexia is the most frequent associated symptom. Nausea and vomiting are more variable. Fever may be present, but up to one-third of patients will be afebrile.
■ Exam:	RLQ point tenderness, tenderness to percussion. Peritonitis is common. Other

Table 5–3 □ CHILD'S CLASSIFICATION OF HEPATIC RESERVE

	Class A (Minimal Risk)	Class B (Moderate Risk)	Class C (Advanced Risk)
Bilirubin (mg/dl)	<2	2–3	>3
Albumin (g/dl)	>3.5	3–3.5	<3.0
Ascites	None	Easy to control	Difficult to control
Encephalopathy	None	Minimal	Advanced
Nutritional status	Excellent	Good	Poor
Mortality in shunting procedures	<2%	10%	50%

findings may include RLQ hyperesthesia, indirect (referred) rebound, or *psoas* or *obturator signs.*

- Studies:

Elevated WBCs, but one-third of patients may have a normal WBC count. Infrequently WBCs in the UA. Ultrasonography is emerging as a valuable tool to diagnose appendicitis and may find a thickened, noncompressible appendix, luminal stones, or rupture. Plain films are not usually helpful but may occasionally show a fecalith in the appendix.

- Differential diagnosis:

See Table 5–4.

- Acuity:

Emergency.

- Treatment:

NPO.

Exploratory laparotomy. If the appendix is found to be normal, it is removed anyway, to avoid future confusion. The presence of a McBurney's incision scar (the most commonly used incision, and used only in appendectomy) will suggest to future examiners that the appendix has been removed. Removing the appendix also eliminates future risk of appendicitis.

- Notes:

Especially difficult to diagnose in the very young (<3 years old) and in the elderly. The orientation of the appendix relative to the cecum may drastically alter the presenting symptoms.

Table 5–4 □ COMMON DIAGNOSES THAT MAY MIMIC APPENDICITIS

Intestinal	Renal
Crohn's disease	Nephrolithiasis
Ulcerative colitis	Pyelonephritis
Gastroenteritis	Perinephric abscess
Mesenteric lymphangitis	Hydronephrosis
Inflamed Meckel's diverticulum	
Diverticulitis	**Gynecologic**
Psoas abscess	Salpingitis
Cecal tumor	Ovarian torsion
Intestinal obstruction	Ovarian cyst
Acute cholecystitis	(ruptured)
Perforated duodenal ulcer	Ectopic pregnancy

Meckel's Diverticulitis

This results from persistence of a portion of the vitelline duct. It is found on the antimesenteric border of the distal ileum. Pain may be caused by inflammation (diverticulitis) or by obstruction and may be difficult to differentiate from acute appendicitis. A technetium-99m pertechnetate scan, which identifies gastric mucosa, may aid in diagnosis if the patient presents with lower GI bleeding.

Acute Diverticulitis

Affects congenital or acquired diverticuli in the large intestine.
- Clues to diagnosis:
  - History: Documented diverticulosis.
  - Pain: Severe ache, crampy pain.
  - Location: Left lower quadrant (LLQ) > RLQ.
  - Other signs and symptoms: Fever and chills.
  - Exam: LLQ tenderness. A mass may be palpable and peritonitis may be apparent if a diverticulum has ruptured resulting in an abscess.
  - Studies: Elevated WBCs. CT scan may show abscess or mass. Contrast enema will fill the diverticuli and may show areas of perforation.
- Acuity: Urgent.
- Treatment: Fluid resuscitation and pain management. Appropriate antibiotic therapy.
                        May be treated as an outpatient, but if the patient is infirm or the inflammation is severe, hospitalization may be required.
                        Emergency surgical management is reserved for perforation with impending sepsis.
- Notes: Surgical options may include exploratory laparotomy with colonic diversion, or transcutaneous drainage of the abscess.

Acute Obstruction of the Small Intestine

Lack of recognition and correction of this problem will lead to bowel infarction. The major etiologies include postoperative adhesions, hernias, tumors, intussusception, strictures, and volvulus.
- Clues to diagnosis:
  - History: Prior abdominal surgery, GI neoplasm.

▪ Pain:	Sudden, crampy, or colicky. The patient may be pain free between bouts.
▪ Location:	Periumbilical or generalized.
▪ Other signs and symptoms:	Vomiting. The character of the vomitus will give clues as to the location of the obstruction. Clear vomitus indicates obstruction proximal to the bile duct. Bilious vomitus indicates obstruction distal to the sphincter of Oddi. Brown or feculent vomitus indicates a distal colonic obstruction and is a late finding.
▪ Exam:	Hyperactive bowel tones with rushes. Distention. Generalized tenderness.
▪ Studies:	Elevated WBCs. Three-way abdominal series is diagnostic and may show dilated loops of bowel or air/fluid levels. The colon distal to the obstruction may be empty of gas or stool.
▪ Differential diagnosis:	Acute appendicitis. Acute cholecystitis. Acute pancreatitis. Ascites. Large-bowel obstruction. Mesenteric ischemia or thrombosis. Paralytic ileus. Peptic ulcer disease.
▪ Acuity:	Urgent.
▪ Treatment:	NPO. NG decompression. Fluid resuscitation. Emergent surgical management is reserved for complications of bowel obstruction such as perforation.

Acute Obstruction of the Large Intestine

Most common causes include carcinoma, diverticulitis, fecal impaction, and volvulus.

▪ Clues to diagnosis:

▪ History:	Age older than 40 years of age. History of prior abdominal surgery.
▪ Pain:	Gradual onset, crampy, and intermittent. Cramps less frequent than in small-bowel obstruction.
▪ Location:	Generalized.
▪ Other signs	Constipation, nausea, and vomiting. Vom-

and
symptoms:

itus may be brown or feculent. Alternating diarrhea and constipation may indicate a partial obstruction.

- Exam:

Distended and tympanitic. Generalized tenderness. Stool may be guaiac positive in cases of carcinoma. A mass may be palpable. "Rushing" bowel tones differentiate obstruction from the quiet abdomen of paralytic ileus.

- Studies:

Elevated WBCs. Three-way abdominal series is diagnostic and may show dilated loops of bowel or air/fluid levels. The proximal small bowel may be normal if the ileocecal valve is competent. A cecum measuring 10 to 12 cm in diameter is an indication of impending perforation.

- Differential
diagnosis:

Metastatic cancer.
Ogilvie's syndrome.
Paralytic ileus.
Endometriosis.

- Acuity:

Urgent.

- Treatment:

NPO.
NG decompression.
Fluid resuscitation.
Sigmoidoscopy may be palliative to relieve pressure. If a lesion is found, diagnosis is possible. A rectal tube may be left in place to facilitate decompression.
Intravenous antibiotics are indicated in settings of fever, leukocytosis, or evidence of perforation.
Emergent surgical management is reserved for complications of bowel obstruction such as perforation. Contrast enema may aid in diagnosis.

Volvulus

This is a form of large-bowel obstruction caused by a twisting of the cecum or the sigmoid colon. The sigmoid is more commonly affected (80–85%). Cecum is more commonly affected in younger patients.
- Clues to diagnosis:
  - History:

Greater than 65 years of age. History of chronic laxative use and chronic constipation.

  - Pain:

Rapid onset, crampy, and intermittent.

- Location: Sigmoid volvulus: generalized to LLQ. Cecal volvulus: generalized to RLQ.

- Other signs and symptoms: Nausea and vomiting. Vomitus may be brown or feculent.

- Exam: Distended and tympanitic. Generalized tenderness.

- Studies: Three-way abdominal films. In sigmoid volvulus, the sigmoid colon looks doubled in a characteristic "bent inner tube" or "omega" sign. The convexity of the loop lies away from the site of obstruction. In cecal volvulus, the gas-filled cecum may be noted in the left upper quadrant (LUQ) and may appear as a "coffee bean" sign with the apex pointing toward the RLQ.

  Contrast enema will show the point of obstruction and may occasionally aid in the reduction of the obstruction.

- Acuity: **Emergency.** Rapid reduction will decrease the risk of infarction.

- Treatment: NPO.

  Fluid resuscitation.

  Sigmoidoscopy. This will be diagnostic and curative in sigmoid volvulus. Cecal volvulus may require contrast enema or surgical reduction.

Mesenteric Ischemia

This may be an acute or chronic disorder. The acute form is usually due to arterial embolization and is associated with a 90 to 95% mortality rate despite surgical resection.

- Clues to diagnosis:

  - History: Known arteriosclerotic disease. Taking medications known to decrease intestinal blood flow (Table 5–5).

  - Pain: Crampy, postprandial, especially after large meals.

  - Location: Epigastric or generalized.

  - Exam: Generalized tenderness, but the pain is usually well out of proportion to the physical findings.

  - Other signs and symptoms: Nausea and vomiting. Weight loss or change in bowel habits. Look for evidence of cardiovascular or peripheral vascular disease. If infarction is present,

Table 5–5 □ **MEDICATIONS KNOWN TO DECREASE INTESTINAL BLOOD FLOW**

Angiotensin	Methoxamine
Digoxin	Norepinephrine
Dopamine (high dose)	Ouabain
Epinephrine	Phenylephrine
Halothane	Prostaglandins E_1, E_2, and F_2 (α or β)
Indomethacin	Vasopressin
Metaraminol	

	then melena and peritonitis will be evident.
▪ Studies:	Elevated WBCs. Angiography may locate the arterial lesion, but degree of occlusion may not correlate with degree of symptoms.
▪ Acuity:	Urgent. **Emergent** if sepsis is evident.
▪ Treatment:	NPO.
	Emergency surgical management is reserved for infarction.
	Arterial reconstruction is curative.

Bowel Infarct

This may be due to intussusception, volvulus, herniation, thrombosis, or ischemic colitis.

- Clues to diagnosis:

▪ History:	Preexisting condition such as inflammatory bowel disease or prior abdominal surgery.
▪ Pain:	Gradual onset, crampy, and sharp.
▪ Location:	Generalized.
▪ Exam:	Distention, generalized abdominal tenderness.
▪ Studies:	Elevated WBCs. Progressive acidemia and shock. Plain films may show stasis or obstruction.
▪ Acuity:	**Emergency.**
▪ Treatment:	NPO.
	Fluid resuscitation.
	Exploratory laparotomy with bowel resection.

Abdominal Abscess

- Clues to diagnosis:

▪ History:	History of diverticulitis or other ruptured

viscus. Recent abdominal procedure, especially biliary, pancreatic, or gastric.

- Pain: Gradual onset, sharp, and constant.
- Location: Depends on the location of the abscess. Pain from subphrenic abscesses may radiate to the shoulders.
- Exam: Distention. Tenderness to palpation. Rupture of an abscess may result in peritonitis.
- Other signs and symptoms: Nausea, vomiting, anorexia, and fever.
- Studies: Elevated WBCs. CT scan or ultrasonogram may localize the mass.
- Acuity: Urgent. Ruptured abscess is an **emergency.**
- Treatment: NPO.
                    Fluid resuscitation.
                    Appropriate antibiotic therapy.
                    Emergency transcutaneous drainage of intact abscesses.
                    Emegency surgical management is reserved for ruptured abscesses.
- Notes: Abdominal abscesses may form even in the setting of broad-spectrum antibiotic therapy. To facilitate the diagnosis, it may be necessary to stop the antibiotics.

Renal Calculi

- Clues to diagnosis:
  - History: Prior renal stones, hypercalcemia, or hypercalciuria.
  - Pain: Sudden, severe, and colicky.
  - Location: Depends on the location of the stone. High ureteral stones are felt in the right or left flank. As they move down the ureter, pain may radiate into the groin, the perineum, or the testicle.
  - Other signs and symptoms: Dysuria, hematuria, and dehydration.
  - Exam: Abdomen may be benign.
  - Studies: RBCs in the UA. 80% of stones are visible on plain films of the abdomen. Intravenous pyelography will determine the degree of obstruction and size of the stone.
- Acuity: Urgent.
- Treatment: Fluid resuscitation.

Pain management.

Strain urine to ensure passage of the stone.

Most stones pass on their own, but stones of >1 cm or stones that do not move with time may need surgical removal, transurethral basket extraction, or lithotripsy.

Pyelonephritis

- Clues to diagnosis:
  - History: Recent UTI.
  - Pain: Gradual, severe, and constant with colicky increases.
  - Location: Right or left flank into back, abdomen, groin, perineum, or testicle.
  - Other signs and symptoms: Dysuria, frequency, hematuria, fever, chills.
  - Exam: Abdomen may be benign. Tenderness over the affected flank.
  - Studies: Elevated WBCs. WBCs and RBCs in the UA. WBC casts may be seen.
- Acuity: Urgent.
- Treatment: Fluid resuscitation.
                    Pain management.
                    Culture urine.
                    Appropriate empirical antibiotic therapy.
                    Focus antibiotic therapy as culture results dictate.

Ruptured Abdominal Aortic Aneurysm

- Clues to diagnosis:
  - History: Known abdominal aneurysm, hypertension, or arteriosclerotic disease.
  - Pain: Sudden, severe, and tearing.
  - Location: Epigastric or periumbilical with sharp radiation to the back or groin.
  - Exam: Hypoactive bowel sounds. Peritonitis. Pulsatile abdominal mass. Decreased femoral and lower extremity pulses. Progressive shock.
  - Studies: CT scan, angiogram, or ultrasonogram will confirm the diagnosis in a stable patient. An unstable patient should be evaluated on the OR table.
- Acuity: **Emergency.**
- Treatment: NPO.

Fluid and pressor resuscitation.

Emergency exploratory laparotomy with repair of the rupture.

- Notes: These patients are critically ill and require immediate surgery. Send a crossmatch immediately for 5 to 10 units of whole blood. Be prepared to transfuse with type O, Rh negative uncrossmatched blood as is necessary until crossmatched blood is available. Advise the blood bank that a "high-volume" case is in progress.

Acute Salpingitis (Pelvic Inflammatory Disease)

- Clues to diagnosis:
  - History: Occurs before menopause, usually just after a menstrual period. History of chlamydial or gonorrheal infection.
  - Pain: Sharp or achy.
  - Location: RLQ or LLQ with radiation to the back and umbilicus.
  - Other signs and symptoms: Nausea, vomiting, fever, and vaginal discharge.
  - Exam: Hypoactive bowel tones. RLQ or LLQ tenderness. Cervical motion tenderness. Possibly adnexal mass.
  - Studies: Elevated WBCs. Ultrasonography may be useful in differentiating ovarian pathology or ectopic pregnancy.
  - Differential diagnosis: Acute appendicitis. Ovarian torsion. Tubal pregnancy.
- Acuity: Urgent.
- Treatment: Fluid resuscitation. Appropriate antibiotic therapy. Emergency surgical management is reserved for tubo-ovarian abscesses.
- Notes: This is best treated by a gynecologist.

Ovarian Cyst

Usually present with pain if in association with torsion or rupture.
- Clues to diagnosis:
  - History: Prior cysts.
  - Pain: Of sudden onset and constant.
  - Location: RLQ or LLQ.

- Exam: Palpable mass on pelvic examination.
- Studies: Ultrasound is diagnostic and is useful in ruling out acute appendicitis.
- Acuity: Urgent.
- Treatment: Fluid resuscitation and pain management. Emergency surgical management is reserved for acute hemorrhage or torsion.
- Notes: This is best treated by a gynecologist.

Ectopic Pregnancy

95% of ectopic pregnancies are tubal.
- Clues to diagnosis:
  - History: Suspected pregnancy.
  - Pain: Sudden onset, sharp, and persistent.
  - Location: RLQ or LLQ.
  - Other signs and symptoms: Occasionally nausea and vomiting. Signs of early pregnancy: softening and cyanosis of the cervix, and amenorrhea.
  - Exam: Mass on abdominal or pelvic examination and point tenderness.
  - Studies: Positive β-hCG. Ultrasonogram is diagnostic. Progressive anemia is possible.
  - Differential diagnosis: Acute appendicitis. Ovarian cyst. Salpingitis.
- Acuity: **Emergency.**
- Treatment: NPO. Exploratory laparotomy or laparoscopy with removal of the conceptus.
- Notes: This is best treated by a gynecologist.

■ SPECIAL SURGICAL CONSIDERATIONS

Postoperative Considerations

1. Table 5–6 lists common postoperative conditions associated with abdominal pain and fever.
2. After antral resection of the stomach, and less commonly with other gastric resections, a "dumping" syndrome results in which partially digested highly osmotic foods are transported into the small intestine. This leads to hypermotility of the small intestine and rapid absorption of carbohydrates. The syndrome presents with early symptoms of abdominal pain after meals and diarrhea, and late symptoms of hypoglycemia due to hypersecretion of insulin in response to the carbohydrate bolus. It is treated by instituting a "postgas-

Table 5–6 □ COMMON CAUSES OF POSTOPERATIVE ABDOMINAL PAIN AND FEVER

Condition	Common Cause	Diagnostic Study	Treatment
Abdominal abscess	Anastomotic leak	CT scan	Drainage, antibiotics
Peritonitis	Anastomotic leak, peritoneal soilage	PE, paracentesis	Antibiotics
Pancreatitis	Surgical trauma	CT scan, amylase	Fluid support, drainage of pseudocyst as necessary
Cholangitis	Surgical trauma	US, transhepatic cholangiogram	T-tube drainage, antibiotics, surgical repair
Perforated peptic ulcer	Stress ulceration	Contrast swallow, endoscopy	Surgical repair
Acute cholecystitis	Perioperative stasis	US, LFTs, scintiscan	Antibiotics, surgical resection
Wound infection	Dehiscence	PE	Debridement, antibiotics

CT = computed tomography; PE = physical examination; US = ultrasonography; LFT = liver function test.

trectomy diet" consisting of frequent, small, low-carbohydrate meals.

3. Diarrhea is also common with onset of feeding after any bowel resection, as there is a measurable loss of absorptive surface. An extensive resection will result in a higher chance of feeding intolerance. Antibiotic-associated diarrhea and *C. difficile* pseudomembranous colitis are common postoperative complications. See Chapter 6.

Remember

- Keep in mind the following "nonabdominal" causes of abdominal pain:
  1. Myocardial infarction
  2. Pneumonia
  3. Diabetes mellitus
  4. Porphyria
  5. UTI
  6. Sickle cell disease
- Female patients should be considered pregnant until proved otherwise.

BOWEL FUNCTION—CONSTIPATION AND DIARRHEA

Phone calls regarding the bowel functions of your patients will be frequent; fortunately, most of these problems can be managed over the phone. Patients usually have major changes in bowel function while hospitalized because of dietary changes, less mobility, narcotic analgesics, and other medications. You should be familiar with the major causes of these changes and feel comfortable with the range of options for treating these problems. Many patients become distressed with bowel function changes and appreciate being made to feel more comfortable.

Constipation

■ PHONE CALL

Questions

1. **Has this patient had surgery? If so, what was the operation and when was it performed?**

   Patients undergoing abdominal surgery develop a functional ileus that lasts 4 to 5 days or more. These patients should *not* be given a laxative. They must wait for their gastrointestinal (GI) function to return. Ambulation appears to help GI function return postoperatively. Also, postoperative appendectomy patients should not receive rectal suppositories. Some surgeons believe that this may cause contractions in the colon and increase the risk of appendix stump leaks.

2. **Why does the patient want a laxative? When was the last bowel movement (BM)? What is the normal bowel routine for this patient?**

   Some people have up to three BMs per day, while others have a BM as seldom as once a week. These ranges are normal. You should know a patient's normal routine before prescribing a laxative.

3. **Is the patient nauseous or has he or she been vomiting?**

   Be hesitant to prescribe a laxative to a patient who has signs of upper GI dysfunction. The patient could have another problem, such as intestinal obstruction or appendicitis. Constipation alone does not lead to upper GI symptoms unless the patient is impacted and has a significant ileus.

4. **Does the patient have abdominal pain?**
   A patient with abdominal pain and who requests a laxative should be examined. An ileus, and hence constipation, results from many serious surgical problems of the abdomen. For example, a perforated viscus often presents with abdominal pain and ileus.
5. **Has a rectal examination been performed on the patient?**
   Fecal impaction is diagnosed by rectal examination. Laxatives do not usually help patients who are impacted.
6. **Does the patient routinely use laxatives?**
   It is becoming more common to see patients who abuse laxatives; these patients develop GI dysfunction.

Orders

Once you have determined that it is safe and appropriate to prescribe a laxative or an enema, you must think about what type of agent to use (Table 6–1). Laxatives can be delivered by mouth or rectum; enemas are delivered by rectum.

Oral Laxatives

Laxatives that are usually considered stool softeners include surface-active agents (docusate sodium [Colace]) and bulk-forming agents (psyllium [Metamucil, Konsyl]). These agents tend to soften the stool for the foodstuffs eaten at about the same time that the agent is taken. For example, a patient with constipation who begins taking Metamucil is unlikely to benefit until the older hard stool has been cleared and the bulk-forming agent can soften the newly formed stool. In a similar fashion, surface-active laxatives such as Colace take a day or more to show significant stool-softening action.

The osmotic laxatives include magnesium citrate. This is a pleasant tasting, carbonated liquid. Most patients have a BM within several hours of taking this agent. You can repeat the dose if no results are obtained with the first dose. Commonly used in bowel preparation before surgery is the osmotic agent GoLYTELY. This agent contains polyethylene glycol, circumvents fluid absorption, and rapidly cleanses the bowel. It is not used routinely as a laxative, but it is a good bowel-preparation agent.

Rectal Laxatives

Glycerin is an osmotic laxative given rectally as a suppository. Onset of action is usually 30 to 60 minutes. Diphenylmethane (bisacodyl [Dulcolax]) is a stimulant of defecation given as a suppository and is popular in hospitals. If the first bisacodyl suppository is ineffective, the dose can be repeated.

Table 6–1 □ COMMON LAXATIVES AND ENEMAS FOR USE IN
SURGICAL PATIENTS

Type of Agent	Name of Agent	Dose	Cautions
Bulk-forming laxative	Psyllium seed Metamucil Konsyl	1 tsp in liquid PO every day to 3 times per day	Some drugs may be bound by the cellulose
Surface-active laxative	Docusate (Colace)	100 mg PO 3 times per day	
Lubricant laxative	Mineral oil	10–15 ml PO twice daily	Decreases fat-soluble vitamin absorption
Osmotic laxatives	Magnesium citrate	100 ml of a 15 g/300 ml solution PO	Do not use in patients with renal dysfunction
	Glycerin	1 preformed suppository	
Stimulant laxatives	Dulcolax	5–15 mg PO or 10 mg PR	
Hypertonic enema	Fleet enema	60–120 ml in disposable container	Do not use in patients with nausea, vomiting, or abdominal pain
Mineral oil enema	Fleet mineral oil enema	60–120 ml in disposable container	Good for fecal impaction

PO = by mouth; PR = rectally.

Enemas

Enemas deliver agents directly to the rectum. This is useful to
help the patient evacuate hard stool. Options include the hypertonic enemas (Fleet enemas), oil-retention enemas, and soapsuds
enemas.

What To Use and When—Some Suggestions

Usually, it is best to put most hospitalized patients on an oral
stool softener, especially if any narcotic analgesic is to be used.
Most patients prefer Colace or a bulk-forming agent such as
Metamucil or Konsyl. Frequently, a stool softener will eliminate
the need for other laxatives.

Many patients who are constipated prefer a stimulatory suppository, such as Dulcolax. This stimulatory suppository is safe
and may be repeated until results are achieved. If the stimulatory
suppository fails, a osmotic agent such as magnesium citrate may

be effective. However, some patients develop some abdominal cramping with osmotic agents.

Finally, enemas can be used if attempts with an osmotic agent are unsuccessful. A Fleet enema or a mineral oil enema usually gives profound evacuation. Mineral oil enemas are especially good for softening impacted feces.

Diarrhea

■ PHONE CALL

Questions

1. **Has the patient had surgery? If so, what was the operation and when was it performed?**
2. **Does the patient have abdominal pain or a fever? Is there blood in the stool?**
   A patient may have infectious diarrhea. Signs that suggest an infectious etiology are abdominal pain, fever, and bloody diarrheal stools. Never give an antidiarrheal agent to a patient you suspect may have an infectious GI process.
3. **Does the patient have a history of diarrhea? Are there any known or suspected medical problems?**
   Perhaps the patient has a history of lactose intolerance, intestinal malabsorption, short-bowel syndrome, Crohn's disease, ulcerative colitis, or ischemic colitis. These are common causes of diarrhea.
4. **Did the patient eat foodstuffs recently that did not agree with him or her?**
   The patient may have developed food poisoning or may have food intolerances.
5. **Does the patient have any flu symptoms?**
   A major cause of diarrhea is viral gastroenteritis.
6. **Is the patient on tube feedings?**
   A major cause of diarrhea in patients taking tube feedings is administration of feedings at a rate or an osmolarity greater than what the small intestine can tolerate.
7. **Is the patient taking broad-spectrum antibiotics?**
   Always suspect *Clostridium difficile* if severe diarrhea begins in a patient taking broad-spectrum antibiotics. Remember that ordinary antibiotic-induced diarrhea is more common than that caused by *C. difficile.*

Orders

Regardless of the cause of diarrhea, make sure that the patient is well hydrated. Ask the nursing staff if the patient has been able to take adequate fluids orally. A good oral fluid for repletion is an isotonic glucose-containing electrolyte solution. Prolonged, severe diarrhea in a patient unable to take oral fluids leads to dehydration. If a patient is unable to take oral fluids and has significant diarrhea, the patient should be rehydrated intravenously.

■ MANAGEMENT

Diarrhea may or may not be associated with abdominal pain. It is not uncommon for the initial resumption of bowel function following an abdominal procedure to be diarrheal stools. This is usually without other symptoms and is self-limited. There are other syndromes of diarrhea, which must be differentiated to appropriately treat the symptom.

- Clues to diagnosis:

  - Pain: Gradual or sudden onset, mild to severe intermittent cramps.

  - Location: Generalized but occasionally will be localized.

  - Other signs and symptoms: Vomiting, fever, and chills may also be present. Diarrhea mixed with blood or mucus suggests a bacterial or parasitic etiology.

  - Exam: Diffuse tenderness. Stool may be guaiac positive.

  - Studies: Elevated WBCs. Stool cultures should be sent for O&P, rotozyme, *C. difficile* toxin titer, and fecal leukocyte studies, as appropriate.

- Acuity: Routine to urgent.
- Treatment: Fluid support.
                    Enteric precautions as indicated.
                    Antibiotics as indicated.
                    See treatments under specific diarrhea etiologies below.

Antibiotic-Induced Diarrhea

A greater understanding of this problem has made this common entity easier to anticipate, diagnose, and treat. This can happen with any antibiotic and is not associated with colitis (tissue invasion).

- Signs and symptoms: May be symptomless or may present with crampy abdominal pain. Evidence of tissue invasion (fever, bloody stool, or leukocytosis) is rarely present.

- Stool characteristics: Watery, rarely bloody or containing fecal leukocytes.

- Treatment: Discontinue the identified antibiotic.

  Fluid support.

  Avoid antidiarrheal and narcotic medications.

Antibiotic-Induced Colitis

This occurs in about 1 per 1000 antibiotic-treated patients and is associated with evidence of invasive disease (fecal leukocytes, fever, and leukocytosis). The most likely antibiotics include ampicillin, clindamycin, and cephalosporins. *C. difficile* toxin–positive colitis represents about 25% of cases of antibiotic-associated colitis. Diagnosis is confirmed by the presence of *C. difficile* toxin in the stool. Sigmoidoscopy may show characteristic pseudomembranes.

- Signs and symptoms: Crampy abdominal pain, fever, and leukocytosis occurring within days after the beginning of antibiotic therapy. Evidence of peritonitis may indicate megacolon or perforation, often associated with marked leukocytosis in excess of 20,000.

- Stool characteristics: Watery, occasionally bloody, fecal leukocytes, and possibly *C. difficile* toxin–positive.

- Treatment:

  - Mild colitis: Discontinue the identified antibiotic.

    Fluid and electrolyte support.

    Avoid antidiarrheal and narcotic medications.

  - Moderate to severe colitis, and *C. difficile* toxin–positive cases: **Vancomycin (Vancocin) 125 to 500 mg by mouth 4 times per day for 7 to 14 days or metronidazole (Flagyl) 500 mg by mouth or intravenously 3 times per day for 10 days.**

    Discontinue the identified antibiotic.

    Fluid and electrolyte support.

    Avoid antidiarrheal and narcotic medications.

    Bowel rest for severe cases.

- Notes: Relapse rate is high, up to 20%, and requires additional treatment.

Noninvasive Gastroenteritis

Usually viral in etiology. The associated risk is of dehydration and electrolyte abnormalities, greatest in pediatric or elderly patients.

- Signs and symptoms: Crampy abdominal pain, fever, and leukocytosis.

- Stool   Watery, rarely with blood or fecal leukocytes,

characteristics:	and may be rotozyme positive if rotavirus is the causative agent.
■ Treatment:	Fluid and electrolyte support.
	Antidiarrheal medications **only** if no intestinal anastomoses are present (Table 6–2).
	NPO if abdominal pain is severe. Clear liquids when tolerated, with slow advancement to a bland diet.
	Avoid milk and milk by-products because lactase is not as readily available in settings of acute gastroenteritis, which increases intraluminal concentrations of milk sugars, contributing to an osmotic diarrhea.
	Enteric precautions as necessary.
	Often treated as an outpatient, but if the patient is infirm or dehydrated or if the inflammation is severe, hospitalization may be required.

Invasive Gastroenteritis

May be bacterial or parasitic. Often there is evidence of invasive disease. Bloody diarrhea is found with acute infections caused by *Shigella*, enterotoxic *Escherichia coli, Campylobacter, Salmonella, Yersinia*, and *Entamoeba*.

■ Signs and symptoms:	Crampy abdominal pain, fever, and leukocytosis.
■ Stool characteristics:	Watery, with blood and mucus. Fecal leukocytes, specific culture, or O&P positivity.
■ Treatment:	Fluid and electrolyte support.
	Appropriate antibiotic therapy.
	NPO if abdominal pain is severe.
	Clear liquids when tolerated, with slow advancement to a bland diet.
	Avoid milk and milk by-products.
	Fluid resuscitation as needed.
	Enteric precautions as needed.

Inflammatory Bowel Disease

Ulcerative colitis and Crohn's disease may reactivate perioperatively and complicate pre- or postoperative care. Usually the patient has a history of prior episodes.

■ Signs and symptoms:	Crampy abdominal pain, fever, and leukocytosis.
■ Stool characteristics:	Watery, occasionally bloody, fecal leukocytes. Negative stool cultures and O&P.
■ Treatment:	Bowel rest as indicated.

Table 6–2 □ ANTIDIARRHEAL THERAPIES

Generic	Brand Name	Dose
Diphenoxylate HCl (2.5 mg) with atropine sulfate (0.025 mg)	Lomotil	2 tablets PO 4 times per day (may take up to 48 hr to work)
Loperamide HCl	Imodium	4 mg PO initial dose followed by 2 mg PO with each unformed stool (not to exceed 16 mg/day)
Difenoxin HCl (1 mg) with atropine sulfate (0.025 mg)	Motofen	2 tablets PO initial dose followed by 1 tablet PO 3 to 4 times per day as needed, or 1 tablet with each unformed stool (not to exceed 8 tablets/day)
Phenobarbital (16.2 mg) with atropine sulfate (0.02 mg) and hyoscyamine sulfate (0.1 mg) and scopolamine hydrobromide (6.5 μg)	Donnatal	1–2 tablets PO every 6–8 hr as needed
Belladonna (16.2) with opium powder (30–60 mg)	B&O Supprette	1 suppository PR every day or twice daily as needed (not to exceed 4 doses/day)
Bismuth subsalicylate	Pepto-Bismol	2 Tbsp or tablets PO every 0.5–1 hr as needed (not to exceed 8 doses/day) (may take up to 24 hr to work)
Morphine (2 mg/5 ml) with anise oil (0.02 ml), benzoic acid (20 mg), camphor (0.2 ml), and alcohol (45%)	Paregoric*	5–10 ml PO 4 times/day as needed
Kaolin (975 mg/5 ml) and pectin (22 mg)	Kaopectate	60–120 ml PO after each loose stool

Notes: Diphenoxylate HCl and difenoxin HCl are related to meperidine HCl; they are considered Schedule V medications and are habit forming. Opium powder is a Schedule II medication and is habit forming. Do not exceed recommended dosage.

PO = by mouth; PR = rectally.

*No brand name.

Corticosteroids. Enemas may be sufficient for localized disease. Oral or intravenous doses may be required for more severe symptoms.
Sulfasalazine (Azulfidine) 1 to 4 g per day by mouth divided into 3 to 6 evenly spaced doses.

Feeding-Associated Diarrhea

This is especially associated with tube feedings. Volumes and concentrations of feedings should be increased slowly, or the bowel will not tolerate the osmotic load.

- Signs and symptoms: May be symptomless or may be associated with crampy abdominal pain.
- Stool characteris-tics: Watery to milky, Clinitest positive.
- Treatment: Slow or stop current feeding regimen. Maintain hydration with intravenous fluids if necessary.

Other Causes of Diarrhea

1. Laxative use.
2. Other malabsorption, e.g., sprue or Whipple's disease.
3. Pancreatic insufficiency.
4. Lactase deficiency (lactose intolerance).
5. Irritable bowel syndrome.
6. Diabetic enteropathy.
7. Visceral scleroderma.

The most common antidiarrheal agents used in the hospital are Kaopectate, Imodium, and Lomotil. These medications are safe and well tolerated by patients. Kaopectate is an absorbent, which decreases stool content. It exerts local action and is not absorbed. Onset is within 30 minutes and duration is 4 to 6 hours. Imodium has a slower onset of action but is well tolerated and effective. The manufacturer does not recommend continuing the maximum dosage of 8 mg/day for >2 days. Lomotil is a highly effective drug that can be titrated to control moderate to serious diarrhea. Although the suggested dose is up to 5 mg every 4 to 6 hours, a patient with chronic diarrhea can usually tolerate higher doses. Safe doses for many patients can be titrated to 10 mg every 6 hours.

Remember that diarrhea in a pediatric patient is a frequent cause of dehydration. Many diarrheal illnesses in pediatric patients are caused by very contagious viruses. Although the diarrhea is usually self-limited, the fluid status of these patients must be monitored carefully and fluid replacement given appropriately.

7

CHEST PAIN

Chest pain is one of the most concerning calls you will receive. Chest pain may represent a nonserious problem such as heartburn or a life-threatening problem such as myocardial infarction (MI). To best handle chest pain calls, follow a logical progression in the evaluation and management of the patient. Always assume that chest pain represents a serious medical problem until proved otherwise.

■ PHONE CALL

Questions

1. **What is the pain like, and how severe is it (on a scale of 1–10)?**

   The greatest concern is that the patient has a life-threatening problem such as myocardial ischemia. Angina pectoris or MI often presents with diverse pain manifestations and severities. However, many types of noncardiac pain can be distinguished by history and pain description. For example, burning chest pain between meals often represents esophageal reflux or peptic ulcer disease, whereas crushing substernal pain after exertion is more suggestive of myocardial ischemia.

   Patients with any significant chest pain, chest pressure, or chest pain radiating to the jaw, neck, shoulder, or arm should have an electrocardiogram (ECG). Always think about a cardiac source of pain, and rule this out before proceeding in the differential diagnosis.

2. **Are there any changes in vital signs?**

   Hemodynamic instability or respiratory compromise associated with chest pain represents a life-threatening emergency. Begin resuscitation efforts immediately.

3. **Is there any shortness of breath (SOB)?**

   SOB is commonly associated with myocardial ischemia. However, SOB may also be the initial symptom of pulmonary problems such as pneumothorax or pulmonary embolus. Ask if the SOB developed before or after the chest pain.

4. **Does the patient have a history of coronary artery disease (CAD), angina, MI, dyspepsia, reflux, or peptic ulcer disease?**

   The best way to ascertain the cause of chest pain is to

obtain a good history. Frequently, patients presenting with chest pain have a history of similar pain episodes already known to be of a cardiac or gastrointestinal (GI) cause. If a postoperative patient has had an MI in the last 6 months, he or she is more likely to have another MI than a patient who has not had a prior infarction.

5. Did the patient have surgery? If so, what operation was performed and when was it performed?

Surgery stresses the heart. Thus, it is understandable that postoperative patients may develop cardiac complications of surgery. Postoperative MIs occur in 0.4% of all patients who have undergone surgery. For some patient groups, the risk is higher. Patients who have significant atherosclerosis of the lower extremities, carotid vessels, or aorta have a risk of postoperative MI in the range of 5 to 10%. Always consider postoperative myocardial ischemia as a cause of chest pain. In general, the longer the duration of the operation and the greater the blood loss, the greater the risk of postoperative MI in patients with CAD.

Orders

Unless the pain is clearly related to a musculoskeletal or GI cause, myocardial ischemia should be suspected until disproved.

1. Obtain an ECG immediately.
2. Obtain a portable chest x-ray immediately if the patient has a chest tube or a history of chest trauma or has had chest surgery.
3. Give **sublingual nitroglycerin 0.4 mg every 5 minutes** until pain resolves. Hold medication for a systolic blood pressure (SBP) of <90 mm Hg.
4. If the pain is severe or associated with vital sign changes, ask the RN to stay with the patient and monitor the vital signs until you arrive.
5. Ask the RN to have the patient's chart at the bedside.

Inform RN

"Will arrive at the bedside in . . . minutes."

You must assume that every chest pain call may represent a medical emergency. Assess the patient immediately, and remember that the best evidence for the cause of the pain will come from the patient's history.

■ ELEVATOR THOUGHTS

What causes chest pain?

There are many possible causes of chest pain. Some of the more common causes are as follows:

- Cardiac
    Angina
    Infarction
    Aortic dissection
    Pericarditis
- Pulmonary
    Pleuritis
    Pneumothorax
    Pulmonary embolus
    Pulmonary contusion
    Severe asthma attack
- GI
    Esophageal reflux
    Esophagitis
    Peptic ulcer disease
    Diaphragmatic hernia
- Musculoskeletal
    Costochondritis
    Rib fracture
    Muscle spasm
    Chest tube–associated pain

■ MAJOR THREAT TO LIFE

- MI
- Pulmonary embolus
- Aortic dissection
- Pneumothorax

It is often difficult to distinguish these serious problems from one another quickly at the bedside. A severe MI leading to cardiogenic shock often is associated with respiratory failure. Pulmonary embolus or pneumothorax may lead to circulatory arrest if not treated appropriately. Frequently, the initial presentation is the best evidence. MI and aortic dissection often begin with pain. Pulmonary embolus and pneumothorax often begin with SOB and hypoxia.

■ BEDSIDE

Quick Look Test

Does the patient look well (comfortable), sick (uncomfortable or distressed), or critical (about to die)?

The overall appearance of the patient provides important evidence to the severity of the problem. A conversant, relatively comfortable patient is more likely to have a nonthreatening cause for chest pain (e.g., costochondritis or reflux). A pale, anxious patient is more likely to have a serious problem (e.g., myocardial ischemia or pulmonary embolism). Evaluating the patient's appearance and taking a quick history will help to best identify and manage the problem.

Airway and Vital Signs

What is the blood pressure (BP)?

Most patients with chest pain will have normal BP. Hypotension suggests cardiogenic shock, pulmonary embolus, cardiac tamponade, or tension pneumothorax, and the hypotension must be treated. Hypertension may be associated with an anxious patient with chest pain. Severe hypertension (systolic BP >180 mm Hg, diastolic BP >110 mm Hg) should also be treated, because it may worsen myocardial ischemia or it may help to expand an aortic aneurysm.

What is the heart rate (HR)?

Bradycardia may be associated with acute MI, in particular an inferior MI. It may also represent cardiogenic shock or a blockade due to drugs (e.g., beta blockers or calcium channel blockers). Treat only if the patient is hypotensive or the HR is <40 beats/min (see Chapter 9).

Tachycardia may be a response to anxiety and pain. However, tachycardia may also represent a tachyarrhythmia. The key tachyarrhythmias to look for include supraventricular tachycardia, wide-complex tachycardia, atrial fibrilliation, atrial flutter, and ventricular tachycardia. Many of these arrhythmias require immediate and emergent treatment (see Chapter 9).

What is the breathing pattern?

Tachypnea associated with hypoxia may signify acute MI, pulmonary edema, pulmonary embolus, or pneumothorax. Patients usually are in distress. Shallow breathing associated with splinting is more suggestive of a musculoskeletal cause (e.g., costochondritis or rib fracture) or of a pleural cause (e.g., pneumothorax or pleuritis).

What does the ECG show?

1. **Normal ECG**

    A normal ECG does not rule out myocardial ischemia. Further workup may be indicated if the chest pain by history is suggestive of a cardiac cause. Compare the new ECG to any previous ECG studies; look for new findings.

2. **An ECG with ST segment changes and T wave changes**

    ST segment changes with peaked upright or inverted T waves suggests acute MI. ST depression may indicate a non–Q wave MI.

3. An ECG with Q waves

New Q waves may suggest MI or prolonged myocardial ischemia.

If an acute MI is suggested by the evaluation, consult with a cardiologist immediately. Begin treatment with oxygen, nitrates, and analgesics. Thrombolytic therapy or coronary angiography with angioplasty is usually managed by the cardiology team. The patient will need continuous ECG monitoring, usually in a cardiac care unit (CCU).

Selective History and Chart Review

Ask the patient if he or she has known heart disease. Include in the brief history questions about angina, MI, reflux problems, and similar episodes of pain in the past. Skim the history and physical examination in the chart, paying special attention to the past medical history, medicines, and current problems.

Selective Physical Examination

The object of the physical examination is to find a cause of the chest pain or any sequelae of the chest pain. Focus on the vital signs, the nature of the pulse, the heart sounds, and the breath sounds.

VS: Measure HR, BP, and respiratory rate. Take the pulse and assess if it is regular or irregular, strong or weak. Evaluate for pulsus paradoxus (associated with cardiac tamponade).

CVS: Evaluate if there is a murmur or rub. Assess the heart sounds carefully.

Resp: Listen for the quality of the breath sounds. Evaluate the symmetry of the breath sounds of right and left lungs. Nonsymmetric breath sounds may indicate pneumothorax or postsurgical change. Listen for regions of nonaeration, hyperaeration, wheezes, rhonchi, and crackles.

Neck: Look for jugular venous distention (JVD). Measure any JVD to assess right-sided heart filling pressures. If there is elevated JVD, consider heart failure, fluid overload, cardiac tamponade, and constrictive pericarditis.

GI: Bowel sounds in the chest are indicative of diaphragmatic hernia. Assess for abdominal tenderness, softness of abdomen, liver edge position, and masses. Some forms of abdominal pain (e.g., epigastric pain) may be described by the patient as chest pain.

■ MANAGEMENT

Initial Management

Initial management includes providing oxygen, relieving ische-mic pain, and preventing and treating life-threatening complica-tions of the major serious causes of chest pain.

1. Place the patient on oxygen. Run oxygen at 4 L/min. If the patient retains CO_2, run oxygen at 2 L/min.
2. Provide **sublingual nitroglycerin 0.4 mg every 5 minutes** until pain resolves.
3. Order a portable chest x-ray (CXR) immediately if there are unequal breath sounds, if the patient has a chest tube or is at high risk for a pneumothorax, or if aortic pathology (aneurysm) is suspected.
4. Provide analgesia, especially during an active MI. Patients with an active MI will not obtain pain relief with nitroglyc-erin alone. **Intravenous (IV) morphine sulfate 2 to 4 mg** is an appropriate starting dosage. You may repeat every 2 to 3 minutes and titrate until pain is relieved.
5. Treat rhythm disturbances that are associated with hemody-namic instability or are at high risk for deteriorating into life-threatening arrhythmia (e.g., ventricular tachycardia) (see Chapter 9).

Definitive Management

This stage of management involves definitive treatment or tri-age after stabilizing the patient.

Myocardial Ischemia

Resolving Angina.   If the chest pain has been relieved with sublingual nitroglycerin and the patient has a history of angina, an adjustment of the patient's cardiac medications may be the only definitive treatment to be rendered. Discuss the case with your chief resident or attending physician. Nonemergent consul-tation with the patient's cardiologist or internist may be appro-priate.

New-Onset or Unstable Angina.   A patient with no prior cardiac history who develops chest pain of cardiac origin must be evaluated by cardiology (CCU/intensive care unit [ICU] team). In addition, a patient who develops angina at rest should be evaluated by a cardiologist whether or not the pain resolved with sublingual nitroglycerin. These consultations should be per-formed promptly.

Order serial ECGs and cardiac isoenzyme tests every 8 hours for a total of 3 times for any patient that you suspect may have had a small infarction not readily detectable on your initial evaluation. Any patient who does not have relief of ischemic cardiac pain with sublingual nitroglycerin or morphine should be transferred to the ICU or the CCU for continuous cardiac monitoring. These patients may need an IV nitroglycerin drip, aspirin administration, and beta-blockade therapy.

Myocardial Infarction.   Patients who are having a suspected MI need emergent evaluation by the cardiology (CCU or ICU) team. The treatment of these patients is variable. Treatment options include noninvasive therapy such as IV nitroglycerin, beta blockers, anticoagulation, and thrombolytic therapy. Invasive treatment options include coronary angiography and angioplasty. Treatment decisions are best made by the attending surgeon and the attending cardiologist.

Pericarditis Associated with MI

Acute Pericarditis.   Patients with large infarctions often develop acute pericarditis. Symptoms include substernal chest pain with pain radiation to the back. Pain is often relieved with sitting up. A pericardial friction rub may be heard. Echocardiography may be useful to diagnose the condition. Unless there is hemodynamic compromise (which is unusual), an echocardiogram may be performed nonemergently to arrive at the definitive diagnosis. Aspirin is useful to relieve pain. Do not use glucocorticoids or other nonsteroidal anti-inflammatory drugs (NSAIDs) because they retard myocardial scar formation and may increase the incidence of ventricular rupture after a large MI. For pericarditis that is *not* associated with MI, the treatment of choice is **indomethacin 50 mg PO three times per day.**

Aortic Dissection

An acute, proximal aortic dissection is a surgical emergency requiring emergent stabilization and antihypertensive therapy. Most of these patients are hypertensive.
1. Start therapy by placing the patient on a sodium nitroprusside drip.
    Start at **0.5 to 1.0 μg/kg/min and titrate the dose** to achieve an SBP of about 100 mm Hg or the minimum BP to maintain organ perfusion. The maximum dose of nitroprusside is about 10 μg/kg/min. Above this dosage, cyanide toxicity can develop, and it is a good idea to check thiocyanate levels if you are going to use higher doses.
2. In addition to nitroprusside, start the patient on a beta blocker.
    The use of nitroprusside alone is inadequate to avoid intimal shearing. Add a beta blocker even if the hypertension is resolved with nitroprusside. Esmolol is a good cardioselective beta-adrenergic antagonist to use. It has a short

half-life (9 minutes). Dosing ranges from 50 to 200 µg/kg/min.

3. If nitroprusside or esmolol is not available, use a single agent, labetalol, to lower BP and intimal shearing.

Dosing of **labetalol** is **20 mg IV every 10 minutes to a total of 300 mg.**

4. Arrange an emergent thoracic computed tomographic (CT) scan or a transesophageal echocardiogram.

A transthoracic echocardiogram provides less information than a CT scan or transesophageal echogram; however, it is better than no diagnostic study if the others are not available.

5. Type and crossmatch the patient for 6 to 8 units of packed red blood cells.

Obtain a platelet count, a prothrombin time, a partial thromboplastin time and electrolytes, and a renal panel.

6. Obtain an emergent surgical consultation.

Be prepared to arrange aortography if the surgical consultant believes it is needed.

Pneumothorax

A pneumothorax can be life threatening when tension or pressure is exerted against the heart, the great vessels, and the lung tissue. In a pneumothorax, air is usually trapped in the pleural space. If there is a parenchymal lung tear or leak, air continues to collect in the pleural space and the pneumothorax worsens. If you suspect a pneumothorax and the patient is stable and well oxygenated, obtain a CXR. Have the patient sit upright for the CXR so that any air in the pleural space can rise to the apex thoracic cavity.

A significant pneumothorax in the presence of a parenchymal air leak requires chest tube drainage (see Chapter 28). If a patient demonstrates agitation, progressive hypoxia, hypotension, or electromechanical dissociation, and you suspect a tension pneumothorax, emergency needle aspiration should be performed before chest tube placement. Insert a 14-gauge catheter or needle into the second or third intercostal space, midclavicular line, to acutely decompress the tension pneumothorax. Once the tension component of the pneumothorax is released, a chest tube can be inserted into the fifth or sixth intercostal space (see Chapter 28).

Pulmonary Embolism

A patient who develops sudden-onset SOB, hypoxia, and chest pain may have a pulmonary embolism. The details of diagnosis and management are presented in Chapter 28. Surgical patients are at high risk for this problem. Pulmonary embolism is common in patients with pelvic trauma, lower abdominal surgery, lower extremity surgery, prolonged immobilization, and venous disease of the lower extremities.

Reflux Esophagitis

Symptoms of reflux include heartburn, chest pain, dysphagia, and sore throat. The following treatments can be useful:
1. Have the patient propped up in bed.
   Keeping at least 30° of head elevation is important.
2. Have the patient avoid alcohol, chocolate, fat, and caffeine.
   These foods frequently make reflux worse.
3. Consider using an antacid.
   Maalox and Mylanta are useful, and both contain aluminum and magnesium hydroxide. These agents may cause diarrhea. The dosage is **30 ml PO every 4 hours as needed.** Amphojel contains only aluminum hydroxide. The dosage is **5 ml PO every 4 hours as needed.** This agent may cause constipation. Tums tablets contain calcium carbonate. The dosage is **500 mg PO as needed.**
4. Patients with ongoing or recurrent reflux problems are best treated with histamine H_2-receptor antagonists. See Chapter 5 for a list of these agents.
5. Metoclopramide improves gastric emptying and increases lower esophageal sphincter tone.
   It is most effective when used in combination with histamine H_2-receptor antagonists.

Musculoskeletal Pain

Costochondritis and rib pain are best treated with NSAIDs. **Ibuprofen 400 to 600 mg PO every 6 to 8 hours** or **naproxen 250 mg PO twice daily** is usually helpful. For more severe musculoskeletal pain, ketorolac (Toradol) is useful. The dosage is a 30- to 60-mg intramuscular (IM) loading dose, followed by 15 to 30 mg IM every 6 hours. Due to the antiplatelet effects of NSAIDs, they should not be given to patients with active peptic ulcer disease or multiple traumatic injuries, or to patients who are anticoagulated. In addition, NSAID use should be avoided in patients with congestive heart failure or renal insufficiency.

8

DRUG REACTIONS

Reactions to medications may be wide-ranging, from complaints of bad aftertaste to more serious problems with allergic reactions and anaphylaxis. Most calls will encompass three major groups of symptoms: rashes, anaphylaxis, and other complaints of patient intolerance of medication. All drugs have side effects, and many calls may be eliminated by explaining to the patient what to expect before administering the drug. This is especially important when the side effects are severe or require additional management to control.

Rashes and Anaphylaxis

Rash is a common manifestation of drug reaction. The first step to management is to rule out anaphylaxis, because urticarial rash is a primary symptom.

■ PHONE CALL

Questions

1. **How long has the rash been present?**
2. **Is the rash urticarial?**
   Rule out anaphylaxis, symptoms of which include an urticarial rash (hives), wheezing, shortness of breath (SOB), and decreased blood pressure.
3. **Is the patient taking any new medications?**
   This includes any recent intravenous (IV) contrast dye.
4. **Does the patient have any known allergies or intolerances?**
5. **Has the patient undergone a surgical procedure, and if so, how long ago?**
6. **Are there any other symptoms?**
   Rashes are also associated with upper respiratory infection symptoms or other irritant exposures.
7. **Are there any changes in vital signs such as hypotension or fever?**

Orders

If the patient has signs of anaphylaxis:
1. Start an IV with normal saline (NS) if not already in place.

2. Have at the bedside the following medications:

   Epinephrine (1:1000) 0.5 ml (0.5 mg) for SC administration and epinephrine (1:10,000) 5 ml (0.5 mg) for IV administration. (Label these carefully by their route of administration, so no mistake is made. Either may be necessary depending on the severity of the reaction.)

   Diphenhydramine (Benadryl) 50 mg for IV administration.

   Hydrocortisone (Solu-Cortef) 250 mg for IV administration.

3. Support SOB with oxygen if necessary as described in Chapter 28.

Degree of Urgency

If the patient is anaphylactic, the patient must be evaluated immediately. Most other rashes may be seen in 1 to 2 hours.

■ ELEVATOR THOUGHTS

Drug eruptions follow patterns specific to their medication class.

Urticaria

Lesion: The lesion is well circumscribed, raised, irregularly bordered, firm, blanching, transient, mobile, and often erythematous with central pallor.

Etiologies include the following:
1. Histamine-releasing drugs
   - IV contrast
   - Narcotics
   - Antibiotics
     a. Beta lactams (penicillins and cephalosporins)
     b. Sulfonamides
     c. Tetracycline
     d. Isoniazid
     e. Polymyxin
   - Anesthetic agents (curare)
   - Vasoactive agents (atropine, amphetamine, and hydralazine)
   - Miscellaneous (thiamine, dextran, deferoxamine)
2. Nonhistamine releasers (aspirin and other nonsteroidal antiinflammatory drugs [NSAIDs])
3. Nondrugs (hereditary angioedema, food allergies, and idiopathic reactions)

Maculopapular (Morbilliform)

Lesion: The lesion may be raised or nonraised, erythematous, irregularly bordered, and firm.

Etiologies include the following:
1. Antibiotics
   - Beta lactams (penicillins and cephalosporins)
   - Sulfonamides
   - Chloramphenicol
2. Antihistamines
3. Antidepressants (amitriptyline)
4. Diuretics (thiazides)
5. Oral hypoglycemics
6. Sedatives (barbiturates)
7. Anti-inflammatory agents (gold and phenylbutazone)
8. Nondrugs (bacterial or viral infection, Reiter's syndrome, inflammatory bowel disease, sarcoidosis, and serum sickness)

Vesicular

Lesion: The lesion is well circumscribed, elevated, and blister-like and may be filled with clear fluid (vesicle) or purulent material (pustule).

Etiologies include the following:
1. Antibiotics (sulfonamides and dapsone)
2. Anti-inflammatory agents (penicillamine)
3. Sedatives (barbiturates)
4. Halogens (iodides and bromides)
5. Nondrugs (bacterial or viral infection, toxic epidermal necrolysis, and inflammatory bowel disease)

Purpuric

Lesion: The lesion is erythematous to purplish, large, macular or papular, and nonblanching.

Etiologies include the following:
1. Antibiotics (sulfonamides and chloramphenicol)
2. Diuretics (thiazides)
3. Anti-inflammatory agents (phenylbutazone, salicylates, and indomethacin)
4. Drug-induced thrombocytopenia, i.e., after heparin administration
5. Vasculitis (sepsis, bacterial or viral infection, and Henoch-Schönlein purpura)

Exfoliative Dermatitis

Lesion: The lesion is typified by flaky patches.

Etiologies include the following:
1. Antibiotics (streptomycin)
2. Anti-inflammatory agents (gold and phenylbutazone)
3. Antiepileptic agents (carbamazepine and phenytoin)

Fixed Drug Reactions

Lesion: The lesion is specific to a region of the body. Repeated administration of the same agent will cause return of the rash in the same region.

Etiologies include the following:
1. Antibiotics (sulfonamides and metronidazole)
2. Anti-inflammatory agents (phenylbutazone)
3. Analgesics (phenacetin)
4. Sedatives (barbiturates and chlordiazepoxide)
5. Laxatives (phenolphthalein)

■ MAJOR THREAT TO LIFE

- Anaphylactic shock
    This is associated with urticaria but not with other forms of skin rash.

■ BEDSIDE

Quick Look Test

A patient in anaphylaxis may be hypoxic (agitated) or in hypovolemic shock (lethargic and comatose).

Airway and Vital Signs

Hypotension is a sign of anaphylaxis. Fever is often associated with drug reactions.

Selective History and Chart Review

- Review the patient's allergy and intolerance profile.
- Review the patient's medications, both current and discontinued.
- Has the patient recently undergone a procedure requiring IV contrast?

Selective Physical Examination

VS:	Repeat now; hypotension (anaphylaxis)
MS:	Agitation (hypoxia) or lethargy (shock)
HEENT:	Facial edema (urticaria)
CVS:	Tachycardia (anaphylaxis)
Resp:	Wheezing or SOB (anaphylaxis)
Skin:	Rash or itching
Neuro:	Decreased mental status (anaphylaxis)

■ MANAGEMENT

Initial Management

- **If the patient is in anaphylaxis**
  1. Have someone notify the resident immediately.
     Anaphylaxis is a medical emergency.
  2. Support respirations. If wheezing is present:
     Supply oxygen to keep oxygen saturation of arterial blood (SaO_2) at 90%.
     Epinephrine 0.3 mg (0.3 ml of 1:1000 solution SC, or 3 ml of 1:10,000 solution IV); may repeat the dosage every 10 to 15 minutes as needed; if the skin is cool or clammy, give epinephrine IV to ensure adequate delivery.
     Albuterol (Ventolin or Proventil) nebulizer treatment, **2.5 mg in 3 ml NS;** may repeat the treatment **every 4 to 6 hours as needed,** more frequently if adequate cardiovascular monitoring is available.
     Diphenhydramine (Benadryl and others) 50 mg IV push.
     Hydrocortisone (Solu-Cortef and others) 250 mg IV push, followed by hydrocortisone 100 mg IV every 6 hours.
  3. Support blood pressure. If hypotension is present:
     Start a large-bore IV and begin aggressive replacement of crystalloid (NS); continue the fluid resuscitation until the patient is normotensive.
     Elevate the patient's legs, which is preferable to having the patient assume Trendelenburg's position.
     Reassess the fluid status frequently.
  4. Correct acidemia as necessary.
     Check arterial blood gases frequently during the resuscitation. If the arterial pH is <7.2, the patient may benefit from a dose of **sodium bicarbonate 0.5 to 1 ampule IV.**
  5. Arrange the transfer of the patient to the intensive care unit or the coronary care unit.
     Anaphylaxis is a potentially fatal, multiorgan disease and should be treated by an experienced team.

- **If the patient is NOT in anaphylaxis**
    1. Treat associated symptoms.
        a. Pruritus

           Cool compresses

           Topical moisturizing creams; topical steroid prepara-
           tions may add some relief if the rash is long-stand-
           ing

           **Diphenhydramine (Benadryl and others) 25 to 50
           mg IV or PO every 6 hours, as needed** or

           **Hydroxyzine (Atarax and Vistaril) 25 to 50 mg PO
           every 6 hours, as needed.**

        b. Secondary lesions, resulting from scratching or if le-
           sions are large bullae resulting in skin loss requires
           wound care lesions.

           Refer to Chapter 32 for principles of wound care;
           treat large erosions as thermal burns.

           The best dressing on a firm blister is the existing
           skin; if the blister is not firm or is leaking, it must
           be debrided and dressed with a burn dressing such
           as bacitracin ointment and xerofom gauze.

           Update the patient's tetanus booster as necessary.

           Watch for evidence of infection; routine antibiotics
           are not necessary for treatment of nonerythema-
           tous erosions, but open skin is a common entry
           site for bacteria and fungi.

    2. Note and document the character of the rash, including
       the following important features:

       Distribution on the body

       Skin color

       Primary lesion (macule, papule, or vesicle)

       Secondary changes (erosion, flaking, crust, and ulcer)

       Special features (annular, groupings, and pruritus)

Definitive Management

- If the rash is urticarial, stop the offending medication and
  treat the associated symptoms.
- If the rash is not urticarial, the medication may be safely
  continued until the morning if necessary for the care of the
  patient, and associated symptoms should be treated.

■ SPECIFIC IMPORTANT RASHES

Urticaria

This is discussed above. Its importance is reiterated because of
its association with anaphylaxis, albeit a rare complication.

Herpes Zoster

Lesion: The lesion is composed of grouped vesicles on an erythematous base, with dermatomal distribution. This disease is especially problematic in immunosuppressed patients such as transplant recipients. To avoid disseminated disease, immediate treatment with IV acyclovir may be indicated.

Petechiae

Lesion: The lesion is composed of pinpoint purple to red macules and is associated with platelet malfunction. Along with searching for and treating the causative agent, patients may also need platelet transfusions.

Purpura

Lesion: This lesion is erythematous to purplish, large, and non-blanching and may be macular or papular (palpable purpura). Purpura may also have a hematologic cause, and complete blood count, prothrombin time, and activated partial thromboplastin time should be obtained as indicated.

Remember

1. History of a drug reaction does not need to be known to make the diagnosis. Drug allergies may present at any time.
2. Drug reactions may be delayed by 1 to 2 weeks after the administration of a drug. Be sure to review the discontinued medication list as well as the active list.
3. Drug reactions may present as almost any type of rash. The rash itself may be polymorphic. Always suspect a medication reaction if rash is present.

Other Drug Reactions

Nonrash reactions range from the harmless (bad aftertaste and dry mouth) to the serious (hepatitis, thrombocytopenia, and leukemia). These symptoms may not be immediately associated with the medication, and they should be considered independently until a clear link is established. Each medication has a variety of side effects and idiosyncratic reactions associated with it, and these may be found in a pharmacology text or by discussion with a pharmacist. These are valuable resources; do not hesitate to use them. It is important to know and anticipate the potential complications of the medications and then the therapies used.

Remember that drugs often interact with each other and polypharmacy is a major cause of drug reactions.

9

DYSRHYTHMIAS

Abnormalities of heart rate (HR) and rhythm include both harmless processes and potentially life-threatening processes. Rate and rhythm disturbances include bradycardias, tachycardias, and irregular rhythms. Bradycardias are rhythms resulting in a ventricular rate of <60 beats/min. Tachycardias are defined as rhythms with an HR of >100 beats/min. As the on-call physician, you must identify the type of rate and rhythm disturbance and the likely cause. This will require that you be familiar with basic electrocardiographic (ECG) techniques and tracings (see Appendix A). The first section of this chapter will cover bradycardias. Tachycardias and irregular rhythms are covered in the second section of this chapter.

Bradycardias

■ PHONE CALL

Questions

1. **What is the HR?**
2. **What is the blood pressure?**
    Hypotension with bradycardia is a medical emergency. A normotensive BP in the presence of a bradycardia may require no acute treatment.
3. **Is the patient taking any medications for HR or BP control?**
    Ask the nurse if the patient is taking digoxin, calcium channel blockers, or beta blockers. These drugs, if taken in overdose, may result in bradycardia.
4. **Does the patient have a history of bradycardia?**
    The patient may have a long-standing, stable bradycardia. If this is the case, ask if the current HR is slower than the past recorded HRs.
5. **Does the patient have a pacemaker?**
    Bradycardia in patients with pacemakers may indicate pacemaker dysfunction. A pacemaker-dependent heart may require external pacing or emergent pacemaker replacement. Postoperative cardiac surgery patients may have epicardial pacing leads in place.

Orders

1. If the patient is hypotensive (systolic blood pressure [SBP] <90 mm Hg), ask the RN to place the patient in Trendelenburg's position.
2. If no intravenous (IV) line is present, have the RN place an IV immediately.
3. Ask the RN to obtain a 12-lead ECG immediately.
4. Have the RN bring the crash cart to the bedside and connect the patient to a continuous ECG monitor.
5. If the HR is <40 beats/min or is <50 beats/min and associated with hypotension (SBP <90 mm Hg), have the RN obtain 1 mg of atropine sulfate and bring it to the bedside.

Inform RN

"Will arrive at the bedside in . . . minutes."

■ ELEVATOR THOUGHTS

What causes slow HR?
1. Sinus bradycardia
   - Drug induced (digoxin, calcium channel blockers, beta blockers, and antiarrhythmic agents)
   - Sick sinus syndrome
   - Vasovagal episode
   - Acute myocardial infarction (MI) (inferior wall)
   - Pacemaker malfunction
   - Conduction system disease
   - Electrolyte abnormalities
2. High level of cardiac fitness (athletic heart)
3. Atrial fibrillation (AF) with slow ventricular rate
4. First-degree heart block
5. Second-degree heart block
   - Mobitz type I (Wenckebach) block
   - Mobitz type II block
6. Third-degree AV block
7. Hypothyroidism
8. Elevated intracranial pressure (ICP)

Sinus Bradycardia: Sinus bradycardia (Fig. 9–1) occurs when the sinus rate slows to <60 beats/min but the activation of atria and ventricles is normal.

First-Degree Atrioventricular (AV) Block: First-degree AV block (Fig. 9–2) is associated with conduction delay through the AV node and a prolonged PR interval on ECG tracings (>200 msec).
Second-Degree AV Block: Second-degree AV block occurs when

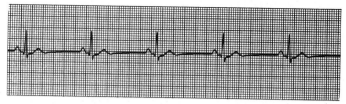

Figure 9–1 □ Sinus bradycardia.

atrial impulses are not conducted to the ventricle during times in which the AV node is not refractory.

Mobitz Type I (Wenckebach) Block: Mobitz type I block (Fig. 9–3) is associated with a progressive elongation of AV conduction before blocking an impulse. ECG tracings show gradual prolongation of the PR interval coming before a nonconducted P wave. Common causes include myocardial ischemia, conduction system abnormalities, drug toxicity, and electrolyte disturbances.

Mobitz Type II Block: Mobitz type II block (Fig. 9–4) is associated with conduction block without conduction delays. No prolongation of PR intervals are noted. Common causes include those of first-degree heart block and acute inferior MI.

Third-Degree Heart Block (Complete Heart Block): Third-degree heart block (Fig. 9–5) results when there is no transmission of atrial impulses to the ventricles. The atrial rate is frequently greater than the ventricular rate. ECG analysis shows no relationship between atrial and ventricular activity. Causes include major MI, conduction system disease, sarcoidosis, amyloidosis, Chagas' disease, aortic valvular disease, trauma, and infection (endocarditis and myocarditis).

■ MAJOR THREAT TO LIFE

- Progression to life-threatening arrhythmia
- Hypotension

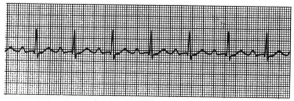

Figure 9–2 □ First-degree atrioventricular block.

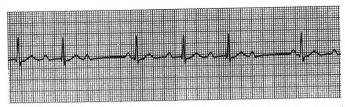

Figure 9–3 □ Second-degree atrioventricular block; Mobitz type I (Wenckebach).

■ MI

Bradycardia may cause hypotension secondary to low cardiac output. Poor perfusion of the myocardium secondary to hypotension may result in myocardial ischemia and infarction. Myocardial ischemia may predispose the patient to life-threatening arrhythmias.

■ **BEDSIDE**

Quick Look Test

Does the patient look well (comfortable), sick (uncomfortable or distressed), or critical (about to die)?

Patients who are bradycardic and hypotensive appear pale and sick. These patients should be monitored with continuous ECG tracings. If the patient is not in an intensive care unit (ICU), connect the patient to a bedside monitor and evaluate rhythm strips. Be prepared to treat symptomatic bradycardia with drugs or pacing techniques.

Airway and Vital Signs

What is the HR?

This absolute rate gives clues to the etiology.

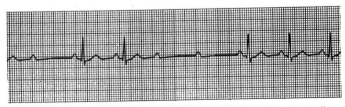

Figure 9–4 □ Second-degree atrioventricular block; Mobitz type II.

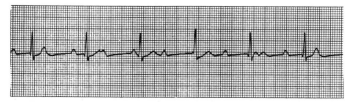

Figure 9–5 □ Third-degree atrioventricular block; complete heart block.

What is the BP?

The BP of the patient determines whether treatment is necessary. A patient who is bradycardic but normotensive requires no treatment. However, a patient who is both bradycardic and hypotensive needs urgent care. Bradycardia and hypotension may precede cardiac arrest.

Selective History and Chart Review

Focus your history and chart evaluation on looking for probable causes for bradycardia. Look for a history of bradycardia, heart block, or ischemic heart disease. Evaluate cardiac medications carefully. Careful attention to the following areas is helpful:
1. Drugs
    Digoxin
    Calcium channel blockers
    Beta blockers
    Antiarrhythmic agents
2. Heart disease
    Silent ischemia
    Acute MI
    History of angina or MI
    Risk factor analysis: diabetes and peripheral vascular disease

Selective Physical Examination

Examination may provide information leading to a likely etiology for the bradycardia.

VS:	HR, BP, temperature (hypothermia may indicate hypothyroidism)
HEENT:	Fundi changes associated with hypertension or diabetes
	Papilledema may suggest increased ICP. Carotid bruits
CVS:	New S_3, S_4, or heart murmur (suggestive of acute MI)

Abd: Evidence of aortic, renal, or femoral bruits (suggestive of atherosclerotic disease with possible concurrent coronary disease)

Extrem: Absent pulses or ischemic changes (diabetes, and peripheral vascular disease with concurrent coronary disease)

■ MANAGEMENT

Sinus Bradycardia

Asymptomatic patients require no treatment. However, the HR should be followed closely. Adjustments in medications or workup may be required if the HR continues to slow or the patient becomes symptomatic. Patients who are symptomatic require **atropine 0.5 to 1.0 mg IV push** (dose may be repeated, as needed, up to 3 mg) or cardiac pacing. External transthoracic pacing or transvenous pacing provides temporary pacing. Cardiac surgery patients may have existing pacing wires. If pacing equipment is not available, a dopamine or epinephrine drip may provide relief of symptomatic bradycardia. Dosing is **5 to 15 μg/kg/min for dopamine** or **2 to 15 μg/min for epinephrine.**

Atrial Fibrillation with Slow Ventricular Response

Asymptomatic patients do not require treatment. Hypotension or hypoperfusion associated with this condition requires ICU or coronary care unit transfer and pacemaker placement. Often, patients with atrial fibrillation are anti-coagulated to prevent blood clot formation in the atrium.

AV Block

First-degree AV block requires no treatment if the patient is asymptomatic. In symptomatic patients, make sure that the electrolytes are within normal limits and that drugs known to cause AV conduction delays are withdrawn (digoxin, calcium channel blockers, and beta blockers). Atropine or cardiac pacing is used to treat symptomatic AV block.

Symptomatic Mobitz I block can be managed with **atropine 0.5 to 1.0 mg IV.** Dose may be repeated as needed, up to 2 mg. Temporary pacing or pressor drips, as described above, may be required if atropine is ineffective. Mobitz II block is treated similarly as Mobitz I block; however, permanent pacemaker placement should be considered early in this condition. In both types of second-degree block, discontinue any medication that might have contributed to the block.

Third-degree AV block should be treated with **atropine 0.5 to 1.0 mg IV** (dose may be repeated), **dopamine (5–15 µg/kg/min),** or **epinephrine (2–15 µg/min).** If a rapidly reversible cause for the complete heart block is not found, pacemaker insertion is appropriate. Cardiac surgery patients may be directly paced via the epicardial leads, if still present.

Drug Overdose

Grossly elevated digoxin levels are associated with bradycardia and toxicity. A single dose of only 2 mg of digoxin is likely to be toxic. If a patient has bradycardia associated with an elevated digoxin level, the patient should be transferred to a monitored bed. Any unabsorbed digoxin may be treated with gastric lavage or charcoal. Serum digoxin levels should be monitored. Digoxin-immune Fab fragments should be given for life-threatening complications of digoxin toxicity, including ventricular tachycardia, ventricular fibrillation (VF), or heart block associated with hypotension.

Tachycardias and Irregular Rhythms

■ PHONE CALL

Questions

1. **What is the HR?**
   Very high HRs may be associated with poor perfusion and hypotension.
2. **Is the rhythm regular or irregular?**
3. **What is the BP?**
   Hypotension with tachycardia is a medical emergency. This could represent either a compensatory mechanism (e.g., hypovolemia) or a life-threatening arrhythmia (e.g., ventricular tachycardia [VT]).
4. **Does the patient have chest pain or shortness of breath?**
   Myocardia ischemia or pulmonary embolism may be associated with tachycardia.
5. **Does the patient have a fever?**
   Fever is a common cause of tachycardia in surgical patients.
6. **Is the patient taking any medications for HR, BP, or rhythm control?**
   Ask the RN if the patient is taking digoxin, calcium channel blockers, beta blockers, procainamide, or other antiarrhyth-

mic drugs. Patients taking these drugs for rate or rhythm control may have subtherapeutic levels or a rebound tachycardia from sudden medication discontinuation.

7. **Does the patient have a history of tachycardia or arrhythmia?**

If the patient has a history of recurrent tachycardia or arrhythmia, see what prior treatments have been effective.

8. **Does the patient have pacing wires or an automatic defibrillation device?**

Pacing wires are placed at the time of cardiac surgery. They are useful when temporary pacing is necessary. Automatic defibrillator devices are implanted in patients with recurrent, life-threatening arrhythmias.

Orders

1. If no IV is present, have the RN place an IV immediately (preferably 16 gauge or greater).
2. If the patient is having chest pain and tachycardia, ask the RN to bring the crash cart into the room and attach the patient to the continuous ECG monitor.
3. Ask the RN to obtain a 12-lead ECG.
4. If otherwise appropriate and if the patient is hypotensive (SBP <90 mm Hg), ask the RN to place the patient in Trendelenburg's position.

Inform RN

"Will arrive at the bedside in . . . minutes."

Tachycardia associated with hypotension or an irregular rhythm requires that you examine the patient immediately. Beware that chest pain associated with tachycardia may represent acute MI or pulmonary embolus. Your rapid intervention may be lifesaving for the patient.

■ ELEVATOR THOUGHTS

What causes rapid HRs or irregular rhythms?
- Tachycardias with regular rhythms
  1. Sinus tachycardia
  2. Atrial tachycardia (supraventricular tachycardia [SVT])
     Paroxysmal atrial tachycardia (PAT)
     Ectopic atrial tachycardia
     Atrial flutter
     AV nodal reentrant tachycardia (AVNRT)
     Wolff-Parkinson-White syndrome (WPW)

3. Ventricular tachycardia (VT)
- Tachycardias with irregular rhythms
  1. Atrial fibrillation
  2. Atrial flutter with variable block
  3. Multifocal atrial tachycardia
  4. Sinus tachycardia with premature atrial contractions (PACs) or premature ventricular contractions (PVCs)
- Irregular rhythms not compatible with life
  1. Ventricular fibrillation (VF) (prolonged)
  2. Asystole (prolonged)

■ MAJOR THREAT TO LIFE

- Arrhythmia progressing to cardiac arrest
- Hypotension
- MI
- Hypoxemia

The tachyarrhythmias may deteriorate to VF and asystole. Rapid diagnosis and treatment of tachyarrhythmias will improve outcome. In addition, it is important to quickly treat any reversible cause of tachycardia associated with hypotension. Hypotension results in coronary hypoperfusion, myocardial dysfunction, and MI.

■ BEDSIDE

Quick Look Test

Does the patient look well (comfortable), sick (uncomfortable or distressed), or critical (about to die)?

With the quick look test, assess tissue perfusion. Patients who are hypoperfused will be pale and lethargic, but patients with a normal BP will have normal color and mental status. Patients who are normotensive with a tachycardia or arrhythmia often look well. However, patients with rapid HRs or abnormal rhythms associated with hypotension usually look sick or critical.

Airway and Vital Signs

What is the HR, and is it regular or irregular?

Assess the HR by taking the patient's pulse and reading the rhythm strip. Feel for the strength of the pulse and its regularity. Also estimate the HR from the strip recording.

What is the BP?

This is the most important issue to consider. If the patient is

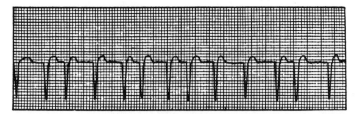

Figure 9–6 □ Atrial fibrillation with rapid ventricular response. (From Marshall SA, Ruedy J: On Call: Principles and Protocols, 2nd ed. Philadelphia, WB Saunders Co, 1993, p 116.)

hypotensive, you must determine if it is related to hypovolemia (compensatory mechanism) or if hypotension is a result of tachycardia.

Compensatory tachycardia is most common after bodily injuries and "third-spacing" of intravascular volume. Bleeding is also a common cause of compensatory tachycardia. Surgical patients may develop hypovolemia and a compensatory tachycardia after major surgery, blunt and sharp trauma, burns, and postoperative bleeding. Tachycardia as a compensatory response to hypovolemia will usually show sinus tachycardia on the rhythm strip. Treat with a crystalloid challenge (**500 ml normal saline or lactated Ringer's solution,** repeat as appropriate) or transfusion.

Tachycardia may cause hypotension. If there is not enough time for diastolic filling of the ventricle, the cardiac output falls. This may lead to hypotension. The most common tachyarrhythmias that are associated with hypotension include the following:

1. AF with rapid ventricular response (Fig. 9–6)
2. SVT (Fig. 9–7)
3. VT (Fig. 9–8)

Accurately diagnose these tachyarrhythmias on rhythm strip or ECG. The treatment for these arrhythmias is outlined below.

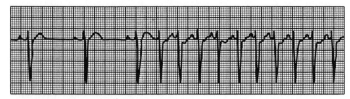

Figure 9–7 □ Supraventricular tachycardia. (From Marshall SA, Ruedy J: On Call: Principles and Protocols, 2nd ed. Philadelphia, WB Saunders Co, 1993, p 117.)

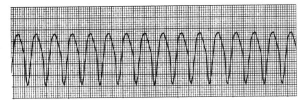

Figure 9–8 □ Ventricular tachycardia.

What is the temperature?

Patients with fever often have a tachycardia. As the body temperature rises, the HR rises. Be aware that persistent fever greatly increases insensible fluid losses. Tachycardia in the presence of infection or sepsis may be a response of both elevated body temperature and hypovolemia.

■ MANAGEMENT

Tachycardia is a HR of >100 beats/min. There are two sites of origin of tachycardias: supraventricular (SVT) and ventricular (VT). These two sites yield very different types of tachycardias, with different treatments and outcomes.

Tachycardias with Regular Rhythms

Sinus Tachycardia

Sinus tachycardia (Fig. 9–9) occurs when the normal sinus mechanism increases its rate of firing under the influence of the autonomic nervous system. Many of the causes of tachycardia are directly or indirectly linked to the autonomic nervous system. Sinus tachycardia may be caused by any of the following:

1. Hypovolemia
2. Hypoxemia
3. Increased sympathetic tone
4. Decreased parasympathetic tone

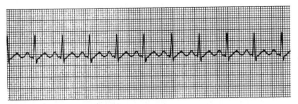

Figure 9–9 □ Sinus tachycardia.

5. Catecholamine release
6. Drugs other than catecholamines (e.g., cocaine and amphetamines)
7. Myocardial ischemia
8. Pain
9. Pulmonary embolism
10. Sepsis or shock
11. Anxiety

The best way to treat sinus tachycardia is to treat the cause. Hypovolemia should be treated with intravenous hydration. Hypoxemia should be treated with oxygen. Use 100% oxygen unless the patient has chronic obstructive pulmonary disease (COPD) and retains CO_2. In these cases, use 30% oxygen. A cause of the hypoxemia should be investigated. Pain should be treated with appropriate analgesics. Myocardial ischemia associated with tachycardia may be treated with oxygen, analgesics, and beta-adrenergic antagonists (see Chapter 7). Sepsis is treated with fluid resuscitation, intravenous antibiotics, and pressor agents as needed.

Atrial Tachycardia

Paroxysmal Atrial Tachycardia (PAT)

PAT frequently occurs in patients with pulmonary disease, coronary artery disease, digoxin toxicity, and acute alcohol overdose. It also may occur due to reentry pathways. Treatment is targeted at the underlying process.

- **If the cause is digoxin toxicity**

    PAT may be due to digoxin toxicity. Stopping digoxin and maintaining normal potassium levels is often all that is needed. If PAT continues, consider loading and treating with lidocaine. Propranolol may also be useful.

- **If the cause is not digoxin toxicity**

    Calcium channel blockers, beta-adrenergic antagonists, or digoxin is helpful in slowing the ventricular response rate.

Atrial Flutter

The ECG (Fig. 9–10) shows a classic sawtooth pattern with an atrial rate of 275 to 350 beats/min.

- Stable hemodynamics

    If the patient is stable (SBP >90 mm Hg), consider IV verapamil. **A dose of 2.5 to 5.0 mg can be given slowly over 2 minutes. The dose may be repeated in 5 to 10 minutes** if there is little or no clinical response. Be aware that verapamil (a calcium channel blocker) is a negative inotropic agent and may worsen congestive heart failure (CHF) or hypotension.

    Digoxin may also be useful in treating atrial flutter. First, rule out that the atrial arrythmia is not due to digoxin toxicity. Once you decide to treat with digoxin, start by loading with

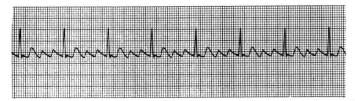

Figure 9–10 □ Atrial flutter.

0.25 to 0.50 mg digoxin IV. Then, give 0.25 mg every 6 hours until a total of 1 mg digoxin is given. A maintenance dose of 0.125 to 0.25 mg PO or IV every day is usually required to maintain therapeutic levels. You will need to lower the digoxin dose for patients with abnormal renal function. Check daily digoxin levels for all patients. Digoxin works by slowing AV nodal conduction and ventricular response.

- Unstable hemodynamics

    Patients with unstable atrial flutter (SBP <90 mm Hg) require cardioversion (Table 9–1).

AV Nodal Reentrant Tachycardia (AVNRT)

AVNRT occurs when there is reentry of two different pathways, one of which is faster than the other. The pathways link the right atrium to the AV node. A narrow complex tachycardia results. The ECG (Fig. 9–11) shows an HR of 150 to 250 beats/min, with the P wave either not visible or inverted in the T wave. The PR interval may be either normal or prolonged.

There are several therapeutic options for the treatment of this type of tachycardia. Vagal maneuvers may help break the tachycardia.

- Valsalva's maneuver

    Ask the patient to take a deep breath and hold it. Have the patient bear down as if having a bowel movement. Holding

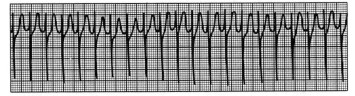

Figure 9–11 □ Rapid regular rhythms; supraventricular tachycardia, atrioventricular nodal reentry, or Wolff-Parkinson-White tachycardia. (From Marshall SA, Ruedy J: On Call: Principles and Protocols, 2nd ed. Philadelphia, WB Saunders Co, 1993, p 120.)

Table 9–1 □ PROTOCOL FOR ELECTIVE CARDIOVERSION

1. Ensure that all antiarrhythmic drugs are at their therapeutic levels.
2. Obtain informed consent.
3. Ensure that a functional IV is present.
4. Connect patient to continuous ECG monitor. Have a crash cart in the patient's room.
5. Check final ECG to ensure that the atrial arrhythmia is still present.
6. Place oxygen (nasal cannula) on the patient.
7. Ensure that intubation equipment and a ventilation bag are at the bedside. If possible, have an anesthesiologist at the bedside to monitor the airway.
8. Place anterior electrode several centimeters to the right of the sternum at the 3rd or 4th interspace. For ventricular arrhythmias, the second electrode should be placed at the cardiac apex or more posteriorly. For atrial arrhythmias, place the second electrode just inferior to the left scapula.
9. Patient should be sedated with IV medications. Consider **midazolam 1–2 mg IV every 2 minutes, maximum 5 mg.** Monitor BP and oxygen saturation.
10. Energy requirements
    Atrial fibrillation usually requires at least 100 J; 200–360 J may be required.
    Atrial flutter often responds to 25–50 J.
    Reentry SVTs respond to 25–100 J.
    Ventricular tachycardia associated with hemodynamic compromise should be cardioverted with 200 J, followed by 360 J if initial shock is unsuccessful.
    Ventricular fibrillation should be treated with a rapid 200-J shock, followed by 360-J shocks.

ECG = electrocardiographic; IV = intravenous; BP = blood pressure; SVT = supraventricular tachycardia.

the breath while bearing down for 10 seconds increases vagal tone and may slow the tachycardia.

- Carotid massage
  This is an effective technique to increase vagal tone. Proceed as follows:
  1. Turn the patient's head to the side.
  2. Locate the carotid sinus.
     The carotid sinus is located between the thyroid cartilage and the sternomastoid muscle (Fig. 9–12).
  3. Apply moderate pressure with several fingers to the neck directly over the carotid pulse.
  4. Massage for about 10 seconds.
  Warning: This maneuver must be done carefully. Always perform carotid massage with ECG monitoring. Have atropine available if a bradycardia results from the massage.

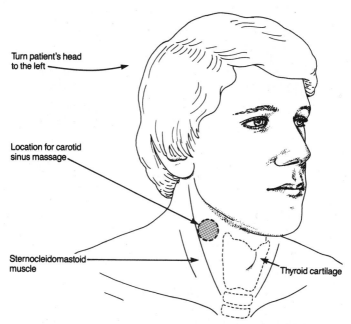

Figure 9–12 □ Carotid sinus massage. (From Marshall SA, Ruedy J: On Call: Principles and Protocols, 2nd ed. Philadelphia, WB Saunders Co, 1993, p 126.)

Never perform this maneuver on a patient with hypotension. The vagal stimulation may lower the HR and further depress the BP. Also, avoid carotid massage in a patient with carotid bruits. It is possible to dislodge a carotid plaque and have it embolize to the brain. Finally, never perform bilateral, simultaneous carotid massage. This may lead to cessation of blood flow to the brain.

Drug therapy options for the treatment of AVNRT include **adenosine (6–12 mg IV)** or **verapamil 5 mg IV every 5 minutes** (may repeat dose once). Remember that before any of these drug regimens are attempted, the patient must have oxygen in place and appropriate monitoring (ECG and oxygen saturation monitors).

Wolff-Parkinson-White Syndrome

WPW syndrome is caused by preexcitation involving a bypass tract or accessory pathway between the atria and the ventricles. ECG findings include a short PR interval (0.12 second), a QRS complex (>0.11 second), and a delta wave (Fig. 9–13).

Delta wave

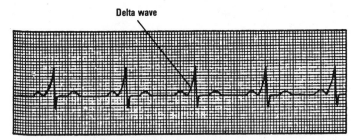

Figure 9–13 □ Wolff-Parkinson-White syndrome. This condition is characterized by a regular rhythm, a PR interval of <0.12 second, a QRS complex of >0.11 second, and a delta wave (i.e., slurred beginning of the QRS complex). (From Marshall SA, Ruedy J: On Call: Principles and Protocols, 2nd ed. Philadelphia, WB Saunders Co, 1993, p 121.)

Treatment of WPW syndrome is similar to the drug treatment for AVNRT. However, much care must be used when giving adenosine, calcium channel blockers, or digoxin to these patients. Atrial fibrillation (AF) or a rapid ventricular response may be triggered, requiring direct current (DC) cardioversion.

Ventricular Tachycardia

VT (see Fig. 9–8) is defined as three or more consecutive premature ventricular beats. The ventricular rate is usually 160 to 250 beats/min. The rhythm is usually regular. Classic ECG appearance includes ventricular complexes with a wide QRS complex (>120 msec) and T waves with an opposite polarity to the QRS complexes. This is the most common life-threatening arrhythmia. MI, electrolyte abnormalities, reentry pathways, cardiomyopathy, myocardial infarction, or inflammation predispose the patient to VT.

A patient with VT may be asymptomatic and normotensive. Symptomatic patients have shortness of breath, presyncope, palpitations, and angina. A patient with VT must be treated immediately and definitively. If untreated, VT commonly degenerates into VF.

Sustained VT associated with compromise requires immediate DC cardioversion (see Appendix A). Compromise includes hypotension, angina, altered level of consciousness, or shortness of breath. Pharmacologic cardioversion may be attempted in patients with clinically stable VT. **Lidocaine (1 mg/kg IV, followed by repeat doses of 0.5 mg/kg every 8 minutes) or procainamide (20 mg/min IV until VT resolves, up to 1000 mg)** may be used. Continuation with lidocaine or procainamide drip is advisable.

Tachycardias with Irregular Rhythms

Atrial Fibrillation

AF is the most common sustained arrythmia (Fig. 9–14; see Fig. 9–6). It is also the most common sustained arrhythmia seen in postoperative patients. AF occurs when multiple waves of activation occur simultaneously in different parts of the atria. The ECG shows ill-defined P waves, with irregular spacing between R waves. The ventricular response is irregular and varies from 80 to 160 beats/min. AF is associated with variable periods of diastolic filling, and thus, each ventricular beat is often not associated with a palpable pulse.

Factors predisposing to the development of AF include atrial stretch (fluid overload and cardiomyopathy), rheumatic heart disease, hypertension, trauma, and cardiac surgery. Complications arising as a result of AF include embolic events such as strokes and peripheral thromboembolisms.

If AF is associated with a rapid ventricular response in conjunction with hypotension, myocardial ischemia, MI, or rapidly worsening CHF, DC cardioversion should be performed (see Appendix A). Patients with stable AF not associated with cardiac decompensation may be loaded with **digoxin (0.25–0.50 mg IV, followed by 0.25 mg IV every 6 hours for total of 1 mg)** or treated with calcium channel blocking drugs. The calcium channel blocking drugs (e.g., **verapamil 5 mg IV**) slow the ventricular rate quickly and may alleviate hypotension due to rapid ventricular rates. However, long-term control of AF or the treatment of AF in patients with heart failure is best done with digoxin.

Multifocal Atrial Tachycardia

Multifocal atrial tachycardia (Fig. 9–15) is characterized by variable P wave morphology and irregular PP intervals. The rate is usually between 100 and 150 beats/min. Patients usually have an underlying pulmonary illness, such as COPD. Treatment for this arrhythmia is best done by treating the underlying cause. Check that the patient does not have the following problems: hypoxia, hypercapnia, hypokalemia, CHF, theophylline toxicity, or acute alcohol toxicity. If the underlying problem has been corrected and

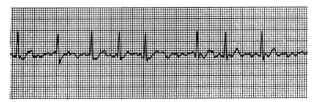

Figure 9–14 □ Atrial fibrillation with slow ventricular response.

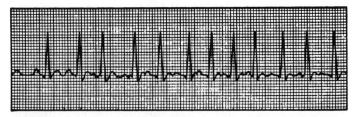

Figure 9–15 □ Rapid irregular rhythms; multifocal atrial tachycardia. (From Marshall SA, Ruedy J: On Call: Principles and Protocols, 2nd ed. Philadelphia, WB Saunders Co, 1993, p 118.)

the patient is still tachycardic, consider **verapamil 5 to 10 mg IV or 80 mg PO.**

Sinus Tachycardia with Premature Atrial Contractions or Premature Ventricular Contractions

Patients with PACs and sinus tachycardia (Fig. 9–16) may not require treatment. However, PACs may degenerate into multifocal atrial tachycardia or AF. Therapy should be directed toward correction of any underlying abnormality (electrolytes and drugs). If desired, a patient with sinus tachycardia and PACs may be treated electively with a calcium channel blocker such as verapamil or diltiazem.

PVCs are premature beats originating in the ventricles (Fig. 9–17). Single PVCs are frequently seen in patients without structural heart disease. However, the presence of complex forms such as couplets and triplets may indicate myocardial ischemia, infection, inflammation, or drug use.

Isolated PVCs require no therapy. If a patient is symptomatic, therapy should be directed at correcting the underlying cause. Common causes of PVCs include the following:

1. MI
2. Myocardial ischemia

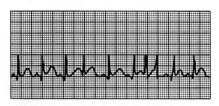

Figure 9–16 □ Rapid irregular rhythms; sinus tachycardia with premature atrial contractions. (From Marshall SA, Ruedy J: On Call: Principles and Protocols, 2nd ed. Philadelphia, WB Saunders Co, 1993, p 118.)

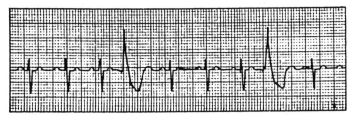

Figure 9-17 □ Rapid irregular rhythms; sinus tachycardia with premature ventricular contractions. (From Marshall SA, Ruedy J: On Call: Principles and Protocols, 2nd ed. Philadelphia, WB Saunders Co, 1993, p 119.)

3. Hypokalemia
4. Hypoxia
5. Acidosis
6. Alkalosis
7. Cardiomyopathy
8. Drug toxicity (antiarrhythmics)
9. Hyperthyroidism
10. Mitral valve disease

If a patient has runs of PVCs (couplets, triplets, and >5 PVCs/min), consider transferring the patient to a cardiac monitored bed. IV lidocaine is effective in suppressing PVCs, but it is associated with toxic effects and is reserved for use in severe cases or in patients with documented VT.

Irregular Rhythms Not Compatible with Life

Ventricular Fibrillation

VF occurs when uncoordinated electrical activity within the ventricle occurs, producing ineffective mechanical contraction. Patients with VF generally have no significant blood pressure and die rapidly unless resuscitated aggressively. Baseline ECG (Fig. 9-18) shows rapid oscillations (250-400 beats/min), without evidence of distinct P waves, QRS complexes, or T waves.

Implement immediate cardiopulmonary resuscitation (CPR)

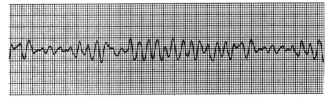

Figure 9-18 □ Ventricular fibrillation.

with bag ventilation or intubation, and immediate unsynchronized DC cardioversion (see Appendix A). If DC cardioversion alone is unsuccessful, IV epinephrine, lidocaine, and bretylium are used one at a time with cardioversion in an attempt to restore a stable cardiac rhythm.

Asystole

Asystole (Fig. 9–19) carries a very poor prognosis for resuscitation. Start resuscitation attempts by beginning CPR and intubation. Then, confirm an ECG reading of asystole in more than one lead. Sometimes, fine VF can appear as asystole. VF has a much better prognosis for resuscitation than asystole. Thus, if VF is suspected or cannot be ruled out, consider attempted unsynchronized cardioversion as per the VF protocol (see Appendix A). If the rhythm strip shows a true asystole, give **1 mg epinephrine IV push.** Follow with **atropine 1 mg IV push.** Consider **high-dose epinephrine (10 mg) IV push** if there is no response to lower dose epinephrine or atropine after 5 to 10 minutes. Consider transcutaneous pacing if early resuscitation of the asystole was initiated.

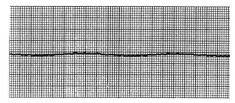

Figure 9–19 □ Asystole.

10

FALLS

When a patient falls it is a serious event. Whether the patient falls from bed or falls elsewhere in the hospital, be mindful of the following two questions after the fall: Is the patient injured? And, what was the cause of the fall?

■ PHONE CALL

Questions

1. **Was the fall witnessed?**
   Anyone who witnessed the fall should be contacted, and his or her story should be documented.
2. **Is there an emergent injury?**
   Head injuries and fractures are particularly worrisome.
3. **Is there a change in the patient's mental status?**
   A computed tomographic (CT) scan of the head immediately is indicated if a significant head injury or change in mental status is apparent.
4. **Was there an obvious identifiable cause?**
   The cause of a fall is often multifactorial.
5. **Has the patient undergone a surgical procedure, and if so, how long ago?**
   Protection from falls is an important part of postoperative management in neurosurgical and orthopedic patients.
6. **Are there any other symptoms?**
7. **Are there any changes in vital signs?**

Orders

1. Ensure the safety of the patient, and respond to any injuries present.
2. Instruct the bedside caregiver to call if there are any further changes in vital signs or mental status.

Inform RN

"Will be at the bedside in . . . minutes."

If there is a significant change in vital signs or symptoms, especially if the patient has an obvious injury such as a fracture or if there is a significant change in mental status, the patient must be evaluated immediately. Also, if the baseline condition of the patient was serious before the fall, it is important to evaluate the situation quickly.

■ ELEVATOR THOUGHTS

What are the causes of falls?

1. Mental status

    Organic causes include Alzheimer's disease, multi-infarct dementia, delirium, confusion, and other organic brain syndromes. Acute changes such as stroke, transient ischemic attack, and epileptic seizure may also cause falls. Patients may also have vasovagal reactions in response to anxiety, severe coughing, or sustained Valsalva's maneuver.

2. Medications

    Medications include sedatives, opiate pain relievers, muscle relaxants, antihypertensive medications, and sleeping aids. Be mindful of any newly started medications.

3. Cardiac events

    Cardiac events include myocardial infarction, dysrhythmias, and hypotension. Be mindful that postoperative patients are often fluid depleted and are predisposed to orthostatic hypotension.

4. Infections

    Infections include sepsis associated with hypotension, delirium associated with fever, or primary central nervous system infections such as meningitis.

5. Respiratory

    Respiratory causes include hypoxia due to pulmonary edema or embolism.

6. Metabolic derangements

    Metabolic derangements include azotemia, liver failure, and electrolyte abnormalities.

7. Environment

    Patients are often unfamiliar with their surroundings, and in addition, they are surrounded by inconvenient obstacles such as intravenous (IV) poles, tubes, wires, catheters, and bed rails. It is amazing that falls do not happen more often. A little preventive organization in the patient's room is helpful, for example, putting the telephone or call button within the patient's reach. Bed rails are a safety measure for alert or comatose patients. They are often a liability for the disoriented or agitated patient. Use them wisely, not fanatically.

■ MAJOR THREAT TO LIFE

Causes of Falls

- Myocardial infarction
- Stroke

- Hypoxia

Result of Falls

- Head injury
  Any patient who has had a fall, especially an unwitnessed fall, must have a full neurologic evaluation. Compare your findings with other documented neurologic examinations in the chart to identify significant changes. Significant changes must be evaluated by CT scan to rule out intracranial bleeding.
- Fractures
  These are especially prevalent in the elderly. Hip fractures carry a high morbidity.

■ BEDSIDE

Quick Look Test

Most patients are well after an uncomplicated fall, although specific complaints are often present. Patients can often tell you exactly what happened.

Airway and Vital Signs

Repeat taking vital signs when at the bedside. Is there a change in the trends?

Is the patient alert and oriented?
Are there symptoms of mental status change?

What is the heart rate, and is there a change in the rhythm?
Perform an electrocardiogram (ECG) as necessary.

What is the blood pressure?
Orthostatic BP and pulse trends may be helpful when assessing fluid status.

How is the patient's breathing, and does the patient appear agitated (a sign of hypoxia)?
Do a spot pulse oximetry reading or chest x-ray as indicated.

Initial Management

1. Look for the cause of the fall.
   Gather as much information as possible. Ask the patient what happened, talk with witnesses, observe the fall site. Be especially mindful of any symptoms the patient noted before

the fall, such as dizziness, palpitations, or pain. These may be clues to the cause.

2. Do a complete neurologic examination on patients who had unwitnessed falls and on those with evidence of head injury.

   If a significant mental status change or a new neurologic sign is present, a head CT scan is indicated immediately.

3. Treat other apparent injuries.

   A patient with mental status changes may not be able to identify other injuries. Have a high level of suspicion, and do a thorough examination.

4. Ensure that the patient is as safe as possible from further falls.

   An identifiable cause may be treated or prevented in the future. If the problem is more unpredictable, such as a delirium, keeping the patient safe may include sedatives or soft restraints, depending on the situation.

Selective History and Chart Review

- Is there a condition predisposing to disorientation, lightheadedness, or postural instability?
  1. Look for previous falls.

     What prior workup has been done? Is there an unidentified trend? Does the patient have a history of nighttime disorientation ("sundowning")?
  2. Are there any new medications?

     Adverse reactions can include BP derangements and mental status changes.
  3. Does the patient have a history of heart disease or arrhythmia?
  4. Look for laboratory abnormalities.

     Is the patient diabetic? A glucose determination immediately by finger stick is useful. Also review any insulin therapy. Are there other treatable metabolic abnormalities?
  5. Does the patient have a seizure disorder?

     Are antiepileptic medication levels within therapeutic range?
  6. Does the patient have nocturia?

     Urinary tract infection, overhydration, diuretic therapy, or prostate enlargement may predispose a patient to urinate at night. Often the route to the bathroom is a maze of tubes and wires.
- Has the patient's surgical procedure contributed to the fall?
  1. Assess the patient's fluid status.

     Is the patient well hydrated? What fluid has the patient already received? If the patient is taking nothing by mouth and has been started on total parenteral nutrition, often glucose abnormalities are present. Check the finger stick.

2. Is the patient taking pain medications?

If disorientation or sedation is too great with the current regimen, consider other combinations of medicines or delivery schemes.

3. Look for other surgery-related changes.

Thyroid or autonomic storm can exacerbate arrhythmias. Pain can slow reflexes and change ambulation patterns.

- Is the patient anticoagulated?

This adds to the danger of any fall. If significant bleeding is present, reversal of the anticoagulation must be considered. It is imperative to reverse anticoagulation if the bleeding is intracranial.

Selective Physical Examination

VS:	Repeat now with orthostatic measurements as necessary.
MS:	Any changes may be significant as a cause or as a result of a fall.
HEENT:	Look for bruises or lacerations to the head indicating significant injury. Tongue or cheek lacerations may be present and may result from seizure activity.
CVS:	Current rate and rhythm should be compared with recent trends.
Resp:	Labored breathing, evidence of hypoxia
Skin:	Bruising or painful regions associated with the fall
Extrem:	Evidence of fracture
Neuro:	A complete neurologic examination is absolutely necessary. Any changes require further evaluation and treatment.
Wound:	Ensure that suture lines are intact and there is no new bleeding.
Tubes:	Are all necessary tubes still in place and secure?
Additional tests:	ECG is indicated to assess rhythm or cardiac symptoms. Finger stick glucose or electrolytes as indicated.
	Radiographs as indicated to assess injury
	Consider checking levels of anticonvulsant or antiarrhythmic medications as necessary.

■ MANAGEMENT

1. Identify a cause for the fall and treat this as necessary.

Sometimes the cause is obvious, but often it is multifactorial. Stop unnecessary medications.

2. Identify all sequelae from the fall and treat these as necessary.

   Patients who are alert and oriented may be embarrassed and only mildly hurt after a fall. They may still require a mild anti-inflammatory and local ice therapy. Other injuries must be evaluated as indicated.

3. Take steps to avoid the next fall.

   Correct identifiable causes, and treat reversible conditions as indicated. If the cause is not apparent or is irreversible, make the patient's environment as safe as possible.

4. Document the fall completely including time, place, circumstances, obvious injuries, complete neurologic examination, and appropriate changes in care and follow-up.

   Falls in an institution are a medicolegal issue. As much as possible, patients are kept in a safe environment, but occasionally accidents happen. Be complete in your documentation!

■ SPECIAL SURGICAL CONSIDERATIONS

Preoperative Considerations

The cause of the fall or any resultant injuries may affect a scheduled procedure. Check with the chief or attending physician if there is any question about needing to reschedule the case.

Postoperative Considerations

1. Postoperative patients are often disoriented because of the combination of intravascular depletion, pain, and pain medication treatment, in addition to whatever underlying causes may already be present. Very sick or febrile patients are also more likely to fall.

2. After intracranial procedures, neurosurgical patients are often neurologically impaired and their mental status changes very quickly. The advantage is that neurologic examinations are performed frequently on these patients, and trends are often readily identifiable. Do not give antiepileptic medications to a postoperative neurosurgical patient unless specifically told to do so by the chief resident or attending physician. Intractable seizures are an indication for a repeat head CT immediately, first, and antiepileptic medication, second. Have a low threshold for considering a head CT scan in these patients.

3. Orthopedic patients who have fractures or repairs of their lower extremities will often have weight-bearing instructions written. Make sure that these were followed. If the patient has walked inappropriately on a cast or dressing, examine the wound and consider x-rays to assess the repair.
4. It is important for most postoperative patients to ambulate. Make sure that the patient is still safe to perform this activity, then encourage it with assistance as necessary.

11

FEVER

All patients with fever warrant clinical investigation. Although most febrile patients in the postoperative period are not infected, the evaluation is directed toward the discovery of infection, as this is the most threatening cause.

■ PHONE CALL

Questions

1. **How high is the temperature?**
   A core temperature of >38.5°C is considered significant.
2. **What was the route of measurement?**
   Temperatures taken orally are about 0.5°C higher than those taken in the axilla or the ear and are about 0.5°C below those taken rectally. Rectal temperature is considered core.
3. **Has the patient been febrile before?**
4. **Has the patient undergone a surgical procedure, and if so, how long ago?**
5. **Are there any other symptoms?**
6. **Are there any changes in vital signs?**
   Be concerned about early sepsis.

Orders

1. If there are changes in vital signs, support hemodynamics and oxygenation.
2. Other orders depend on other symptoms.

Inform RN

"Will be at the bedside in . . . minutes."
The patient should be evaluated usually within the hour if the patient is stable. If there is a significant change in vital signs or symptoms, then the patient must be evaluated immediately.

■ ELEVATOR THOUGHTS

The timing of the fever relative to the postoperative day will indicate the most likely cause (Table 11–1). Noninfectious causes must be considered with infectious causes in the postoperative patient.

Table 11–1 □ **THE TIMING OF COMMON CAUSES OF POSTOPERATIVE FEVER**

	POD 1	POD 2–3	POD 3 and Up
Infectious			
Respiratory	Atelectasis	Pneumonia	Pulmonary embolus
Wound	*Streptococcus* sp.	*Clostridium* sp.	*Staphylococcus* sp., mixed aerobic and anaerobic species
GU	—	UTI	UTI, pyelonephritis
IVs, drains	—	Staph./Strep.	Staph./Strep.
Surgical bed	—	—	Abscess
Noninfectious*			
Malignant hyperthermia			
Thyroid storm			
Multiple trauma			
Hematoma			
Devitalized tissue			
Contaminated IV fluids			
Blood product transfusion			
Deep venous thrombosis			
Malignancy			
DT			
Drug fever			

POD = postoperative day; GU = genitourinary system; IV = intravenous; UTI = urinary tract infection; Staph./Strep. = *Staphylococcus/Streptococcus;* DT = delirium tremens.

*Noninfectious etiologies may occur at any time.

■ MAJOR THREAT TO LIFE

- Sepsis
- Other life-threatening infection
    Pneumonia
    Meningitis
- Pulmonary embolus

■ BEDSIDE

Quick Look Test

Most patients will be comfortable. If early sepsis is present, then the patient may appear agitated or delirious.

Airway and Vital Signs

Is the patient in shock?
Note the heart rate (HR) and the blood pressure (BP).

What is the patient's fluid status?
Note the perfusion and the respiratory rate (RR).

Selective History and Chart Review

- Does the patient have specific complaints?
  This often leads to the source of the infection.
- Surgical procedure, if any
- Postoperative complications
- Medications including antibiotics, immunosuppressants, chemotherapeutics, and antipyretics
  Especially note any recent change in antibiotic therapy.
- Temperature curve pattern
  Patients with abscess complications often have repetitive, high, spiking fevers.
- Recent cultures and blood work
  The primary care team may have a plan outlined if a patient has continued fevers.
- Any underlying condition that may have fever as a component, such as colitis, collagen vascular disease, and malignancy
- Recent blood product administration
- What lines, tubes, or foreign bodies are present, and how long have they been in?
  This includes any prosthetic joints or devices.
- Is the patient diabetic (uncontrolled)?
  This condition increases the susceptibility to bacterial and yeast infection.
- Is the patient otherwise immunosuppressed, e.g., an acquired immunodeficiency syndrome (AIDS) patient or transplant recipient?
- Does the patient have an existing seizure disorder?
  Seizure activity (witnessed or unwitnessed) can raise temperature, but rarely above 38.5°C.

Selective Physical Examination

VS:	Repeat now
MS:	Delirium or agitation; think of early sepsis or hypoxia
HEENT:	Headache. Is a nasogastric tube in place? Check for evidence of sinusitis, otitis, pharyngitis, or parotitis. Look for dental abscesses. Look for meningeal signs including nuchal rigidity or photophobia.
CVS:	Tachycardia, possible flow murmur, and skin perfusion

Resp:	Tachypnea, aeration, rales, rhonchi, and wheezes
Abd:	Evidence of distention and peritonitis
GU:	Bladder discomfort, dysuria, and flank pain. Is a urinary catheter in place?
Extrem:	IV sites, redness or swelling, and calf tenderness
Wound:	Redness, induration, tenderness, drainage, or purulence
Tubes:	Redness, induration, tenderness, drainage, or purulence
Special examinations:	Check IV fluids for evidence of contamination.
	Special examinations for meningitis; as follows:

> *Brudzinski's sign:* Positive if a patient flexes at the hip or knee in response to flexion at the neck.
>
> *Kernig's sign:* Positive if pain response is elicited with passive straightening of the knee from a position of 90° flexion at the hip.

■ MANAGEMENT

Initial Management (If the Patient Is Unstable)

1. Order oxygen and pulse oximetry.
   Fever shifts the oxygen saturation curve such that a given arterial partial pressure of oxygen (PaO_2) results in a lower hemoglobin saturation.
2. Order cardiovascular monitoring.
3. Support hemodynamics with fluids and inotropes as necessary.
4. Provide adequate intravenous (IV) access.
5. Prevent shivering.
   Fever is a already a high metabolic state. Further muscle contractions may result in increased myocardial oxygen demand and increased HR and RR and may produce metabolic acidosis. Cooling blankets are not as useful in this setting as judicious use of paralytic agents.

Definitive Management

For the first episode of fever without an obvious source (preoperative or postoperative), an ardent search for the site of infection is undertaken and the following preliminary measures are begun:

1. Obtain a complete blood count with differential analysis.
2. Take blood cultures; two distant sites.
3. Obtain a urinalysis (UA), microscopic analysis, and culture.
4. Obtain a wound or a drain site culture.

    IV sites may be "milked" by gently stroking from proximally to distally, to attempt to express purulence.

5. Obtain a sputum analysis and culture as indicated.

    If the patient is intubated, obtain a Gram stain of the endotracheal tube aspirate. This site will be chronically colonized, so culture only if there are significant white blood cells (WBCs) present. A suction lavage may be useful to obtain a deeper pulmonary sample.

6. Obtain a chest x-ray.
7. Consider a finger stick glucose measurement.

    Often early septic patients will exhibit glucose instability.

8. Consider a lumbar puncture as symptoms dictate.

    This is especially important to consider in the obtunded patient. Also consider computed tomographic (CT) scan of the head to rule out central nervous system (CNS) abscess if fevers are prolonged and unremitting in an unconscious patient.

9. Perform a vaginal examination with cervical cultures as indicated.
10. Obtain a throat culture.
11. Change IV and central line sites.

    Some hospital protocols advocate changing central lines over a wire, maintaining the original site. This is useful when IV access is problematic. The safest approach is the removal of central access catheters and replacement at a clean site after the resolution of the fevers. This is especially important if there is purulence evident at the IV site. When a central line is removed, send the tip for culture by sterilely clipping the distal inch or so off and placing it in a sterile container (e.g., a urine specimen cup). Suspect any IV line that is still in place after a documented positive blood culture.

12. Remove the urinary catheter as indicated.

    Expect that patients with urinary catheters in place for >3 days will be colonized with bacteria. Use the presence of WBCs and leukocyte esterase in the UA to interpret the significance of a positive culture.

13. Perform a pulmonary toilet as indicated.

    Especially in the intubated or the obtunded patient, improving mobilization and expulsion of secretions will decrease the risk of pulmonary infection. This includes the use of mucolytics such as acetylcysteine, bronchodilators, and chest physical therapy (CPT) as indicated. In awake patients, hourly use of incentive spirometry will decrease atelectasis. Make sure postoperative patients have adequate pain control to ensure comfort during CPT or incentive spirometry.

14. Use antipyretics as a comfort measure only.

Their use may obscure the temperature curve and may mask other symptoms.

15. Antibiotic therapy as outlined below.

Patients Who Require Empirical Broad-Spectrum Antibiotic Therapy

1. Febrile patients without a source who are becoming more ill, which especially applies to early septic, hypotensive, or hypermetabolic patients, require empirical broad-spectrum antibiotic therapy.

Start with broad-spectrum antibiotic coverage, and narrow the therapy if the microorganism, specificities, and site of infection become known.

2. Patients with suspected serious infections such as meningitis or pneumonia with associated hypoxia also require broad-spectrum antibiotic therapy.

Narrow the therapy as the microorganism, sensitivities, and site become known.

3. Immunocompromised patients such as transplant recipients, patients with AIDS, or patients treated with high-dose steroids or chemotherapy also require broad-spectrum antibiotic therapy.

Remember that patients with low absolute neutrophil counts may have fever without a documentable source. This does not preclude them from empirical treatment. It is prudent to assume infection in these patients.

Patients Who Require Directed Antibiotic Treatment

Those patients with an identifiable source and who are currently stable require directed antibiotic treatment. A choice of antibiotic coverage can be made based on a knowledge of common pathogens and based on Gram stain information when available. See Table 11–2 for typical sites, pathogens, and antibiotic regimens for common infections. As each hospital has a different spectrum of bacteria that are common to wards and intensive care units, it is wise to check with the clinical microbiology division to find out the local nosocomial flora and any sensitivity idiosyncrasies.

Table 11–2 □ EMPIRICAL TREATMENT FOR COMMON INFECTIONS

Site	Common Pathogens	Empirical Treatment
Lungs		
Community acquired	*Streptococcus pneumoniae* *Haemophilus influenzae*	Penicillin, ampicillin, co-trimoxazole, or 2nd-generation cephalosporin
	Mycoplasma pneumoniae *Legionella pneumophila*	Erythromycin
Hospital acquired	*Escherichia coli* *Klebsiella pneumoniae* *Proteus* sp. *Pseudomonas aeruginosa* *Enterobacteriaceae*	Synthetic penicillin, carbapenem, or 3rd-generation cephalosporin **plus** aminoglycoside (or aztreonam)
	Staphylococcus aureus *Bacteroides*	Add clindamycin, synthetic penicillin, or 1st-generation cephalosporin
Urine	*Enterobacteriaceae* (including *E. coli*)	Aminoglycosides (or aztreonam) with or without ampicillin; co-trimoxazole, fluoroquinolone
	Enterococci	Penicillin **plus** aminoglycoside
Wound	*Streptococcus* sp. *Staphylococcus* sp. *Clostridium* sp.	1st-generation cephalosporin, synthetic penicillin, or clindamycin

Patients Who Require No Antibiotic Therapy Immediately

1. Nonsick patients in whom no source is readily identifiable and those for whom a fever workup is in progress require no antibiotic therapy immediately.

   These may include patients with a cause of fever other than infection such as malignancy, but it must be emphasized that infection must still be ruled out.

2. Patients with temperature spikes of <38.5°C require no antibiotic therapy immediately.

3. Patients with suspected atelectasis require no antibiotic therapy immediately.

Patients with Fever Already Taking Antibiotics

1. If a source has been identified, consider the natural history of the disease.

Patients with abscesses and severe infections such as pyelonephritis and meningitis often have spikes of fevers for several days after initiation of appropriate therapy.

2. Make sure that the current antibiotic therapy is appropriate for the pathogens identified (type of antibiotic, dose, and dosing interval).

3. Nonbacterial sources of infection (especially yeast) must be considered in the very ill or immunosuppressed patient, the patient on prolonged antibiotic therapy, and the patient treated with total parenteral nutrition.

Patients with Fever in Whom Surgical Intervention Should Be Considered

1. Any acute abdomen patient with fever should be considered for surgical intervention.

2. Patients who have undergone abdominal surgery in whom there is a question of bowel viability should be considered for surgical intervention.

3. Those with documented abscesses should be considered for surgical intervention.

   These abscesses may often be drained by transcutaneous catheter placement under ultrasonographic or CT guidance by interventional radiology.

4. Those patients with infected foreign bodies such as septic prosthetic joints should be considered for prosthesis removal.

■ SPECIAL SURGICAL CONSIDERATIONS

Preoperative Considerations

1. A remote infection increases the risk of subsequent wound infection postoperatively; so, fever in the elective preoperative patient will most likely preclude the planned procedure pending evaluation of the symptoms.

2. A change in condition associated with fever, such as development of an acute abdomen, can require emergent surgery.

3. Consider the following factors, which predispose for infection in the preoperative patient:
   Immunosuppressants
   Protein malnutrition
   Inadequate hydration
   Uncontrolled diabetes
   Prolonged hospitalization
   Alcoholism
   Remote infection

Postoperative Considerations

1. Cardiopulmonary bypass is a frequent cause of fever in the postoperative cardiac patient.
2. Large spiking fevers 5 to 7 days after a surgical procedure may indicate abscess formation.
3. Devitalized tissue such as massive crush injuries and necrotic bowel can be a source of fever and may require repeat surgery for resection.
4. In transplant recipients, fever can be a sign of rejection.

Malignant Hyperthermia

- It generally occurs intraoperatively but may occur up to 25 hours after delivery of anesthesia.
- The incidence is 1:16,000 anesthetics and is higher in children (1:12,000).
- The most likely causes are volatile agents such as halothane, enflurane, or isoflurane, or the paralytic agent succinylcholine.
- Mortality is 10% even in appropriately treated patients.
- Symptoms include the following:
  Increased temperature, as high as 43°C at times. This may be a late finding. Do not wait for it to initiate therapy.
  Increased RR, HR, and BP
  Agitation
  Hypoxia
  Skin mottling
- Damage is to the CNS, and it occurs rapidly because of cerebral edema and hypermetabolism. When the diagnosis is suspected, the following treatment is emergent:
  Provide fluid support
  Discontinue anesthetic agents.
  Hyperventilate with 100% O_2.
  Administer dantrolene (Dantrium) 1.0 mg/kg IV immediately and **every 5 minutes up to 10 mg/kg** until symptoms abate.
  Treat metabolic acidosis.
  Watch for evidence of muscle breakdown products. Maintain urine output with adequate hydration and furosemide. Check urine for myoglobin.
  Check serial creatine phosphokinase (CPK) levels.
  Watch for and treat disseminated intravascular coagulation.
  Watch for and treat arrhythmias.
  Control pyrexia.

12

FLUIDS, ELECTROLYTES, AND ACID–BASE STATUS

Surgical disease and treatment is often associated with aberrations in fluids, electrolytes, and acid–base status. Rapid fluid status assessment is a constant exercise in the management of surgical patients, as well as the application of therapies best suited to treat respective abnormalities. The common denominator in all fluid management is the avoidance of shock or inadequate end-organ perfusion. Poor end-organ perfusion may lead to hypoxia and irreversible damage. This chapter will discuss normal fluid distributions and describe the more frequent causes of changes in volume distribution, biochemical abnormalities, and their treatments. The chapter is organized to address aberrations in intravascular volume. The intravascular space is the smallest fluid compartment but is the most dynamic (i.e., changeable) and is of critical importance to the maintenance of end-organ perfusion.

■ NORMAL FLUID DISTRIBUTION

The body is composed mostly of water (Fig. 12–1). Total body water represents up to 60% of the weight of an adult male. This percentage is higher in infants and lower in adult women, elderly, and obese persons. Total body water can be thought of as residing in two separate compartments; *intracellular* and *extracellular* compartments. The extracellular compartment is further divided into *interstitial fluid*, which bathes the cells and tissues, and *intravascular fluid* which is in the blood and lymphatic vessels of the body. Fluid can be thought to be freely flowing between the compartments, constrained mostly by the ionic strength or osmotic pressure of the respective compartment. Intravascular fluid makes up only about 8 to 10% of the total body water and is essentially the only site at which fluid replacement can take place.

In addition to the compartments listed above, there is a potential space that is loosely termed the "third space." The third space is a pathologic expansion of the interstitial space in response to injury and illness. The size of the third space is proportional to the severity of the illness or injury. It is the shift of fluid between the intravascular space and the third space that is most important in the evaluation and care of surgical patients. The shift between

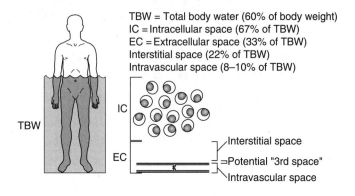

TBW = Total body water (60% of body weight)
IC = Intracellular space (67% of TBW)
EC = Extracellular space (33% of TBW)
Interstitial space (22% of TBW)
Intravascular space (8–10% of TBW)

Figure 12–1 □ Normal body distribution of water.

intracellular and extracellular fluid spaces also becomes important in the management of some electrolyte imbalances.

Normal daily fluid requirements are about 1500 ml/m². This volume replaces the sensible (measurable) losses of urine, feces, and drain outputs, and the insensible (unmeasurable) losses from respiration, skin, and open wounds. Fluid resuscitation often refers to the replacement of fluid losses in addition to these normal daily requirements. Remember that various metabolic states such as fever, tachypnea, diarrhea, and large open wounds greatly increase insensible losses and will increase the daily requirement. Renal failure may decrease the sensible losses and may require and reduce the daily maintenance fluid requirements.

■ POSTOPERATIVE FLUID CHANGES

After surgery, especially major surgery, there are physical and endocrine causes for changes in intravascular volume. The most common abnormality is a depletion of intravascular volume leading to inadequate perfusion of end-organs. This may be a total body depletion due to underhydration, or there may be functional depletion by fluid shifts away from the intravascular space. Various surgical factors influencing intravascular volume are listed in Table 12–1. The longer the surgical procedure, the greater the fluid losses. The anesthesiologist will do most of the fluid replacement intraoperatively, but there is often need for continued fluid replacement postoperatively. In addition to intraoperative losses, there are often postoperative losses through open wounds, nasogastric (NG) or drainage tubes, or postoperative bleeding. These

**Table 12–1 □ PERIOPERATIVE FACTORS RESULTING IN
DECREASED INTRAVASCULAR VOLUME**

Inadequate preoperative resuscitation
Insensible loss through an open surgical field
Blood loss
Suction loss (from nasogastric tube and from the surgical field)
Insufficient intraoperative fluid replacement
Postoperative antidiuretic hormone secretion
Medications (including diuretics)
Postoperative fluid shifts ("third spacing")

ongoing losses represent depletion of electrolytes as well as
fluid.

■ RAPID FLUID STATUS ASSESSMENT

The assessment of fluid status should be second nature, and it
should be practiced daily on rounds on ill and non–ill appearing
patients. Soon it will become a comfortable skill. The assessment
is based on observation, examination of the patient and the chart,
and vital signs and laboratory data. The following are the three
basic states of total body fluid status: *normal, fluid overloaded,* and
fluid depleted. The state of intravascular volume is described as
normovolemic, hypervolemic, and *hypovolemic.* The intravascular volume is important in determining perfusion of organs, and a
depletion of this space has readily apparent signs. The three most
apparent signs are changes in the perfusion of the skin, the
kidneys, and the brain. Confirm the following:

1. **The skin is warm and moist.**
   One response to hypovolemia is to decrease perfusion of
   the peripheral vascular beds. Skin that is cool, blue, and dry
   is poorly perfused.
2. **The urine output (UO) is adequate.**
   Generally this is considered >20 ml/hr. Less urine volume
   than that is considered oliguria and may be due to hypovolemia.
3. **The patient is mentating well or at least at the baseline
   level.**
   Hypovolemia is a cause of delirium and confusion.
These signs individually may have many causes but when
considered together represent a rapid, effective scan of the adequate functional intravascular volume. Remember that the fluid
may not be missing from the body; it may be displaced from the
intravascular space into the interstitial space. That is, a patient

does not need to be total body volume depleted to be hypovolemic.

Common Fluid Imbalances: The Fluid-Overloaded Patient

■ ELEVATOR THOUGHTS

What causes fluid overload?
1. Sequestration of fluids
    - Systemic infection
    - Pancreatitis
    - Severe injuries, polytrauma, or burns
    - Ileus
2. Overzealous hydration
3. Renal failure
4. Hepatic failure

■ MAJOR THREAT TO LIFE

- Pulmonary edema (increased intravascular volume)
- Myocardial infarction (MI) (increased intravascular volume)

■ BEDSIDE

Quick Look Test

Patients with minor fluid shifts may be asymptomatic, but patients who are severely fluid overloaded may present with pulmonary edema causing tachypnea and hypoxia. Patients with hypoxia will be quite agitated and distressed.

Airway and Vital Signs

The first step in evaluating fluid status is to check the vital signs. Tachypnea may be present in settings of pulmonary edema. If you suspect pulmonary edema, check the oxygenation of the patient with pulse oximetry.

Tachycardia may also be present in fluid overload as the heart attempts to unload the fluid accumulation in the lungs.

Selective History and Chart Review

- Check the input and output measurements (I/Os) for the last day or so. Do not forget the output from drains and tubes.
  These measurements are notoriously inaccurate but may supply clues.
- Has the patient had aggressive fluid resuscitation?
- Does the patient have a disease that would predispose to fluid sequestration?
- How are the renal function and the liver function?
- Is the patient taking medication or therapy that might alter fluid distribution?
- Is the patient improving?
  After a serious illness or major surgery a patient may sequester several liters of fluid. This will return to the vascular space during the recovery phase and may cause fluid overload.
- Is the patient worsening, or is there a change in fluid status, indicating MI or systemic infection?

Selective Physical Examination

VS: Tachycardia (pulmonary edema)

MS: Decreased mental status (hypoxia)

HEENT: Moist mucous membranes

Full neck veins

Evaluation of neck veins is often a reasonable assessment of central venous pressure (CVP). When the patient is evaluated while lying down, note the fullness of the external jugular vein. Then slowly raise the head of the bed until the neck veins lose their fullness and pulsations are noted. Note the distance between the point of pulsation and the approximate position of the right atrium on a vertical axis (measure to the sternal notch and add 5 cm; Fig. 12–2). The distance is a gross estimate of the CVP in centimeters of H_2O. A measurement of 2 to 3 cm above the sternal notch is normal in adults. Patients with fluid overload may have jugular venous distention (JVD) at >3 cm; <2 cm or consistently flat neck veins despite lying flat indicates fluid depletion.

Resp: Rales and decreased aeration (fluid overload, congestive heart failure [CHF])

CVS: S_3

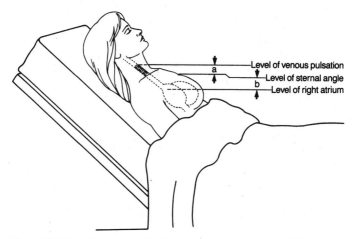

Figure 12–2 □ Measurement of jugular venous pressure. *a*, The perpendicular distance from the sternal angle to the top of the column of blood; *b*, the distance from the center of the right atrium to the sternal angle, commonly accepted as measuring 5 cm, regardless of inclination. (From Marshall SA, Ruedy J: On Call: Principles and Protocols, 2nd ed. Philadelphia, WB Saunders Co, 1993, p 12.)

Abd:	Hepatomegaly (CHF)
Skin:	Dependent edema, especially over the sacrum in supine patients or in the calves of ambulatory patients; edematous skin may be taut
Additional tests:	
1. UA:	Low specific gravity supports fluid overload if the kidneys are functioning normally
2. Electrolytes:	To assess for metabolic derangement and elevations in blood urea nitrogen (BUN) and creatinine
3. Urine Na$^+$:	Assessment of renal function (see Table 31–2)

■ MANAGEMENT

See Chapter 31 for a complete discussion of the fluid-overloaded patient.

Initial Management

1. Support oxygenation as necessary.
2. Order intravenous (IV) access if not already available.

Definitive Management

1. Correct the underlying cause if known.
2. Limit ongoing fluid replacement regimens.
3. If the patient is in respiratory distress, maintain oxygenation and monitor with pulse oximetry. Consider intubation if necessary. Notify your resident.
4. Consider diuretic therapy as outlined in Chapter 31.
5. Rarely, if diuretic therapy is ineffective, hemodialysis is required.

Common Fluid Imbalances: The Fluid-Depleted Patient

■ ELEVATOR THOUGHTS

What causes fluid depletion?
See Tables 12–1 and 12–2.

■ MAJOR THREAT TO LIFE

- Hemodynamic shock

■ BEDSIDE

Quick Look Test

Patients with minor fluid shifts (<10%) may be asymptomatic. Greater losses are associated with stupor and drowsiness. Major fluid deficit can cause hypotension and shock. (See Chapter 17.)

Airway and Vital Signs

The first step in evaluating fluid status is to check the vital signs. Orthostatic vital signs are the most useful in determining a deficiency in intravascular volume. Orthostatics are heart rate (HR) and blood pressure (BP) taken while the patient is lying flat, while the patient is sitting, and while the patient is standing. Allow a minute or two to pass between each change in position so the patient may equilibrate. A rise in HR of 15 beats/min or a drop in systolic blood pressure (SBP) of 15 mm Hg or any drop in diastolic blood pressure with a change in position is evidence of a significant intravascular deficit and may require fluid replace-

Table 12–2 □ ETIOLOGIES OF FLUID DEPLETION

GI losses	Vomiting
	Diarrhea
	Nasogastric suction
Urinary losses	Diuretics
	Diabetes mellitus
	Diabetes insipidus
	Osmotic agents (mannitol and hypertonic fluid)
	Postobstructive diuresis
	Adrenal insufficiency
	Mobilization of third-spaced fluid
	Recovery phase of acute tubular necrosis
Insensible losses	Open wounds (e.g., burns; large defects may lose up to 5 L/day)
	Respiratory tract (unhumidified oxygen; hyperventilation may lose up to 1.5 L/day)
	Increased sweating (may lose up to 3 L/day)
Third spacing	Systemic infection
	Pancreatitis
	Ileus
	Burns
	Postoperative
Blood losses	Perioperative
	GI bleeding
	Trauma
Iatrogenic	Insufficient maintenance fluids
	Insufficient replacement of losses
	Frequent blood sampling
Other	Poor PO intake

GI = gastrointestinal; PO = by mouth.

ment. Also be mindful of any symptoms that the patient exhibits during changes in position. Dizziness on standing may also indicate loss of intravascular volume. In a young individual, BP is tightly controlled and may be maintained easily with only an increase in pulse rate despite dangerous hypovolemia. In these patients, tachycardia with a stable BP may be the last step before complete cardiovascular collapse. Also, beta blockade may mask increases in HR and result in profound drops in BP on changes in position.

Tachycardia itself is not sufficient to make the diagnosis of intravascular depletion, as it may also be present in fluid overload states.

Selective History and Chart Review

- Check the I/Os for the last day or so.
  This measurement is notoriously inaccurate but may sup-

ply clues. Remember that UO is an indication of renal perfusion. Look carefully at the most recent changes in UO.

- Has the patient had inadequate maintenance fluid replacement?
- Does the patient have a disease that would predispose to fluid loss?
- How is the renal function? (See Chapter 31.)
- Is the patient taking medication or therapy that might alter fluid distribution?
- Is the patient worsening, or is there a change in fluid status, indicating sepsis or another form of shock?

Selective Physical Examination

VS:	Tachycardia or postural BP changes (dehydration)
MS:	Decreased mental status (decreased perfusion)
HEENT:	Dry or sticky mucous membranes and flat neck veins (dehydration)
Skin:	Decease in warmth or turgor and dry axilla (dehydration).
Tubes and drains:	Is the output from these tubes high? Is the output volume being added to replacement fluids?

Additional tests:

1. UA	High specific gravity supports fluid deficit if the kidneys are able to concentrate normally.
2. Electrolytes	To assess for metabolic derangement and elevations in BUN and creatinine (Cr). A BUN/Cr ratio of >12 is an indication of dehydration.
3. CBC	Hemoconcentration
4. Urine Na$^+$	Assessment of renal function (see Table 31–2)

■ MANAGEMENT

Also see Chapter 17 for treatment of shock and hypovolemia.

Initial Management

1. Support perfusion and oxygenation as necessary.
2. Order orthostatics if not already done.
3. Order IV access if not already available.

Definitive Management

1. Correct the underlying cause if known (see Table 12–2 for a list of common etiologies).
2. Choose an appropriate fluid to replace the loss.
   - Gastric loss   5% dextrose in one-half normal saline (NS) + 30 to 40 mEq/L KCl.
   - Biliary loss   Lactated Ringer's (LR).
   - Pancreatic loss   LR + supplemental HCO_3.
   - Small bowel loss   LR.
   - Diarrheal losses   LR or one-half NS + 20 mEq/L KCl + 25 mEq/L HCO_3.
3. Replace fluids with the goal of maintaining adequate end-organ perfusion.
4. Choose a rate of rehydration that the patient can tolerate and reevaluate frequently with examinations of respiratory rate (RR), lung fields for rales, skin for adequate perfusion, and I/Os for consistent UO.

■ REPLACEMENT OF FLUID DEFICITS

The major goal in replacement of fluids to the intravascular space is to maintain an adequate preload. This helps ensure end-organ perfusion and oxygenation to decrease the risk of ischemia or infarction. Remember that there are other aspects of delivery of oxygen to the end-organs, of which intravascular volume is one. Be sure to optimize the oxygen delivery to the patient, the cardiac output, and the vascular bed tone in addition to replacing the intravascular fluid.

When replacing fluids, there are a variety of products to choose from, and the correct choice is a matter of the pathophysiology of the fluid deficit, the goals of fluid replacement, and the preferences of the primary care team. In general, it is reasonable to rehydrate with a fluid whose characteristics closely match those of the fluid that is being lost. See Table 12–3 for a listing of common gastrointestinal (GI) fluids and their electrolyte compositions. If there is a question, consult the resident or attending physician.

The timing in which the fluid should be replaced is variable, depending on the severity of the deficit, the type of fluid lost, and the ability of the patient to tolerate large volumes of fluid replacement. Shock should be treated aggressively and rapidly until hemodynamics stabilize. Thereafter, further fluid deficits are generally replaced over 24 to 48 hours with the first 50% of the loss being replaced in the first 6 to 8 hours.

Monitoring the progress of the resuscitation is very important. The goal is to find the balance between adequate rehydration and

Table 12–3 □ ELECTROLYTE COMPOSITIONS OF GASTROINTESTINAL FLUIDS

Type	Na⁺ (mEq/L)	K⁺ (mEq/L)	Cl⁻ (mEq/L)	HCO₃⁻ (mEq/L)	Volume per day (L)
Saliva	30	20	35	15	1.5
Gastric					
pH >3.0	100	10	100	—	2.0
pH 1.0–2.0	25	15	140	—	
Bile	140	5	60–120	30–50	1.5
Pancreatic	140	5	60–90	90–115	1.0
Small bowel					
Proximal	140	5	130	30	
Distal	90	10	90	40	
Diarrhea	25–130	10–60	20–90	20–50	3.5

119

overhydration. Rapid fluid replacement can be associated with peripheral and pulmonary edema and with electrolyte abnormalities. Underhydration may lead to shock. Large-volume fluid resuscitation should always be accompanied by adequate hemodynamic monitoring and frequent serum electrolyte determinations.

Types of Fluid Replacement

Red Blood Cells

If the fluid deficit is due to ongoing blood loss, the correct fluid to replace is generally packed red blood cells (RBCs). Whole blood, which replaces plasma volume and RBCs, may not be available at all hospitals but may be reconstructed by the blood bank from packed RBCs and fresh frozen plasma. Always check with the resident before replacing blood or blood products.

Advantages
- Volume replacement
- Oxygen-carrying capacity (lower in banked blood than in fresh blood)

Disadvantages
- Preparation time: requires type and cross, except in cases of an emergency, such as trauma, in which uncrossmatched O type, Rh-negative blood may be used.
- Infectious risks: hepatitis C and cytomegalovirus (CMV), rarely bacteria
- Costly

Blood Products

These include fresh frozen plasma, cryoprecipitate, albumin, and platelets. They are used as a colloid source of volume expansion and may also replace or fulfill specific deficiencies such as specific blood coagulation factors or thrombocytopenia.

Advantages
- Volume replacement
- Replacement of osmotic pressure
- Concurrent replacement of clotting factors

Disadvantages
- Preparation time: some require special screening in the blood bank
- Infectious risk
- Costly

Colloid

These include dextran 40 or 70, and hetastarch. The goal of colloid administration is to replace fluid and osmotic elements to the intravascular space. Colloids serve to draw fluid from the interstitium by exerting osmotic pressure. They do not carry the risks of infection that blood products do and are more rapidly available. Some colloids are also used to enhance microcirculation by reducing blood viscosity, which may be desirable after revascularization procedures.

Advantages

- Volume replacement
- Replacement of osmotic pressure
- No risk of infection
- Reduction of blood viscosity

Disadvantages

- Preparation time: requires ordering from the pharmacy
- In settings of leaking capillaries, colloid will not remain in the vascular bed, resulting in peripheral or pulmonary edema.
- No improvement in oxygen-carrying capacity
- Costly
- May interfere with coagulation

Crystalloid

Crystalloid is the most widely used option because it is available and inexpensive. Even if another fluid is ultimately desirable, it is often worth beginning the volume expansion with crystalloid until the other product becomes available. Because of its easy passage from the intravascular space into the extravascular space, crystalloid replacement tends to take 4 times the volume to achieve the same expansion of the intravascular space as does colloid. A list of available crystalloid products and their electrolyte compositions is presented in Table 12–4.

Advantages

- Volume replacement
- Inexpensive
- Rapidly available
- No risk of infection

Disadvantages

- In settings of leaking capillaries, crystalloid will not remain in the vascular bed, resulting in peripheral or pulmonary edema
- Poor replacement of osmotic pressure
- No improvement in oxygen-carrying capacity

■ SPECIAL SURGICAL CONSIDERATIONS

Burn Patients

Adequate fluid resuscitation of patients with severe burn injuries is an important surgical consideration. Fluid losses are

Table 12-4 □ COMMONLY USED CRYSTALLOID FLUIDS

Type	Glucose (g/L)	Na (mEg/L)	K (mEq/L)	Cl (mEq/L)	Ca (mEq/L)	Lactate (mEq/L)	Osm (mOsm/L)
D5W	50	—	—	—	—	—	252
D10W	100	—	—	—	—	—	505
D20W	200	—	—	—	—	—	1010
D50W	500	—	—	—	—	—	2525
NS	—	154	—	154	—	—	308
LR	—	130	4	109	3	28	272

D5W = 5% dextrose in water; D10W = 10% dextrose in water; D20W = 20% dextrose in water; D50W = 50% dextrose in water; NS = nornal saline; LR = lactated Ringer's.

tremendous and are due to leakage across capillary membranes into the extravascular space (including into the lungs) and to surface evaporation. IV fluid replacement is indicated in those patients whose burn involves 15% or more of the body surface area (BSA) (10% in children).

There are a variety of resuscitation techniques, and most are based on the patient's body weight and the percentage of BSA involved in the burn. The major difference between the techniques is the timing of colloid administration. The goal of therapy is to supply daily fluid requirements and to replace ongoing losses, to maintain an adequate cardiac output.

A rapid estimation of BSA may be made by following the "rule of nines" (Fig. 12–3), in which body surfaces are roughly divided into 9% regions. Another simple technique is to remember that the palm is roughly 1% of the patient's BSA.

The fluid resuscitation is divided into two time frames, the acute phase (<48 hours) and the subacute phase (>48 hours). In the acute phase, fluid replacement is rapid (Table 12–5). LR solution is commonly used. Some centers advocate the addition of sodium bicarbonate (0.5 ampule/L) to the LR. The absolute volume (2–4 ml/kg/% of burned BSA) depends on which actual formula is used (2–3 ml/kg/% of BSA = Brooke's revised technique; 3 ml/kg/% of BSA = Duke University technique; 4 ml/

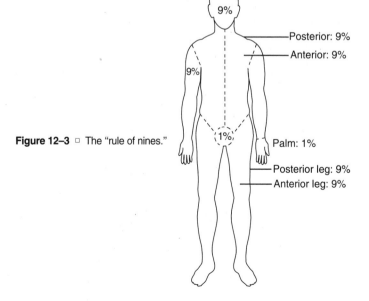

Figure 12–3 □ The "rule of nines."

9%

Posterior: 9%

Anterior: 9%

9%

1%

Palm: 1%

Posterior leg: 9%

Anterior leg: 9%

Table 12–5 □ **FLUID RESUSCITATION TECHNIQUE FOR INITIAL TREATMENT OF BURN PATIENTS DURING FIRST 24 HOURS**

Fluid	Volume	Rate of Administration
Lactated Ringer's	2–4 ml/ kg/% BSA	1/2 over the 1st 8 hr (postburn, **not** postadmission) 1/2 over the next 16 hr

kg/% of BSA = Baker and Parkland techniques). As most severe burn patients are initially behind in fluids, it is best to err on the high side (4 ml/kg/% of BSA) and decrease the rate later as UO dictates.

Deliver the first half of the replacement volume over the first 8 hours postburn (note that the clock starts at the time of the burn, not the time of admission). Deliver the second half of the fluid over the next 16 hours. Over the second 24 hours, attempt to reduce the fluid delivery rate. Do so slowly (25% drop in rate over 3 hours, as tolerated), until the rate equals a volume adequate to deliver maintenance fluids and replace ongoing losses. If the UO drops below 30 ml/hr, return to the higher rate and bolus with crystalloid as necessary.

The adequacy of the fluid resuscitation must be closely monitored in the acute phase after a burn:

1. Measure hourly UO.
   - An indwelling urinary catheter is required for severe burns.
   - Maintain the UO at 30 to 50 ml/hr. Adjust the fluid rate based on the UO.
   - If the sodium delivery is too great, consider combining LR therapy with 5% dextrose in water (electrolyte-free fluid) to maintain UO.
2. Measure daily body weights.
   - Expect an increase of 10 to 20% of the admission body weight in the first 48 hours after resuscitation.
   - During the subacute phase, expect a loss of 1 to 2% of body weight per day for the next 7 to 10 days.
3. Measure pulmonary artery pressures with a Swan-Ganz catheter in selected patients, including the following:
   - Those who do not respond appropriately to initial attempts at resuscitation
   - Those with known cardiopulmonary disease
   - The elderly
4. Use electrolyte and hematologic laboratory data appropriately.
   - The hematrocrit will vary due to surface blood loss, to the

dilutional effects of the fluid resuscitation, and to the relative bone marrow aplasia due to acute illness; hematocrit is not a very accurate measurement of the adequacy of the fluid resuscitation.

- Electrolytes should be checked at least every 6 hours during the acute phase of the burn.

  Follow also the base deficit from the arterial blood gas (ABG) data. This is a reflection of the serum lactate level and is a good way to follow the efficacy of the resuscitation.

The subacute phase (>48 hours) of burn management still requires fluid replacement. This is due to the ongoing insensible surface losses. The volume of surface losses (in ml/hr) may be estimated by the following formula:

$$\text{Total BSA (in m}^2) \times (25 + \% \text{ of burned BSA})$$

Continue to administer maintenance fluids in addition to replacement fluids for ongoing losses. Follow physiologic parameters of UO, end-organ perfusion, and serum electrolytes.

Colloid is generally withheld in the first 24 to 48 hours because of the severity of the capillary leak. This avoids extravasation of the osmotic agent into the extravascular space. When capillary leakage begins to abate, consider the addition of colloid to the fluid replacement:

1. Confirm that the serum albumin is <2.5 g/dl.
2. 50 g albumin/L of NS is equivalent to physiologic levels of protein (5 g/dl).
3. The rate of colloid delivery is also dependent on the severity of the burn; as follows:

   30 to 50% BSA = 0.3 ml/kg/% of BSA over 24 hours
   50 to 70% BSA = 0.4 ml/kg/% of BSA over 24 hours
   >70% BSA = 0.5 ml/kg/% of BSA over 24 hours

Burn care is very difficult and requires appropriate initial management as well as complicated long-term therapies. Severe burns are best treated in specified burn units. Indications for referral to a burn facility include the following:

1. Adults with >20% of BSA burns
2. Children with >10% of BSA burns
3. Full-thickness burns of >10% of BSA
4. Burns involving regions of great functional or cosmetic value (face, hands, feet, eyes, ears, and perineum)
5. High-voltage electrical injuries
6. Inhalation injuries
7. Burns associated with other trauma
8. Burns in patients with other severe medical conditions
9. Circumferential limb burns, which are at risk for compartmental syndrome

Remember

1. Rapid infusion of glucose-containing fluid will result in hyperglycemia and may cause an osmotic diuresis, which will be counterproductive to the resuscitative effort.
2. Rapid infusion of NS can result in hyperchloremic metabolic acidosis.
3. Fluid poured into a patient during a resuscitation effort will at some point need to be excreted during the resolution phase of the illness. Anticipate this shift, and be mindful that it may contribute to the cardiac complications of those patients who have marginal myocardial reserve.

Common Electrolyte Abnormalities

■ SODIUM (Na⁺)

Normal range: 135 to 147 mmol/L.

Sodium Metabolism

The serum concentration of sodium is not an indication of total body sodium; it is an indication of fluid status. Disturbances in water balance are evident by derangements in sodium levels. Hyponatremia is an indication of fluid overload, and hypernatremia, of fluid depletion. The signs and symptoms of sodium concentration derangements are more dependent on the rate of change of serum sodium levels than the actual level. Likewise, the rate of correction should be slow, unless severe symptoms are present.

Oral intake of sodium generally more than satisfies the needs of the body. Only about 30 mEq of sodium is lost through stool and sweat per day. The remainder is excreted through urine under the control of aldosterone. In settings of severe water deprivation, sodium is resorbed in exchange for potassium under the control of antidiuretic hormone (ADH). Free water is resorbed with the sodium. The physiologic stimulus for ADH secretion is increased serum osmolality.

Hypernatremia

Etiology

1. Inadequate intake of water
   a. Unconscious patient

    b. Hypothalamic disorder
2. Excessive water loss
    a. Renal losses of water
        (1) Diabetes insipidus (pituitary or renal origin) (U_{Na} variable)
        (2) Osmotic diuresis (hyperglycemia, urea, and mannitol administration) ($U_{Na} > 20$ mEq/L)
    b. Extrarenal losses of water ($U_{Na} < 10$ mEq/L)
        (1) Vomiting and NG suction
        (2) Diarrhea
        (3) Insensible losses (sweating, open wounds, and respiration)
3. Excessive sodium gain ($U_{Na} > 20$ mEq/L)
    a. Iatrogenic (excessive sodium administration)
    b. Primary hyperaldosteronism
    c. Cushing's syndrome
    d. Salt tablets
    e. Hypertonic dialysis

Selective Physical Examination

Symptoms of hypernatremia are the result of cellular dehydration in the brain. Other symptoms are secondary to extracellular fluid deficit (see The Fluid Depleted Patient section above).

MS:	Confusion, restlessness, irritability, and obtundation
Resp:	Respiratory paralysis
GU:	Polyuria and polydipsia
Neuro:	Muscular irritability, hyperreflexia, ataxia, and seizures

Additional tests:
1. Serum Na: Determine severity
2. Serum osmolality: Aids in diagnosis
3. Urine Na: Aids in diagnosis

Management

1. Determine the severity.
    The therapy is dependent on the patient's condition and symptoms and the results of laboratory studies listed above. Also the rate of development of hypernatremia must be taken into account. Serum osmolality may be measured in the laboratory or may be estimated from other laboratory data using the following formula:

Serum osmolality (mOsm) =

$$2[Na\ (mEq/L)] + \frac{[glucose\ (mg/dl)]}{[18]} + \frac{[BUN\ (mg/dl)]}{[2.8]}$$

Normal range: 280 to 295 mOsm.

In the absence of fluid deficit or other significant symptoms, and if the serum Na is <150 mEq/L, specific therapy may not be warranted.

2. Assess the patient's fluid status.

The effects of hypernatremia are due to cellular dehydration as water is drawn from the cell toward the high osmolality of the extracellular fluid. This is most likely due to an extracellular fluid deficit. An estimation of free water deficit in liters is given by the following formula:

Water deficit (L) =

$$\frac{[\text{serum Na (observed)} - \text{serum Na (normal)}]\ [0.6]\ [\text{Wt (kg)}]}{[\text{serum Na (normal)}]}$$

Assume serum Na (normal) = 140 mEq/L. The 0.6 represents the volume of distribution of sodium, which may be assumed to be the same volume as total body water. Another rapid key to determine fluid deficit is shown in Table 12–6.

3. Correct the fluid deficit.

The rate of fluid deficit replacement is dependent on the rate of development of the hypernatremia. Rapid onset with prominent symptoms should be corrected in several hours. A more chronic development of hypernatremia should be corrected no faster than 2 mOsm/hr to avoid formation of cerebral edema. The fluid of choice is NS until the patient is hemodynamically stable. Then reassess and switch to a more hypotonic solution, such as 5% dextrose in water + one-half NS, until the remainder of the extracellular volume depletion is corrected.

4. Correct the underlying cause.

In a very rare case, hypernatremia is noted in settings of fluid overload. In this case, a loop diuretic such as furosemide (Lasix) may be used to stimulate the excretion of both salt and water.

Special Surgical Considerations

Hypernatremia in surgical patients most likely results from underestimation of free water losses.

Table 12–6 □ ESTIMATION OF FREE WATER DEFICIT IN SETTINGS OF HYPERNATREMIA

Serum Na (Observed)	Estimated Free Water Deficit
150 mEq/L	50 ml/kg
160 mEq/L	90 ml/kg
170 mEq/L	140 ml/kg

Hyponatremia

Low serum sodium is a common postoperative problem. A normal physiologic response to surgery is the secretion of ADH from the pituitary gland. This occurs in the absence of hyperosmolar stimuli and may result in mild hemodilution due to the retention of water. This typically lasts for 3 to 5 days after an uncomplicated surgical procedure. This resolves without specific therapy with a physiologic diuresis. In settings of severe hyponatremia (<130 mEq/L), further diagnostic measures are warranted. The first step to diagnosis is to rule out spurious causes such as increased plasma glucose, proteins, or lipids.

Etiology

Hyponatremia may be present in either fluid excess or fluid deficit conditions.

1. Decreased extracellular volume
   a. Renal losses of sodium ($U_{Na} >20$ mmol/L)
      (1) Diuretic medications
      (2) Mineralocorticoid deficiency
      (3) Salt-losing nephritis
      (4) Osmotic diuresis
      (5) Renal tubular acidosis
      (6) Metabolic acidosis
      (7) Ketonuria
      (8) Bartter's syndrome
      (9) Diuretic phase of acute tubular necrosis
   b. Extrarenal losses of sodium ($U_{Na} <20$ mmol/L)
      (1) GI losses (vomiting, diarrhea, and NG suctioning)
      (2) Sequestration (pancreatitis, peritonitis, and "third spacing")
      (3) Burns
      (4) Traumatized muscle
      (5) Sweating
2. Increased extracellular volume
   a. Acute and chronic renal failure ($U_{Na} >20$ mmol/L)
   b. Other causes ($U_{Na} <20$ mmol/L)
      (1) Nephrotic syndrome
      (2) Cirrhosis
      (3) Cardiac failure
3. Normal volume to moderate volume excess ($U_{Na} >20$ mmol/L)
   a. Glucocorticoid deficiency
      (1) Addison's disease
      (2) Inadequate steroid replacement in a steroid-dependent patient
   b. Hypothyroidism
   c. Pain
   d. Emotional stress

e. Medications
f. Syndrome of inappropriate ADH secretion (SIADH)
   (1) Tumors (small cell carcinoma of the lung, pancreatic carcinoma, and duodenal adenocarcinoma)
   (2) Central nervous system (CNS) disorders (tumor, trauma, meningitis, and encephalitis)
   (3) Pulmonary disorders (pneumonia and tuberculosis)
   (4) Medications (chlorpropamide, clofibrate, cyclophosphamide, vincristine, carbamazepine, narcotics, and tricyclic antidepressants)
g. Pseudohyponatremia
   (1) With normal serum osmolality
      (a) Hyperlipidemia
      (b) Hyperproteinemia
   (2) With increased serum osmolality
      (a) Hyperglycemia
      (b) Urea
      (c) Mannitol administration
      (d) Alcohol (ethanol, methanol, and isopropyl alcohol)
      (e) Ethylene glycol

Major Threat to Life

It is the overly rapid correction of hyponatremia that is a threat to life. One response to hyponatremia is the export of solute from the cell to maintain volume. If the extracellular fluid in the brain becomes too hypertonic relative to the cells during correction, a net shift of fluid outward can cause cellular dehydration. The result can be central pontine myelinolysis. A slow correction is necessary to avoid cerebral damage. Do not exceed a rate of 2 mEq/L/hr.

Selective Physical Examination

MS:	Lethargy, apathy, disorientation, agitation, and coma
Neuro:	Weakness, decreased deep tendon reflexes (DTRs), and seizures

Additional tests:
1. Serum Na:	Determine severity
2. Serum osmolality:	Aids in diagnosis
3. Serum glucose:	Rule out pseudohyponatremia (Each increase in serum glucose of 100 mg/dl above normal decreases serum Na by 0.4 mEq/L.)
4. Serum protein:	Rule out pseudohyponatremia
5. Serum lipids:	Rule out pseudohyponatremia
6. Urine Na:	Aids in diagnosis

Management

1. Determine the severity.

    The therapy is dependent on the patient's condition and symptoms and the results of laboratory studies listed above. Also the rate of development of hyponatremia must be taken into account. In the absence of fluid deficit or other significant symptoms, specific therapy may not be warranted.

2. Assess the patient's fluid status.

3. Correct fluid deficit (if present).

    The rate of fluid deficit replacement is dependent on the rate of development of the hyponatremia. Initial correction of severe hyponatremia (<110 mEq/L) should not go beyond 120 to 125 mEq/L and should not exceed a correction rate of 2 mEq/L/hr to avoid cerebral dehydration and irreversible brain damage. The fluid of choice is NS until the patient is hemodynamically stable. If the patient is hyponatremic with a metabolic acidosis, consider replacement with sodium lactate (M/6 fluid). Then reassess and switch to a more hypotonic solution, such as 5% dextrose in water + one-half NS, until the remainder of the extracellular volume depletion is corrected.

4. Replace sodium if necessary.

    Especially useful in settings of fluid deficit. Estimation of sodium deficit is calculated by the following formula:

[serum Na (desired) − serum Na (observed)] [0.6] [Wt (kg)]

Use 135 mEq/L as the serum Na (desired) as it represents the low end of normal serum sodium concentration. The method and rate of sodium replacement is dependent on the severity of the hyponatremia. In general, replace one-half of the deficit over 8 hours and the remaining one-half over the next 16 hours. Table 12–7 shows the sodium concentration of various preparations of saline. In rare cases, such as seizure associated with hyponatremia, it may be necessary to treat with hypertonic saline. Administer 3% saline at a rate of 2 mEq/L/hr until the serum sodium

Table 12–7 □ SODIUM CONCENTRATIONS IN VARIOUS SALINE PREPARATIONS

Normal saline (0.9%)	154 mEq/L
Sodium lactate (M/6)	167 mEq/L
Lactated Ringer's	130 mEq/L
3% saline	500 mEq/L
5% saline	850 mEq/L

concentration is >125 mEq/L or until the seizure activity stops.
5. Treat fluid excess (if necessary).

This may be accomplished with fluid restriction and the administration of diuretics. In settings of hyponatremia, a minimally salt wasting diuretic such as **spironolactone (Aldactone) is recommended. An initial dose of 100 mg is recommended, with daily doses ranging from 25 to 200 mg PO.** The diuretic effects may be delayed by 2 to 3 days.
6. Correct the underlying cause.

Specific disorders that require further treatment include SIADH and forms of pseudohyponatremia.

■ SIADH

This is a condition in which nonosmotic stimuli are responsible for the release of ADH. The possible causes are listed under the etiology of hyponatremia. The diagnosis is dependent on the following criteria:
1. Hyponatremia with low serum osmolality
2. Nonmaximal urine dilution despite serum hypo-osmolality
3. U_{Na} >20 mmol/L
4. Normally functioning kidneys
5. Normally functioning thyroid
6. No diuretic therapy

Management measures include
1. Correction of the underlying cause
2. Water restriction to less than insensible losses (500–1000 ml/day)
3. In settings of severe hyponatremia (<115 mEq/L)
   - Diuretic therapy with **furosemide (Lasix) 20 to 40 mg IV every 2 to 4 hours**
   - **Demeclocycline (Declomycin) 300 to 600 mg PO twice daily** may be useful in patients with chronic SIADH in which water restriction has not been effective.

Pseudohyponatremia

The many causes of pseudohyponatremia are listed under the etiologies of hyponatremia. The diagnosis is made by identifying the agent that is displacing sodium from the blood stream. This may be associated with a normal serum osmolality as with hyperproteinemia or hyperlipidemia; or it may be associated with an increased serum osmolality. Look for an "osmolar gap." Osmolar gap is the difference between the laboratory measured osmolality and the osmolality calculated by hand using glucose and BUN concentrations. If the osmolar gap is >10 mmol/L, look for other osmotically active agents in the serum. Note that there may be an osmolar gap even if the serum osmolality is normal. The treatment of pseudohyponatremia depends on the underlying disease.

Of special note is hyperglycemia. In such cases, the true serum sodium concentration may be determined using the following formula:

$$\text{Actual serum Na} = \frac{[\text{glucose (observed)} - \text{glucose (normal)}]\,[1.4]}{[\text{glucose (normal)}]} + \text{serum Na (observed)}$$

Correction of the hyperglycemia will tend to correct the hyponatremia.

Special Surgical Considerations

Surgical procedures that may be associated with postoperative hyponatremia include the following:
1. Spinal fusion surgery (20%)
2. Subtotal gastrectomy (67%)
3. Enterocutaneous biliary drainage (22%)
4. Mitral valve surgery (30%)
5. Trauma surgery (40%)

■ POTASSIUM (K^+)

Normal range: 3.5 to 5.0 mmol/L.

Potassium Metabolism

Total stores of potassium are in the range of 50 to 55 mEq/kg; 98% of the potassium is intracellular. Intracellular concentrations are about 150 mEq/L, and extracellular concentrations are about 3.5 to 5 mEq/L with this gradient maintained by the Na^+/K^+-ATPase pump. Normal intake averages about 100 mEq/day with 95% excretion through the kidneys, and 5% loss through stool and sweat. Most of the potassium filtered through the glomerulus is resorbed in the proximal renal tubule. The site of potassium control is at the distal renal tubule where selective resorption and secretion takes place. Potassium excretion is under the control of aldosterone, plasma potassium levels, and glomerular filtration rates.

Acid–base imbalance also exerts a control on the ratios of intracellular and extracellular potassium. Alkalosis enhances excretion of potassium in exchange for resorption of H^+ and Na^+ ions in the distal renal tubule. Acidosis enhances renal conservation of K^+ in the distal tubule. High concentrations of H^+ ion also may displace intracellular K^+, causing an apparent hyperkalemia.

Hyperkalemia

Etiology

1. Excessive intake
   a. Iatrogenic supplementation (IV or PO)
   b. Salt substitutes
   c. High-dose potassium penicillin therapy
   d. Blood transfusions
2. Decreased excretion
   a. Renal failure (acute or chronic)
   b. Potassium-sparing diuretics (amiloride, spironolactone, and triamterene)
   c. Addison's disease
   d. Hypoaldosteronism
   e. Distal tubular dysfunction
3. Fluid shifts of intracellular to extracellular
   a. Acidemia
   b. Insulin deficiency
   c. Tissue destruction (hemolysis, crush injuries, rhabdomyolysis, burns, and tumor lysis)
   d. Medications (arginine, beta blockers, digoxin, and succinylcholine)
   e. Hyperkalemic periodic paralysis
4. Factitious
   a. Prolonged tourniquet application before blood draw
   b. Hemolysis of blood sample
   c. Leukocytosis
   d. Thrombocytosis

Major Threat to Life

Cardiac arrhythmias are the major threat to life.

Selective Physical Examination

CVS:	Fatal arrhythmias
Neuro:	Weakness, paresthesias, depressed DTRs

Additional tests:

1. ECG: The rhythm manifestations progress relative to the severity of the hyperkalemia (Fig. 12–4).

   Peaked T waves
   Depressed ST segments
   Decreased R wave amplitude
   Prolonged PR interval
   Small or absent P waves
   Wide QRS complexes
   Sine wave pattern

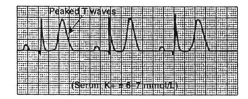

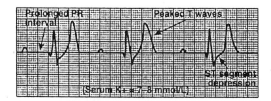

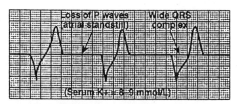

Figure 12–4 □ Progressive electrocardiographic manifestations of hyperkalemia. (From Marshall SA, Ruedy J: On Call: Principles and Protocols, 2nd ed. Philadelphia, WB Saunders Co, 1993, p 310.)

Management

1. Assess the severity.

   Perform a 12-lead electrocardiogram (ECG) and serum potassium level immediately. The degree of hyperkalemia dictates how aggressive the therapy should be.

2. Perform continuous cardiac monitoring.

   This should be continued for 24 hours after the resolution of the hyperkalemia. Fatal arrhythmias may occur at any time during therapy and at seemingly small increases in serum potassium.

3. Correct the underlying cause, if known.

4. Remove potassium from IV fluids, if present.

Discontinue or replace potassium-containing medications.
5. If the hyperkalemia is mild (<6.5 mEq/L)
   - Consider continuous cardiac monitoring.
   - Recheck the serum potassium every 4 to 6 hours until stabilized.
6. If the hyperkalemia is moderate (6.5–8 mEq/L)
   - Perform continuous cardiac monitoring.
   - Recheck the serum potassium every 1 to 2 hours until the serum potassium level stabilizes at <6.5 mEq/L.
   - Administer one or more of the following:
     a. **NaHCO$_3$, 1 ampule (44.6 mmol) IV**
        This shifts the potassium from the extracellular space into the intracellular space. The effect is immediate and lasts 1 to 2 hours.
     b. Glucose and insulin
        50% dextrose in water, 50 ml IV, followed by **regular insulin 5 to 10 units IV.** This therapy shifts potassium from the extracellular space into the intracellular space. The effect is immediate and lasts 1 to 2 hours.
     c. The glucose, insulin, and bicarbonate may be administered together as a cocktail.
        Add **3 ampules of NaHCO$_3$ and 20 units of regular insulin to 1000 ml 20% dextrose in water.** Administer at 75 ml/hr as other therapies are being instituted.
     d. **Sodium polystyrene sulfonate (Kayexalate)**
        15 to 30 g (4–8 tsp) in 50 to 100 ml of 20% sorbitol or **20% dextrose in water administered PO every 3 to 4 hours,** or **50 g in 200 ml 20% sorbitol** or **20% dextrose in water administered as a retention enema for 30 to 60 minutes every 4 hours.** This is the only therapy that removes potassium from the body. The resin exchanges potassium for sodium.
7. If the hyperkalemia is severe (>8 mEq/L)
   - Perform continuous cardiac monitoring.
   - Notify your resident.
   - Recheck the serum potassium every 1 to 2 hours until the serum potassium level stabilizes at <6.5 mEq/L.
   - Administer one or more of the following:
     a. **NaHCO$_3$, 1 ampule (44.6 mmol) IV**
     b. Glucose and insulin
        50% dextrose in water 50 ml IV followed by **regular insulin 5 to 10 units IV.**
     c. Glucose, insulin, and bicarbonate cocktail
        Add **3 ampules of NaHCO$_3$** and 20 units of regular insulin to 1000 ml 20% dextrose in water. Administer at 75 ml/hr as other therapies are being instituted.
     d. **Sodium polystyrene sulfonate (Kayexalate)**
        15 to 30 g (4–8 tsp) in 50 to 100 ml of 20% sorbitol

or **20% dextrose in water** administered **PO every 3 to 4 hours,** or **50 g** in **200 ml 20% sorbitol** or **20% dextrose in water** administered as a retention enema for **30 to 60 minutes every 4 hours.**

   e. **Calcium gluconate 5 to 10 ml 10% solution IV over 2 minutes**

     This temporarily stabilizes the myocardial and neuromuscular effects of the hyperkalemia. Note that this therapy will not affect the serum potassium level.

- Hemodialysis therapy is reserved for patients in renal failure or for whom the above measures have proved ineffective.

Hypokalemia

Etiology

1. Renal losses (U_K >20 mEq/day)
   a. Diuretic therapy
   b. Osmotic diuresis
   c. Antibiotic therapy (aminoglycosides, amphotericin, carbenicillin, nafcillin, and ticarcillin)
   d. Renal tubular acidosis (type I)
   e. Hyperaldosteronism
   f. Glucocorticoid excess
   g. Magnesium deficiency
   h. Chronic metabolic alkalosis
   i. Bartter's syndrome
   j. Fanconi's syndrome
   k. Ureterosigmoidostomy
   l. GI losses (vomiting and NG suctioning) due to the loss of hydrogen ions resulting in alkalosis
2. Extrarenal losses (U_K <20 mEq/day)
   a. Diarrhea
   b. Intestinal fistulas
3. Inadequate potassium intake
4. Fluid shift from extracellular space to intracellular space
   a. Acute alkalosis (hyperventilation, GI losses, intestinal fistulas)
   b. Insulin therapy
   c. Vitamin B_{12} therapy
   d. Hypokalemic periodic paralysis
   e. Medications (lithium and salbutamol)

Major Threat to Life

Cardiac arrhythmias are the major threat to life.

Selective Physical Examination

CVS: Premature atrial contractions (PACs)

	and premature ventricular contractions (PVCs); digoxin toxicity
Abd:	Paralytic ileus
Neuro:	Weakness, parasthesias, and depressed DTRs
Additional tests:	
1. ECG:	The following findings may be present (Fig. 12–5):
	T wave flattening
	U waves
	Depression of ST waves
2. ABG:	Metabolic alkalosis
3. Serum Ca^{2+}:	Hypokalemia and hypocalcemia may coexist
4. Serum Mg^{2+}:	Hypokalemia and hypomagnesemia may coexist

Management

1. Assess the severity.
    Obtain a 12-lead ECG and a serum potassium level immediately.
2. Consider cardiac monitoring, especially if there is coexistent hypocalcemia.
3. Correct the underlying cause, if known.
    If the hypokalemia coexists with another electrolyte derangement, failure to correct the other deficiency will complicate the correction of the low serum potassium.
4. If the hypokalemia is mild (3.1–3.5 mEq/L, without severe cardiac arrhythmias)
    ▪ Give oral potassium supplementation (Table 12–8 for options).
    ▪ Recheck serum potassium in the morning.
5. If the hypokalemia is moderate (<3.0 mEq/L, with PACs but infrequent PVCs)
    ▪ Notify your resident.

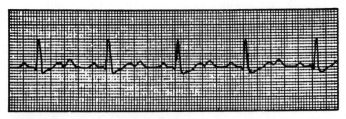

Figure 12–5 □ Electrocardiographic manifestations of hypokalemia. (From Marshall SA, Ruedy J: On Call: Principles and Protocols, 2nd ed. Philadelphia, WB Saunders Co, 1993, p 313.)

Table 12–8 □ ORAL POTASSIUM SUPPLEMENTS

Slow-K	8 mEq/tablet
Micro-K Extencaps	8 mEq/tablet
Micro-K 10 Extencaps	10 mEq/tablet
Kay Ciel liquid	20 mEq/15ml
K-Lyte	25 mEq/packet
Banana	1 mEq/inch

- Give oral potassium supplementation.
- Give IV potassium supplementation.
   Reserve this option for severe hypokalemia or for those patients who are unable to tolerate oral potassium.
- Recheck serum potassium in the morning.
6. If the hypokalemia is severe (<3.0 mEq/L, with frequent PVCs or digoxin toxicity)
- Notify your resident.
- Obtain continuous cardiac monitoring.
- Give bolus IV potassium replacement.
   Give **10 mEq KCl in 100 ml 5% dextrose in water administered over 1 hour.** IV potassium in high concentrations is best delivered through central venous access, as severe burning and thrombophlebitis can occur if it is delivered through a peripheral vein.
- Give continuous IV potassium replacement.
   KCl may be added to intravenous fluids (IVF) to final concentrations of **40 to 60 mEq/L, which may be delivered at rates up to 20 mEq/hr.**
- Recheck serum potassium levels after every 20 to 30 mEq replaced and in the morning.
   Frequent monitoring is required to avoid iatrogenic hyperkalemia.

■ CALCIUM (Ca^{2+})

Normal range (total): 2.2 to 2.6 mmol/L.
Normal range (ionized): 1.12 to 1.23 mmol/L.

Calcium Metabolism

Calcium is absorbed from the GI tract under control of vitamin D. Once absorbed, Ca^{2+} is deposited and resorbed from the bones under the control of vitamin D and parathyroid hormone (PTH).

Approximately 40% of serum calcium is bound by albumin. An additional 10% is bound as a complexing ion. The remaining 50% is free ionized Ca^{2+}, which is the physiologically available form. Hypoalbuminemia can result in factitious hypocalcemia if the **total** Ca^{2+} is measured. Measurement of **ionized** Ca^{2+} will circumvent this problem. To correct for aberrations in albumin level, use the following formula:

Add 0.2 mmol/L Ca^{2+} to the measured total Ca^{2+} value for every 10 g/L hypoalbuminemia (assume a normal albumin to be 4.0 g/L).

Hypercalcemia

Etiology

1. Increased intake or absorption
   a. Vitamin D or A intoxication
   b. Excessive calcium supplementation
   c. Milk-alkali syndrome (excessive antacid ingestion)
   d. Sarcoidosis or other granulomatous disease
2. Increased mobilization from bone
   a. Primary hyperthyroidism
   b. Severe secondary hyperthyroidism associated with renal failure
   c. Neoplasm
      (1) Bony metastasis (prostate, breast, thyroid, kidney, and lung)
      (2) PTH-like substance secreted by tumor (lung, kidney, ovary, and colon)
      (3) Increased bony resorption mediated by prostaglandin E_2
      (4) Osteoclast-stimulating factor (due to multiple myeloma and lymphoproliferative disorders)
   d. Paget's disease
   e. Long-term immobilization
   f. Hyperthyroidism
   g. Adrenal insufficiency
   h. Acromegaly
   i. Sarcoidosis; in addition to increased absorption from the GI tract, sarcoidosis increases conversion of 25-(OH) vitamin D to 1,25-$(OH)_2$ vitamin D
   j. Chronic lithium use
3. Decreased excretion
   a. Thiazide diuretics
   b. Familial hypocalciuric hypercalcemia

Major Threat to Life

Bradycardia and complete heart block are the major threats to life.

Selective Physical Examination

VS:	Bradycardia
MS:	Insomnia, restlessness, delirium, dementia, lethargy, and coma
HEENT:	Corneal calcification
CVS:	Bradycardia
	Dysrhythmias, hypertension, and digoxin sensitivity
Abd:	GI upset, anorexia, nausea, vomiting, constipation, and pancreatitis
GU:	Polyuria, polydipsia, and nephrolithiasis
Neuro:	Muscle weakness, hyporeflexia, bone pain, and pathologic fractures

Additional tests:

1. ECG: Shortened QT interval and prolonged PR interval (Fig. 12–6)
2. ABG: May show hyperchlorhydric metabolic acidosis
3. PTH: If no known malignancy is found, a serum PTH should be drawn. A high PTH is indicative of hyperparathyroidism; a low PTH requires workup for occult malignancy.

Management

1. Determine the severity.

   Treatment is determined by the absolute calcium level. Severe symptoms generally appear above total Ca^{2+} levels of 3.2 mmol/L. Be mindful of recent trends or symptoms. A rapid or continuous rise in Ca^{2+} will require immediate treatment, as will a symptomatic patient.
2. If the hypercalcemia is mild (2.6–2.9 mmol/L)

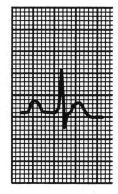

Figure 12–6 □ Hypercalcemia (short QT interval, prolonged PR interval). (From Marshall SA, Ruedy J: On Call: Principles and Protocols, 2nd ed. Philadelphia, WB Saunders Co, 1993, p 287.)

- Expand volume.

    Administer a **500 ml NS bolus IV** as rapidly as possible. Expansion of the intravascular space will bring the Ca^{2+} level down by hemodilution. Further fluid boluses may be given depending on the patient's fluid status. Take care in rehydrating a patient with a history of CHF.

- Recheck the serum calcium in the morning.

3. If the hypercalcemia is moderate (2.9–3.2 mmol/L)

    - Expand volume.
    - Induce diuresis (UO of >2500 ml/day is sufficient).

        Furosemide (Lasix) in doses of **20 to 40 mg IV every 2 to 4 hours** should be sufficient to ensure UO should be >2500 ml/day. Continue to maintain volume expansion during the diuresis; do not get behind in fluid administration. Furosemide has the additional advantage of inhibiting calcium absorption in the renal tubule. Thiazide diuretics are not desirable, as they will elevate serum calcium levels.

    - Closely follow serum K^+ and Mg^{2+} levels.
    - Recheck serum calcium in 4 to 6 hours and in the morning.

4. If the hypercalcemia is severe (>3.2 mmol/L, or if the patient is symptomatic)

    - Expand volume.
    - Induce diuresis.
    - Perform dialysis, useful for severe hypercalcemia (>4.5 mmol/L).
    - Give medications.

        One or more of the following medications are useful in the treatment of severe hypercalcemia:

        a. **Disodium etidronate** (EHDP) **(Biphosphonate)** inhibits bone resorption of Ca^{2+} **(5 to 10 mg/kg/day IV over 2 hours for 3 days),** followed by a repeat course in 7 days if necessary; longer term therapy may be maintained with **20 mg/kg/day PO for 30 days.**

        b. **Plicamycin (Mithracin)** inhibits bone resorption of Ca^{2+} **(15 to 25 μg/kg in 1 L NS over 3 to 6 hours).** (This is not an acute acting medication; the onset of action is delayed by 48 hours.)

        c. **Phosphate (Fleet Phospho-Soda)** causes Ca^{2+} to be removed from the blood and deposited in extravascular tissues; it should be given to any patient whose serum PO_4^- is less than 1 mmol/L, and whose kidneys are working well **(5 ml PO 3 to 4 times daily** until serum PO_4^- is 1.6 mmol/L).

        d. **Prednisone** decreases Ca^{2+} absorption in malignancy and may have antitumor effects **(10 to 25 mg PO every 6 hours).** (This is not an acute acting medication; effects are noted in 2 to 3 days.)

      e. **Calcitonin** decreases bone resorption **(4 U/kg IV followed by 4 U/kg SC every 12 hours).** (Not effective in 25% of patients.)

      f. **Indomethacin (Indocin)** is used for hypercalcemia associated with malignancy, and it inhibits the synthesis of prostaglandin E_2 **(50 mg PO every 8 hours).**

- Recheck serum Ca^{2+} and PO_4- levels as well as other appropriate laboratory studies to monitor hydration.

Hypocalcemia

Etiology

1. Decreased intake or absorption
   a. Malabsorption
   b. Intestinal bypass surgery
   c. Short bowel syndrome
   d. Vitamin D deficiency
2. Decreased production or mobilization from bone
   a. Hypoparathyroidism (after subtotal thyroidectomy or parathyroidectomy)
   b. Pseudohypoparathyroidism
   c. Vitamin D deficiency [decreased production of 25-(OH) vitamin D or 1,25-$(OH)_2$ vitamin D]
   d. Acute hyperphosphatemia (tumor lysis syndrome, acute renal failure, and rhabdomyolysis)
   e. Acute pancreatitis
   f. Hypomagnesemia
   g. Alkalosis (hyperventilation, GI losses, and intestinal fistulas)
   h. Neoplasm
      (1) Paradoxical hypocalcemia associated with osteoblastic metastases from lung, breast, or prostate cancer
      (2) Medullary carcinoma of the thyroid (calcitonin-producing tumor)
      (3) Tumor lysis syndrome
3. Increased excretion
   a. Chronic renal failure
   b. Medications (aminoglycosides and loop diuretics)

Major Threat to Life

Fatal arrhythmia is the major threat to life.

Selective Physical Examination

MS:	Confusion, irritability, and depression
HEENT:	Papilledema and diplopia
	Stridor (laryngospasm)
Abd:	Abdominal cramping

Neuro:	Paresthesias of the fingers and toes
Special examinations:	Increased DTRs, carpopedal spasm tetany, and seizures
1. Chvostek's sign:	Facial muscle spasm elicited by light tapping on the facial nerve at the angle of the jaw; may be a normal finding in about 10% of the population despite normal calcium levels
2. Trousseau's sign:	Carpal spasm elicited by placement of a blood pressure cuff on the arm and inflation to above SBP for 3 to 5 minutes (This is often a painful test for the patient.)
Additional tests:	
1. ECG:	Prolonged QT interval without U waves (Fig. 12–7).

Management

1. Assess the severity.

   Measure serum calcium and albumin levels. Correct for low albumin as above. Asymptomatic patients do not require aggressive therapy.

2. Measure the serum phosphate level.

   If the level is severely elevated (>6 mmol/L), correct the hyperphosphatemia with glucose and insulin therapy, as described with hyperkalemia above, before replacing calcium. The calcium and phosphate in the blood stream can ionically bind and deposit into tissues. This is most often associated with renal failure, and nephrology service consultation may be required.

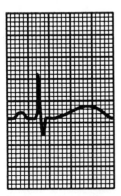

Figure 12–7 □ Hypocalcemia (long QT interval). (From Marshall SA, Ruedy J: On Call: Principles and Protocols, 2nd ed. Philadelphia, WB Saunders Co, 1993, p 290.)

3. If the hypocalcemia is mild (total calcium = 1.9–2.2 mmol/ L)
   - Give oral replacement of **calcium with 1000 to 1500 mg/ day PO.**
   - Recheck serum calcium at daily to weekly intervals.
4. If the hypocalcemia is moderate (total calcium = 1.5–1.9 mmol/L)
   - Give oral replacement of **calcium with 1000 to 1500 mg/ day PO.**
   - Recheck serum calcium at daily to weekly intervals.
   - Evaluate further as warranted.
5. If the hypocalcemia is severe (total calcium <1.5 mmol/L, or if the patient is symptomatic)
   - Perform continuous cardiac monitoring.
     Special caution is required for patients taking digoxin as calcium will potentiate its effects.
   - Contact your resident.
   - Confirm a normal to low serum PO_4^-.
   - Give bolus IV replacement of calcium.
     Give calcium gluconate (10–20 ml of 10% solution [1–2 g] in 100 ml 5% dextrose in water given IV over 30 minutes). This dose may be given without dilution as rapidly as over 2 minutes if symptoms of tetany or laryngospasm are apparent.
   - Perform continuous IV replacement of calcium.
     If the serum calcium level is still <1.9 mmol/L after 6 hours, start a continuous drip with **calcium gluconate (10 ml of a 10% solution [1 g] diluted into 500 ml 5% dextrose in water, infused IV over 6 hours).**
     If the serum calcium has not normalized after 6 hours of the continuous infusion, add **15 ml of the 10% solution (1.5 g) to the next 500 ml 5% dextrose in water and infuse IV over 6 hours.**
   - Give oral replacement of calcium.
     Give **200 mg elemental calcium PO every 2 hours for 4 doses.** This may be started at the same time as the bolus IV injection.
   - Recheck serum calcium levels every 6 hours.

Special Surgical Considerations

The patient who has undergone subtotal thyroidectomy or parathyroidectomy may require replacement of **1 to 1.5 g calcium gluconate/hr. This may be achieved by continuous drip of calcium gluconate. Add 100 ml of a 10% solution (10 g) to 500 ml 5% dextrose in water and run at 50 ml/hr (1 g/hr).**
Often thyroidectomy patients can manage their own mild postoperative hypocalcemia by taking an oral supplement made available at the bedside (such as 1 or 2 chewable Tums) when they

notice symptoms of circumoral or fingertip tingling. Make sure to have the bedside caregiver monitor the quantity of calcium consumed. Long-term calcium supplementation is rarely required.

■ MAGNESIUM (Mg^{2+})

Normal range: 1.3 to 2.1 mEq/L.

Magnesium Metabolism

Magnesium is required for proper function of many cellular mechanisms including the Na^+/K^+-ATPase pump. Derangements in magnesium levels should be sought in conditions associated with abnormalities in potassium or calcium concentrations.

Hypermagnesemia

Etiology

1. Medications
    a. Lithium
    b. Magnesium-containing drugs in settings of renal failure
2. Tumor metastases to bone
3. Hypothyroidism
4. Viral hepatitis
5. Acidosis

Major Threat to Life

Respiratory depression is the major threat to life.

Selective Physical Examination

Symptoms generally do not become apparent until the level is >4 mEq/L.

VS:	Bradycardia
CVS:	Hypotension
Resp:	Respiratory depression
Abd:	Nausea and vomiting
Skin:	Flushing
Neuro:	Loss of DTRs, and muscular paralysis

Management

1. Identify and eliminate the magnesium source.
2. Give **calcium gluconate (or $CaCl_2$) (100–200 mg IV over 5–10 minutes).** Effects are immediate but transient.
3. Provide dialysis for cases of severe hypermagnesemia, especially in settings of renal failure.
4. Avoid magnesium in the future.

Hypomagnesemia

Etiology

Hypomagnesemia is most commonly due to urinary or GI losses.

1. Diminished PO intake
   a. Malabsorption
   b. Malnutrition (prolonged IV therapy, and alcoholism)
2. GI losses
   a. Chronic diarrhea (laxative abuse, gastroenteritis, and inflammatory bowel disease)
   b. High outputs from fistulas and NG drainage
   c. Emesis
3. Medications that increase urinary losses
   a. Cisplatin
   b. Digoxin
   c. Aminoglycosides
   d. Amphotericin B
   e. Diuretics

Major Threat to Life

Ventricular arrhythmia is the major threat to life.

Selective Physical Examination

MS:	Confusion, mood alteration, psychosis, and coma
HEENT:	Nystagmus
CVS:	Arrhythmias and digoxin toxicity
Abd:	Anorexia, vomiting, and difficulty swallowing
Neuro:	Paresthesias, tremors, weakness, vertigo, ataxia, and seizures

Management

1. Treat acute magnesium deficiencies.
   Give **$MgSO_4$ 2 g (8 mEq/g as a 20% solution) IV over 2 to 5 minutes, followed by 10 g IV over the next 24 hours, followed by 4 to 6 g/day IV or PO for the next 4 to 5 days.** Kidneys must be functioning normally.
2. Treat chronic magnesium deficiencies.
   Give **$MgSO_4$ 3 to 6 g/day IV or PO for the next 3 days.** Kidneys must be functioning normally.
3. Provide prophylactic therapy.
   $MgSO_4$ 1 to 2 g/day may be added to IV fluids. Kidneys must be functioning normally.

Common Acid–Base Abnormalities

The normal buffering systems of the body (bicarbonate, hemoglobin, phosphate, and protein) are frequently overwhelmed by

Table 12–9 □ THE HENDERSON-HASSELBALCH EQUATION

$$pH = 6.1 + \log \left(\frac{HCO_3^- \; (mEq/L)}{0.03 \times P_{CO_2} \; (mm \; Hg)} \right)$$

disease states. The differentiation of respiratory causes from metabolic causes is often easily achieved by proper interpretation of the ABG data. Recall that the bicarbonate data on an ABG are calculated values derived from the Henderson-Hasselbalch equation (Table 12–9). If accurate diagnosis is desired, a serum bicarbonate level should be sent to the laboratory in addition to the ABG.

Acid–base abnormalities may occur singly or in combination (mixed disorders). An algorithm describing the common findings in various simple acid–base states is detailed in Table 12–10. For each primary aberration (change in partial pressure of carbon dioxide [P_{CO_2}] or bicarbonate [HCO_3^-] concentration) there is a compensatory response by the body, which abates the effects of pH. Rapid responses occur in the lung with alterations of the respiratory rate (RR); slower responses occur in the kidney with alterations in the absorption or excretion of bicarbonate.

■ **ACIDOSIS**

A small volume of acid (approximately 70 mEq) is added to the body daily. This is generally excreted by the kidney. The major load of total body acid is the result of oxidative metabolism (approximately 22,000 mEq/day) and is excreted as CO_2 by the lungs. An additional 50 to 100 mEq soluble acid/day is created as H_3PO_4 and H_2SO_4 during protein catabolism. Conversion of the soluble acid to volatile acid is according to the following equation:

$$CO_2 + H_2O \leftrightarrow H_2CO_3 \leftrightarrow H^+ + HCO_3^-$$

Table 12–10 □ BLOOD GAS DATA IN VARIOUS SIMPLE ACID-BASE ABNORMALITIES

	Initial Finding	Compensatory Finding	Resultant pH
Acidosis (pH <7.35)			
Metabolic	↓ [HCO_3]	↓ P_{CO_2}	↓
Respiratory	↑ P_{CO_2}	↑ [HCO_3]	↓
Alkalosis (pH >7.45)			
Metabolic	↑ [HCO_3]	↑ P_{CO_2}	↑
Respiratory	↓ P_{CO_2}	↓ [HCO_3]	↑

Acidosis is defined as arterial pH of <7.35. Causes include respiratory etiologies such as hypoventilation and metabolic etiologies such as excess acid or decreased bicarbonate in the serum. Rapid compensation to acidosis is respiratory with an increased respiratory rate. More chronic compensation occurs in the kidneys where bicarbonate is synthesized. The renal response takes 12 hours to become apparent and is maximum at 3 to 5 days.

Respiratory Acidosis

Etiology

Respiratory acidosis results from the accumulation of CO_2 in the blood stream due to hypoventilation. Etiologies include the following:
1. CNS depression
   a. Medications (residual anesthesia, narcotics, and benzodiazepines)
   b. Primary brain lesions in the respiratory centers
2. Neuromuscular disorders
   a. Medications (paralytics)
   b. Primary muscular disease
   c. Hypokalemia and hypophosphatemia
   d. Primary neuropathies
3. Respiratory disorders
   a. Acute airway obstruction (sleep apnea or aspiration)
   b. Severe lung parenchymal disease (especially with oxygen delivery, which may inhibit respiratory drive)
   c. Pleural effusion
   d. Pneumothorax
   e. Pulmonary edema
   f. Aspiration
   g. Limitation of inspiration motion (i.e., due to postoperative pain)
4. Cardiac arrest

Major Threat to Life

- Ventricular arrhythmias
- Hypotension

Selective Physical Examination

Signs and symptoms are generally nonspecific. Acidemia is generally associated with hypoxia.

VS:	Decreased RR
MS:	Drowsiness and confusion
HEENT:	Papilledema
Neuro:	Asterixis

Management

1. Assess the severity.

Mild	pH = 7.30 to 7.35
Moderate	pH = 7.20 to 7.29
Severe	pH < 7.20

2. Treat reversible causes.

   Mild acidemia may be observed cautiously. Moderate to severe acidemia requires intervention to avoid respiratory arrest.

3. Notify your resident if acidemia is severe.

   If hypoventilation is present, consider intubation of the patient and transfer to the intensive care unit (ICU)/cardiac care unit (CCU).

4. Monitor serial blood gases to follow therapy.

Special Surgical Considerations

A common cause of respiratory failure in postoperative patients is overmedication with narcotic pain relievers. Look at the pupils, which will be pinpoint, and review the medication delivery logs. Reverse narcosis with **naloxone (Narcan) 0.4 to 2.0 mg IM or IV every 2 to 3 minutes to a maximum dose of 10 mg.**

Metabolic Acidosis

Etiology

Metabolic acidoses are caused by accumulation of acids in the serum. These fall into two categories: normal anion gap (or hyperchloremic) acidosis or increased anion gap (or normochloremic) acidosis.

The anion gap is defined by the following equation:

$$\text{Anion gap} = (Na + K) - (Cl + HCO_3)$$

Normal values range from 10 to 12 mEq/L and reflect the unmeasured anionic role of plasma proteins. Hypoalbuminemia must be corrected for in this equation by adding 4 mEq/L to the calculated anion gap for each decrease in albumin of 1 g/dl. (Assume a normal of 4 g/dl.)

1. Normal anionic gap acidosis
   a. Loss of HCO_3
      (1) Diarrhea, paralytic ileus, and intestinal fistula
      (2) High-output ileostomy
      (3) Renal tubular acidosis
      (4) Carbonic anhydrase inhibitors
   b. Addition of acid

      (1) NH_4Cl
      (2) HCl (as with administration of arginine or lysine as HCl salts in total parenteral nutrition)
      (3) Rapid NaCl administration
      (4) Blood transfusions
2. Increased anionic gap acidosis
   a. Lactic acidosis
   b. Ketoacidosis (diabetes mellitus, starvation, or alcohol)
   c. Renal failure
   d. Medications (aspirin, ethylene glycol, methanol, and paraldehyde)
   e. Rhabdomyolysis

Major Threat to Life

- Ventricular arrhythmias
- Hypotension

Selective Physical Examination

Signs and symptoms are generally nonspecific.

VS:	Increased RR
MS:	Confusion, stupor, and coma
CVS:	Decreased cardiac contractility; peripheral vasodilation leading to hypotension
Neuro:	Fatigue

Management

1. Assess the severity.

Mild	pH = 7.30 to 7.35
Moderate	pH = 7.20 to 7.29
Severe	pH < 7.20

2. Treat reversible causes.
    Mild acidemia may be observed cautiously. Moderate to severe acidemia requires intervention to avoid respiratory arrest.
3. Notify your resident if acidemia is severe.
    If hypoventilation is present, consider intubation of the patient and transfer to the ICU/CCU.
4. Monitor serial blood gases to follow therapy.
5. $NaHCO_3$.
    IV sodium bicarbonate should be reserved for patients who are in acute, severe acidemia. At HCO_3 levels of <10 mEq/L, and pH of <7.1, the buffering capacity of bicarbonate is exhausted and hydrogen ion builds up rapidly in the serum.
    - The amount of bicarbonate to replace may be calculated by the following formula:

$$HCO_3 \text{ to be replaced (in mEq)} = Wt \text{ (in kg)} \times$$
$$(0.4) \text{ } (15 - \text{measured bicarbonate})$$

or

$$HCO_3 \text{ to be replaced (in mEq)} = \frac{(\text{base deficit}) \text{ } (Wt \text{ in kg})(0.4)}{2}$$

The goal of therapy is not to normalize bicarbonate levels, but to bring the pH to >7.2 and the bicarbonate to about 15 mEq/L.

- The rate of replacement depends on the severity of the acidemia.

  In general, a slower approach is preferred to avoid complication of fluid overload (for example, over 8 to 12 hours). In cases of severe, life-threatening acidemia, i.e., pH of <7.0, it may be necessary to administer a **rapid bolus of 150 mEq NaHCO₃ by IV push.**

- Unless given in a code situation, always dilute bicarbonate in a large volume of fluid (such as 50–150 mEq/L of 5% dextrose in water); rapid infusion can cause cardiac dysrhythmias.

- Renal tubular acidosis responds well to oral administration of bicarbonate; consult a nephrologist for appropriate care of these disorders.

- Complications of bicarbonate administration include
    a. Fluid overload
    b. Hypernatremia
    c. Shift of potassium ion to intracellular, causing hypokalemia
    d. Drop in ionized calcium, leading to tetany
    e. Cardiac dysrhythmias with rapid infusion

■ ALKALOSIS

Alkalosis is defined as arterial pH of >7.45. Causes include respiratory etiologies such as hyperventilation and metabolic etiologies such as loss of acid or increased bicarbonate in the serum. Rapid compensation to alkalosis is respiratory with a decreased RR. This compensatory response is limited by the hypoxic drive to ventilation. More chronic compensation occurs in the kidneys where bicarbonate is actively excreted. This causes a measurable drop in serum bicarbonate. The drop in bicarbonate is greater in metabolic alkalosis (0.6 mEq/L) when compared with respiratory alkalosis (0.2–0.4 mEq/L). The renal response takes 12 hours to become apparent and is maximum at 3 to 5 days.

Respiratory Alkalosis

Etiology

Respiratory alkalosis results from decreased CO_2 in the blood stream due to hyperventilation. Etiologies include the following:
1. Physiologic oxygen need (pregnancy or high altitude)
2. Hypoxia
3. CNS states or disorders (anxiety, pain, fever, tumor, trauma, and infection)
4. Medications (aspirin, nicotine, and progesterone)
5. Respiratory disorders
   a. CHF
   b. Pulmonary embolism
   c. Asthma
6. Hepatic failure
7. Hyperthyroidism
8. Sepsis or other hypermetabolic states

Major Threat to Life

Major threat to life depends on the underlying cause.

Selective Physical Examination

Signs and symptoms are generally nonspecific.

MS: Confusion and lightheadedness
Neuro: Numbness, tingling, and perioral or acral paresthesias; tetany, in severe cases

Management

1. Assess the severity.

   Mild   pH = 7.45 to 7.55
   Moderate   pH = 7.56 to 7.69
   Severe   pH > 7.70

2. Treat reversible causes.
   Mild alkalemia may be observed cautiously. Moderate to severe alkalemia may require intervention. Symptomatic treatment, such as antipyretics for fever, may be all that is required. Moderate alkalemia with symptoms of tetany may be treated with a rebreathing bag, which will recirculate exhaled CO_2. Take care in correcting chronic alkalemia in this fashion, as increasing CO_2 may precipitate an acidemia.
3. Notify your resident if alkalemia is severe.
4. Monitor serial blood gases to follow therapy.

Metabolic Alkalosis

Etiology

Metabolic alkalosis results from a loss of acid from the serum or an accumulation of base. The etiologies may be divided into chloride-responsive alkalemia and chloride-resistant alkalemia.

1. Chloride responsive ($U_{Cl} < 20$)
   a. GI losses (NG suction and emesis)
   b. Chloride deficiency (diuretics and villous adenoma of the colon)
   c. Posthypercapnea
   d. Contraction alkalosis due to fluid depletion or diuretic use
   e. Excessive $NaHCO_3$ administration, or administration of agents that are metabolized to bicarbonate, such as citrate (in blood products), lactate, or acetate
   f. Medications (penicillin, carbenicillin, and ticarcillin)
2. Chloride resistant ($U_{Cl} > 20$)
   a. Severe K^+ deficiency ($K^+ < 2$ mEq/L)
   b. Magnesium deficiency
   c. Mineralocorticoid excess
      (1) Primary aldosteronism
      (2) Cushing's syndrome
      (3) Exogenous steroid replacement
      (4) Licorice ingestion
      (5) Renal artery stenosis
   d. Bartter's syndrome
   e. Poststarvation feeding

Major Threat to Life

Major threat to life depends on the underlying cause.

Selective Physical Examination

Signs and symptoms are generally nonspecific.

MS: Apathy, confusion, and stupor

Management

1. Assess the severity.

Mild	pH = 7.45 to 7.55
Moderate	pH = 7.56 to 7.69
Severe	pH > 7.70

2. Treat reversible causes.
   Mild alkalemia may be observed cautiously. Moderate to severe alkalemia may require intervention.
3. Notify your resident if alkalemia is severe.
4. Monitor serial blood gases to follow therapy.
5. Administer fluids.
   Chloride-responsive alkaloses generally are associated with fluid deficit and respond well to replacement using NS with supplemental KCl.
   Chloride-resistant alkaloses are associated with a concurrent deficiency in K^+ and therefore do not respond to NaCl replacement. Usually the underlying cause must be corrected.

6. Provide histamine H_2 blockade.

   If gastric losses are the cause of alkalosis, diminishing the production of acid in the stomach may decrease the net loss of chloride.

7. Administer acid therapy.

   This is reserved for cases of severe alkalemia. Notify your resident before administration of any of these agents.

   ■ **Arginine HCl (50 mEq HCl/100 ml)**

   Use this therapy with caution as arginine can move to the intracellular space. This displaces intracellular potassium, and life-threatening hyperkalemia can result.

   ■ NH_4Cl

   Ammonium chloride must be converted to H^+ and NH_3 in the liver and is therefore contraindicated in patients with liver disease.

   ■ **0.1 M HCl**

   This is the safest of current options. Still, it is best administered through central venous access over 8 to 12 hours.

8. **Acetazolamide (Diamox) 250 to 500 mg PO or IV every 8 hours** may be useful to decrease excess fluid in cases of fluid overload.

   This diuretic also enhances renal excretion of bicarbonate.

■ MIXED ACID–BASE DISORDERS

Many disorders of acid–base status are combinations of simple situations. These may be identified by noting that the magnitude of biochemical derangement is greater than expected from a simple abnormality alone (a simple acid–base disorder will never overcompensate). A breakdown in the normal relationship between P_{CO_2}, pH, and HCO_3 (as in the Henderson-Hasselbalch equation) suggests a mixed disorder. See Figure 12–8 for a graphic depiction of various pH value and P_{CO_2} relationships in various simple acid–base disorders. Frequently encountered examples include the following:

Chronic Respiratory Acidosis Plus Metabolic Alkalosis

This is encountered in patients with chronic obstructive pulmonary disease (COPD) who are concurrently treated with gastric suction, diuretics, or a low-salt diet. The blood pH may be normal, but the P_{CO_2} and HCO_3 will be abnormal or changed from the patient's baseline. The goal of therapy is to normalize the pH and not the P_{CO_2}.

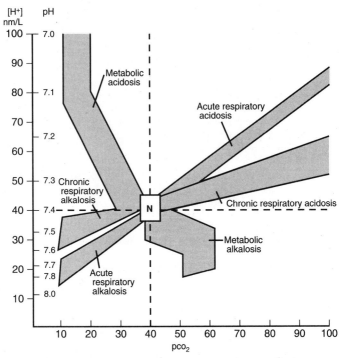

Figure 12–8 □ Acid–base map determination of usual compensatory responses to primary acid–base disturbances.

Acute Respiratory Acidosis Superimposed on Chronic Respiratory Acidosis

In severe COPD patients who retain CO_2, a pulmonary decompensation such as pneumonia, sedative medication, or oxygen administration may lead to this finding.

Acute Respiratory Acidosis Superimposed on Metabolic Acidosis

This is often seen after cardiac arrest, where there is accumulation of lactic acid from hypoperfusion and accumulation of CO_2 due to hypoventilation. The acidemias may be additive and may be very dangerous.

Respiratory Alkalosis plus Metabolic Alkalosis

This finding is characteristic of early sepsis and aspirin intoxication.

13

GASTROINTESTINAL BLEEDING

Gastrointestinal (GI) bleeding is a stressful on-call problem to manage. It is common in hospitalized patients, and it includes a broad spectrum of disorders. GI bleeding can represent a minor problem or a life-threatening emergency. Initial management involves resuscitation and stabilization. History taking, evaluation, and definitive treatment should follow in rapid sequence.

■ PHONE CALL

Questions

1. **Where is the blood coming from, and what does it look like?**

    It is important to have the RN describe to you what the bleeding looks like. This will help you better delineate what type of GI bleeding the patient may have. **Melena** (passage of black or tarry stools) indicates blood entering the GI tract at any point from the mouth to the cecum. The dark color is the result of oxidation of heme by bacterial and digestive enzymes. **Hematochezia** is the passage of bright-red blood from the rectum. It usually indicates bleeding from the colon, the rectum, or the anus. **Hematemesis** of bright-red or dark blood indicates a bleeding source proximal to the ligament of Treitz.

2. **How much blood has been lost?**

    Ask the RN to estimate the amount of blood lost. This will give you an idea as to whether the GI bleeding represents a life-threatening problem. Remember that rapid GI bleeding is an emergency.

3. **What are the vital signs?**

    Rapid GI hemorrhaging may be associated with hypotension and tachycardia.

4. **Did the patient have surgery, and if so, what was the operation and when did it occur?**

    The stress of surgery may precipitate acute GI bleeding. Stress gastritis in the perioperative period may occur in patients undergoing major surgery. In addition, patients undergoing surgery on the GI tract may develop GI bleeding if a suture line has broken down or if a major blood vessel has ruptured.

5. What are the major medical problems?

Some conditions such as liver disease, esophageal varices, and gastric or duodenal ulcer predispose patients to either more frequent or more serious GI bleeding.

6. Is the patient taking ulcerogenic medications, anticoagulants, or thrombolytic agents?

Patients taking nonsteroidal anti-inflammatory drugs (NSAIDs) or steroids are more likely to develop gastric ulcers and GI bleeds. Patients taking anticoagulants such as warfarin (Coumadin), aspirin, and heparin may develop severe GI bleeding refractory to conventional treatment. Often, anticoagulant medications must be discontinued or reversed if severe bleeding occurs. Thrombolytic agents such as streptokinase or urokinase may require discontinuation in an actively bleeding patient.

Orders

For any significant GI bleed:

1. Ask the RN to stay at the bedside with the patient and to get help from additional nursing staff.
2. Order immediate placement of two large-bore intravenous (IV) lines with 14- to 16-gauge catheters in large peripheral veins. Antecubital veins are preferred if available. Large peripheral lines are preferred to central lines.
3. Ask the RN to draw an immediate hematocrit and prothrombin time (PT), partial thromboplastin time (PTT), and platelet counts, at the time of IV placement if possible. If not already done, have the RN also draw an immediate type and cross-match. Always have 6 units of packed red blood cells (PRBCs) available in a major GI bleed (stay ahead by 6 units).
4. Once the hematocrit is drawn, start rapid infusion of isotonic saline, lactated Ringer's solution (LR), or Hespan. The rate of volume infusion should correlate with the patient's condition and the volume of blood lost.
5. If a massive upper GI bleeder is suspected, order an Ewald nasogastric (NG) tube (32–36 Fr) or a Minnesota tube (if esophageal variceal bleeding) to the bedside.
6. Ask the RN to have the patient's chart at the bedside.

Inform RN

"Will arrive at the bedside in . . . minutes."

Significant upper or lower GI bleeding or bleeding associated with changes in vital signs (hypotension or tachycardia) requires immediate evaluation of the patient.

■ ELEVATOR THOUGHTS

What causes GI bleeding?

- Upper GI bleed
    1. Peptic ulcer
        Duodenal ulcer
        Gastric ulcer
    2. Esophageal varices
    3. Esophagitis
    4. Gastritis
    5. Duodenitis
    6. Mallory-Weiss tear
    7. Upper GI neoplasm
- Lower GI bleed
    1. Hemorrhoids
    2. Rectal fissures
    3. Polyps
    4. Lower GI neoplasms
    5. Ulcerative or infectious colitis
    6. Ischemic colitis
    7. Dead bowel
    8. Diverticulosis
    9. Meckel's diverticulum
    10. Angiodysplasia

■ MAJOR THREAT TO LIFE

- Hypovolemic shock/exsanguination

    Patients with rapid GI hemorrhaging will quickly deplete their intravascular volume and become hypotensive. Sympathetic activation (tachycardia and vasoconstriction) occurs in an attempt to maintain blood pressure (BP). Continued GI bleeding rapidly overcomes the body's attempts to maintain BP, and hypovolemic shock ensues. Shock can be prevented by aggressive fluid resuscitation using adequate IV access. The rate of fluid resuscitation should be dictated by the amount and the rapidity of blood loss. Crystalloid (normal saline [NS] or LR) should be used until blood products are available. If ongoing massive GI hemorrhaging occurs and there is a significant delay in obtaining crossmatched blood, consider replacement of crystalloid infusion for O-negative blood. The best way to prevent shock in GI bleeding patients is to restore intravascular volume.

■ BEDSIDE

Quick Look Test

Does the patient look well (comfortable), sick (uncomfortable or distressed), or critical (about to die)?

Patients with minor GI bleeding look comfortable and well perfused. Patients with significant GI bleeding are often pale, uncomfortable, tachycardic, tremulous, and apprehensive.

Airway and Vital Signs

Airway

It is imperative that the airway be protected in patients with upper GI bleeding. It is common for a debilitated patient to aspirate during ongoing upper GI bleeding. Consider endotracheal intubation in the presence of shock, diminished mental status, hepatic encephalopathy, massive hematemesis, or active variceal hemorrhage.

Vital Signs

Assess the BP and the heart rate (HR) carefully. Hypotension and tachycardia while the patient is in the supine position signal severe hypovolemia. In patients with GI bleeding and less pronounced vital sign changes, check orthostatics. Start by measuring the HR and BP with the patient in the supine position, and then compare those measurements with the HR and the BP while the patient sits with legs dangling off the side of the bed. If there are no significant changes with this positional change, measure the BP and the HR with the patient standing. A fall in systolic blood pressure (SBP) by >15 mm Hg or an increase in HR of >15 beats/min indicates orthostatic change and significant hypovolemia.

Selective Physical Examination I

The initial evaluation is for assessing the patient for evidence of hypovolemia or shock.

VS: Repeat now; pay particular attention to BP and HR
CVS: Assess perfusion; note skin color and temperature
Neuro: Note level of consciousness and mental status

Patients who demonstrate inadequate tissue perfusion in the presence of GI bleeding may be in shock. These patients generally have an SBP of <90 mm Hg and a urine output (UO) of <20 ml/hr or 250 ml/8-hour-shift. As BP falls in the presence of significant GI bleeding, cerebral perfusion decreases. Patients with hypovolemia from GI bleeding may become lethargic, somnolent, delirious, or unconscious.

Initial Management

1. Fluid resuscitation with crystalloid
2. Placement of Foley catheter

3. Close monitoring of vital signs
4. Transfusion of PRBCs, fresh frozen plasma (FFP), and platelets as necessary
5. Monitor O_2 saturation with pulse oximetry.

The first step in management is to replenish intravascular volume. For a patient with significant GI bleeding associated with hypovolemia and hypotension, give a **500- to 1000-L bolus of NS or LR** through large-bore peripheral IVs. Watch the effect that the fluid challenge has on the BP. For massive bleeds, consider repeating the bolus two or three times to maintain normotensive BPs. Patients with congestive heart failure or pulmonary disease may develop cardiopulmonary complications of rapid fluid resuscitation. Such complications may worsen heart failure and cause pulmonary edema.

Fluid status is best managed with a Foley catheter. UO is a sensitive measure of end-organ perfusion.

While crystalloid boluses are being given, check on the availability of PRBCs. If at least 6 units of PBRCs are not available, send for a type and crossmatch immediately. You must always stay ahead of the bleed by at least 6 units of PRBCs.

It may also be useful to see if the hematocrit sent earlier is available. Remember that hematocrit results in the presence of acute GI bleeding may be a relatively unreliable indicator of the extent of blood loss. This is because it takes time for the acute changes in intravascular space to equilibrate with fluid from the extravascular space. Remember this when evaluating hematocrit results obtained during periods of acute bleeding.

Crystalloid is useful and expands the intravascular compartment, but it does not raise the oxygen-carrying capacity of blood. With continued crystalloid administration, blood cells become hemodiluted. Patients who have significant blood loss should be resuscitated initially with crystalloid and, when available, transfused with appropriate volumes of blood. Maintain a hematocrit of at least 30 in elderly patients or in patients with heart disease. Young, otherwise healthy patients can easily tolerate hematocrit values of <20 to 25 without transfusion, unless there is risk of rebleeding. Use good judgment in determining what hematocrit is satisfactory. Your goal is to transfuse to avoid shock, to provide adequate perfusion of tissues, and to keep the patient from becoming symptomatic (orthostatic). If there is a significant likelihood of rebleeding, it is a good idea to resuscitate the patient adequately, such that he or she has a reserve if acute rebleeding occurs.

Remember to record BP, pulse, central venous pressure (if central line), hematocrit, and UO hourly. You must document the need for blood transfusions in the medical record.

Check the results of coagulation studies. If a patient with significant GI bleeding has significant coagulopathy from elevated

PT or PTT, consider transfusion with FFP. Two units of FFP are usually required for any significant clinical effect on bleeding. For many patients, 2 to 4 units of FFP are required to correct coagulopathy to the extent that clotting is significantly enhanced.

Low platelet count or platelet dysfunction may cause or worsen GI bleeding. Patients with thrombocytopenia may develop spontaneous upper GI bleeding. GI bleeding associated with platelet counts of $<40,000/mm^3$ requires platelet transfusion. A patient with a normal platelet count may develop severe GI bleeding, or existing bleeding may be exacerbated if significant platelet dysfunction is present. Uremia, Willebrand's disease, recent ingestion of NSAIDs, and other conditions may prolong bleeding time and result in bleeding that is difficult to control without platelet transfusion. Consider platelet transfusion if bleeding is uncontrollable and the patient has a significant risk for platelet dysfunction. If time allows, an IVY bleeding time test will provide evidence of bleeding dysfunction. A bleeding time of >7 minutes indicates abnormal platelet function.

Selective History and Chart Review

Once the patient is stabilized, review the history and medications as indicated in the medical record. If the patient is able to converse, ask about previous bleeds, medications, and known diagnoses that may cause GI bleeding. These data will help you diagnose the likely cause of bleeding and help with management.

Has the patient had an episode of GI bleeding during this admission or at any time recently?

Is there a known condition that predisposes the patient to GI bleeding?

Is the patient taking any medications that predispose to bleeding?

The following several common medications are known to interfere with normal coagulation function: heparin, warfarin (Coumadin), and NSAIDs.

Selective Physical Examination II

This examination focuses on identifying whether the bleeding is from the upper or the lower GI tract. If possible, the site of bleeding is identified.

VS:	Repeat now.
HEENT:	Look for nosebleed.
Abd:	When melena or coffee-ground emesis is present, pass NG tube into stomach. Perform gastric aspiration.

Evaluate for epigastric tenderness (bleeding gastric or duodenal ulcer).

Look for left lower quadrant tenderness (diverticulitis, ischemic bowel, angiodysplasia, or bleeding colon cancer.)

Rectal: Note hematochezia, melena, and hemorrhoids.

■ DEFINITIVE MANAGEMENT

The goal of the second stage of management is to maintain adequate fluid resuscitation and oxygen-carrying capacity (hemoglobin), to slow or stop the bleeding if possible, and to identify the lesion responsible for the bleeding.

It is important to understand the differences in management between upper and lower GI bleeding.

Upper GI Bleeding

1. Peptic ulcer, acute gastritis, esophageal varices, and Mallory-Weiss tear account for >90% of upper GI bleeds.

   These sources are proximal to the ligament of Treitz. They generally present with hematemesis, coffee-ground emesis, or melena.

2. Insert a large-bore NG tube (>16 Fr).

   Perform gastric aspiration to determine if bleeding is from the stomach. An Ewald tube may be needed if large amounts of clot are present. Most gastric bleeds and >75% of bleeding duodenal ulcers will give positive gastric aspirates for blood.

3. Lavage the stomach free of blood and clots.

   Irrigate the stomach with a large syringe and several liters of iced saline. Continue lavage until blood no longer returns. Iced saline is very effective at slowing or stopping small to moderate GI bleeds.

4. If bleeding continues or if the patient becomes hemodynamically unstable despite fluid and blood replacement, urgent esophagogastroduodenoscopy (EGD) is indicated.

   Contact the GI fellow or the attending gastroenterologist to perform the EGD. Sclerosis of varices, electrocoagulation, or epinephrine injections can be performed through the scope to stop bleeding. Stabilized patients who stop bleeding may benefit from elective EGD 24 hours after the bleeding episode.

5. Management for particular lesions
   - Esophageal varices

     For esophageal varices, **IV vasopressin infusion (100 U in 250 ml 5% dextrose in water)** may help slow bleeding. Start infusion at 0.4 U/min (60 ml/hr). If life-threatening bleeding occurs from known esophageal varices, insertion of a Sengstaken-Blakemore tube or a Minnesota tube may be helpful (Fig. 13–1). Although these tubes may balloon tamponade bleeding varices, they also carry the risk of causing airway obstruction, aspiration, and esophageal rupture.

- Mallory-Weiss tears

  Mallory-Weiss tears are often self-limited and respond to conservative therapy. However, if life-threatening bleeding occurs, angiographic embolization may be indicated.

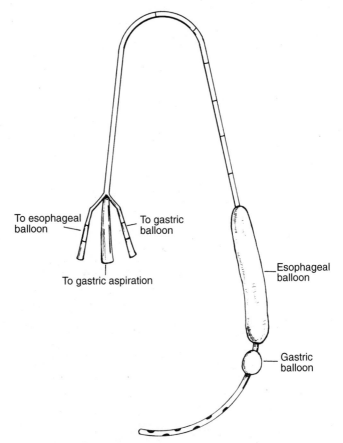

Figure 13–1 □ The Sengstaken-Blakemore tube. The Minnesota tube is similar; it has an additional port for esophageal aspiration. (From Marshall SA, Ruedy J: On Call: Principles and Protocols, 2nd ed. Philadelphia, WB Saunders Co, 1993, p 102.)

- Ulcers

    Ulcers may be treated with antacids via NG tube every 1 to 2 hours. Ulcer rebleeding may be minimized with cimetidine (300 mg IV every 6 hours) or ranitidine (50 mg IV every 8 hours). Stress gastritis often responds to antacids.

6. Consider surgery for any patient with >6 units of blood loss in a day or any patient with uncontrollable bleeding.

    Other lesions frequently requiring surgery include ulcers with visible large vessels at the ulcer base and ulcers that rebleed significantly during the same hospital stay. Obtain surgical consultation early. It is helpful to have the surgical team following the patient.

Lower GI Bleeding

1. Lower GI bleeds are associated with dark to bright-red blood from the rectum.

    The color of the blood is associated with the length of time in the GI tract. These bleeds occur distal to the ligament of Treitz. Bright-red blood from the rectum may be associated with a proximal lesion, such as a duodenal bleed, if the transit time through the gut is short.

2. Perform digital rectal examination, anoscopy, or sigmoidoscopy.

    A general surgery consultation may be appropriate. Treat any bleeding lesion noted on examination (e.g., bleeding hemorrhoid).

3. Insert an NG tube and check aspirate.

    Gross blood, coffee-ground blood, and occult blood should be noted. Blood in the stomach indicates an upper GI bleed. EGD should be performed.

4. If EGD is negative and sigmoidoscopy and anoscopy show that bleeding is coming from above the sigmoid colon, consider the following steps:

    - Perform radionuclide scanning; if the radionuclide scan is positive for bleeding, consider colonoscopy or angiography; if the radionuclide scan is negative, consider colonoscopy.
    - Proceed immediately with colonoscopy if EGD is negative and sigmoidoscopy suggests colonic bleeding.
    - Colonoscopy by an expert endoscopist may allow electrocoagulation or other treatment of the bleeding lesion.

5. Surgical consultation should be obtained if bleeding persists despite all conservative measures.

14

GLUCOSE MANAGEMENT AND SURGICAL NUTRITION

This chapter covers briefly the nutritional needs of surgical patients. They differ from other patients in the hospital in that in addition to basal metabolic demands and the increased nutritional requirements of disease and immune defense, surgical patients also have demands that result from the surgical procedure and wound healing. In many cases the normal enteral route of feeding is not available.

■ BASIC METABOLIC REQUIREMENTS

The average (70-kg) resting patient has a basal requirement of 1800 to 2000 kcal/day. Those calories must include approximately 180 g of glucose to supply the needs of obligate glucose-requiring tissues such as brain, red blood cells (RBCs), white blood cells (WBCs), and renal medulla. The fasting patient will generally have sufficient stores in muscle and adipose tissues to maintain protein and glucose needs for a short time perioperatively. Unless the patient is severely malnourished or is expected to be fasting for a long period of time, only glucose and crystalloid fluids are replaced routinely. This is generally accomplished with sufficient maintenance fluid volumes of 5% dextrose in water.

Various disease states will increase caloric requirements well above the basal state. These are summarized in Table 14–1. In addition, the patient's activity level will affect the caloric requirements. A patient undergoing physical therapy will use more energy than one restricted to bed rest.

Patients known to be at risk for requiring supplemental enteral or parenteral nutrition are those patients undergoing major bowel resection, severely ill patients, and patients identified as malnour-

Table 14–1 □ METABOLIC RATES OF VARIOUS DISEASE STATES

Basal metabolic rate	100%
Elective surgery	124%
Skeletal trauma	132%
40% burn	134%
Head trauma (with steroid use)	161%
Sepsis	179%

Table 14–2 □ **HORMONES AFFECTING METABOLISM**

Anabolic	Catabolic
Insulin	Cortisol
Growth hormone (early)	Epinephrine
	Glucagon
	Growth hormone (late)
	Vasopressin
	Somatostatin

ished preoperatively (15% documented weight loss or albumin level of <3.0 mg/dl).

■ CHANGES IN METABOLIC NEEDS RELATED TO SURGERY

Patients after serious injury or a major surgical procedure are in a "stress state" of metabolism. This state differs from simple starvation. The metabolic needs increase well above the basal requirements, and there are changes in the origin and consumption of proteins, lipids, and carbohydrates. A variety of neuroendocrine influences affect substrate availability and utilization. These are summarized briefly in Tables 14–2 and 14–3. The sum total of responses depends on the severity of the injury or illness and the general health and nutrition of the patient. Wound healing occurs as a "priority" even in severely injured or ill individuals, but additional stress (which may include malnutrition or concomitant injury elsewhere) will delay or abrogate normal wound healing. If you have a question regarding the nutritional status of a patient, a nutritional consultation may be obtained, but this is generally not an on-call issue.

Other high-metabolic stress states to be mindful of include major burns, sepsis (and other sources of fever), polytrauma, and frequent seizure activity.

Table 14–3 □ **FACTORS INFLUENCING NEUROENDOCRINE EFFECTS ON METABOLISM**

Changes in circulating blood volume
Changes in substrate availability
Changes in tissue levels of oxygen, hydrogen ion, and carbon dioxide
Changes in body temperature
Pain
Infection
Emotional state

Protein

After major stress, patients are in an obligate protein catabolic state in which nitrogen excretion increases from a basal level of 5 to 7 g/day to a level of 8 to 11 g/day. Negative nitrogen balance occurs despite adequate delivery of glucose and amino acids. Protein wasting lasts until the wounds are closed, adequate circulating volume has been established, pain is well controlled, and infection is eliminated. This may take several days to several weeks. Some energy needs during stress are met through gluconeogenesis with a net catabolism of 300 to 500 g of lean body mass/day. But most energy in a stress situation is derived from fat, and replacement of amino acids is needed to minimize the negative nitrogen balance. In general, 10 to 15% of the daily calories should be delivered as protein (optimally, 1.5–2.5 g/kg/day). The most efficient use of protein occurs when a ratio of 150 to 250 nonprotein calories (carbohydrates and fats) for each protein calorie is given. This may increase to a ratio of 400–500 to 1 in settings of severe illness or hepatic or renal decompensation.

Nitrogen balance is defined by the following formula:

$$N_2 \text{ balance} = \frac{24\text{-hour protein intake}}{6.25} - [(24\text{-hour UUN}) + (4)]$$

where 24-hour UUN is urinary urea nitrogen excretion (in g/day), 4 is obligatory loss (in g/day), and 6.25 is the number of grams of protein that yield 1 g N_2. The goal of therapy is +4 g/day balance.

Lipid

Recovery from injury is fueled mostly by fats. There is net increased lipolysis despite increased insulin concentrations. In the liver there is increased free fatty acid synthesis. The fatty acids are used primarily for oxidation. Ketogenesis is increased in minor injury or stress, but it is nearly absent in major injury or stress. The high fat content of the average American diet makes it unnecessary to supplement fats routinely, but for prolonged nutritional replacement, fats are the most concentrated source of calories. Replacement of lipids is indicated to supply calories and to avoid depletion of essential fatty acids.

Carbohydrate

The hallmark of injury or stress is hyperglycemia. This sets stress apart from fasting or starvation. Blood sugar rises in response to catabolic neuroendocrine hormones. Initially, the hyperglycemia is due to decreased circulating insulin secondary to beta-cell insensitivity to insulin. Soon, insulin levels become normal or elevated, and persistent hyperglycemia is probably due in part to peripheral resistance to insulin. Despite the insulin resistance, the increased glucose in the blood stream allows greater uptake of glucose into the tissues during stress. Healing wounds must be thought of as obligate glucose-requiring tissues like brain and RBCs. This requirement may be due to the large number of infiltrating WBCs in the wound.

■ MEANS OF DELIVERING CALORIES

Simple replacement of maintenance fluids, salt, and glucose is the most frequent and the most simple of approaches. When it is determined that a patient does need supplemental calories, there are a variety of avenues available for use, depending on the needs and constraints of the particular patient.

Enteral

If the patient has adequate bowel function, the enteral route is the best route to use. It allows physiologic use of the bowel, decreases bacterial translocation across the bowel wall, which may be a significant source of sepsis, and allows normal glucose use. The delivery of enteral feeds depends on the patient.

Oral. The oral route is available to awake, alert patients whose gastrointestinal (GI) continuity is intact. Patients who have had esophageal or gastric procedures, or those with fresh anastomoses in the proximal GI tract, may not be the best candidates for the oral approach.

Feeding Tubes. Feeding tubes are useful for patients who are not able to take food by mouth or for those in whom an anastomosis must be protected. Feeding tubes may be temporarily placed through the oral or the nasal passageway or may be surgically or endoscopically placed. Either the stomach (gastrostomy) or the proximal small intestine (jejunostomy) may be used. If the jejunum is used, bolus feedings are not possible.

Parenteral

In patients in whom the bowel is not functioning properly or in whom the absorptive surface is insufficient to maintain adequate nutrition, enteral feeds may be supplemented with or replaced by parenteral delivery of nutrition. This may be delivered as complete nutritional replacement, in which case it is termed total parenteral nutrition (TPN). TPN uses a hypertonic solution delivered through a central venous catheter that consists of adequate glucose, protein, and lipid replacement to facilitate wound healing and anabolism (Table 14–4). Another approach does not require central venous access and is termed peripheral parenteral nutrition (PPN). The fluids used in PPN are of a low enough osmolarity to allow delivery through peripheral veins, but they will not deliver adequate calories when used alone. They must be coupled with enteral feeds or with body stores of nutrients. Each hospital has specific guidelines as to safe and effective delivery of parenteral nutrition. The concentrations of glucose and lipid must be increased slowly to avoid complications of hyperglycemia and hyperlipidemia; the electrolytes and the blood glucose concentrations must be followed closely; and the central access must be well protected from infection, as the nutrients delivered make this site more vulnerable to bacterial and yeast infection. There are often printed TPN delivery orders that may be followed. Consult with your resident, the pharmacy, or the specific dietary department before starting or stopping TPN.

When adequate calories are delivered with TPN, the concentration of glucose is high, and the pancreas becomes acclimated to the rate of glucose delivery. The maximum rate can reach 5 to 8 mg/kg/min. This puts a patient at risk for hypoglycemia if the TPN infusion is discontinued abruptly. If a central line becomes unusable, a peripheral line may be used for concentrations as high as 10% dextrose in water for a short period of time. Periodic glucose checks must be made to ensure adequate blood sugar levels. When TPN is no longer needed, the infusion is released slowly over 1 to 2 days, and care is taken to make sure that adequate blood sugar levels are maintained.

Vitamins and trace elements should be provided as directed by the TPN guidelines in your institution. In general, an ampule of multivitamins should be added to the formulation per day. Additional **vitamin K (10–20 mg)** should be administered to the patient, **intramuscularly (IM) or subcutaneously (SC) once per week**. Additional vitamin and mineral supplementation is outlined below and in Table 14–5.

Electrolyte administration will vary with each patient; reasonable guidelines are listed in Table 14–6. The patient must be followed closely with daily electrolyte, phosphorus, and glucose levels until the administration of TPN has stabilized (usually 1–2

Table 14–4 □ CALORIC CONTENT OF TPN CONSTITUENTS

Dextrose (10% solution)	0.34 kcal/ml
Lipid (10% solution)	1.1 kcal/ml
Amino acids	3.33 kcal/g

6.25 g amino acids = 1 g nitrogen.
TPN = total parenteral nutrition.

Table 14–5 □ VITAMIN AND MINERAL SUPPLEMENTATION TO SUPPORT WOUND HEALING IN PATIENTS WITH CHRONIC STEROID USE

Vitamin A	50,000 IU PO/IV every day
Vitamin C	1000 mg PO every day
Zinc sulfate	220 mg (50 mg elemental Zn) PO every day or 10 mg IV every day

PO = by mouth; IV = intravenously.

weeks) and then 3 times per week thereafter. Weekly liver function tests and triglyceride levels should be monitored.

Complications of TPN delivery are common and can be severe. They are divided into physical, metabolic, and infectious complications. The physical complications are related to placement and maintenance of the central line. The metabolic complications are influenced by the formulation of the TPN solution, the rate of delivery, and the underlying biochemistry of the patient. The infectious risks are nearly inevitable with long-term administration but can be minimized by close adherence to sterile technique during placement and by following the TPN line protocols of your institution. A summary of complications is listed in Table 14–7.

■ SPECIAL SURGICAL CONSIDERATIONS

Normal Return of Bowel Function After Abdominal Procedures

The loss of function of the intestines after surgery is a physiologic protective measure termed paralytic ileus. Paralytic ileus is poorly understood and most likely multifactorial. Influences include anticholinergic medications, pain medications, and irritation of the peritoneum. It is prolonged with major surgery, infection, or electrolyte or acid–base abnormalities. Consider starting

Table 14–6 □ GUIDELINES FOR DAILY ELECTROLYTE REPLACEMENTS IN TPN

Sodium	75–100 mEq/day
Potassium	75–100 mEq/day
Calcium	10–20 mEq/day
Magnesium	10–20 mEq/day
Phosphate	5–40 mEq/day

TPN = total parenteral nutrition.

Table 14–7 □ POTENTIAL COMPLICATIONS OF TPN ADMINISTRATION

Physical	Metabolic	Infectious
Pneumothorax	Hyperglycemia	Insertion site infection
Hemothorax	Hypoglycemia	Phlebitis
Hemomediastinum	Electrolyte	Systemic infection
Arterial injury	derangement	Bacterial
Venous injury	Vitamin deficiency	Yeast
Thoracic duct injury	Mineral deficiency	Line sepsis
Brachial plexus injury	Essential fatty acid	
Venous thrombosis	deficiency	
Superior vena cava	Hyperlipidemia	
syndrome	Metabolic acidosis	
Air embolism	Respiratory failure	
Pulmonary embolism	Hepatic disorders	
Catheter embolism	Anemia	
Catheter malposition	Bone demineralization	
Horner's syndrome		

TPN = total parenteral nutrition.

TPN by the second postoperative day if there is a <50% chance of normal bowel function by the fifth postoperative day.

The uncomplicated return of bowel function occurs in stages as summarized in Table 14–8. It is not a synchronous event. First to return is the small bowel function, which generally occurs in 5 to 8 hours; often the small bowel is seen to undergo peristalsis during return of the bowels to the abdomen following a surgical procedure. Bowel tones are present with small bowel function. Next to return is gastric motility, which occurs in 24 hours. A decrease in nasogastric tube output, mild abdominal bloating, or a subjective increase in patient belching may be noted. The last to return is colonic motility. This normalizes in 24 to 60 hours and is preceded by the passage of flatus. It is safe to wait for the passage of gas before the introduction of oral food. The introduction of oral food may be further delayed by the creation of a new

Table 14–8 □ TIMING OF UNCOMPLICATED RETURN OF BOWEL FUNCTION

Structure	Timing	Hallmark
Small intestine	5–8 hr	Bowel tones
Stomach	24 hr	Decreased nasogastric tube output, abdominal bloating
Large intestine	24–60 hr	Passage of flatus

anastomosis or a major loss of absorptive surface, as with extensive bowel resections.

The Diabetic Patient

Patients with diabetes have a higher risk of coronary disease, renal insufficiency, and peripheral vascular disease. These patients also require surgical therapy more frequently than nondiabetics. Poor diabetic control will predispose a patient to a higher risk of bacterial and fungal infections and poor wound healing.

The stress of surgery will exacerbate insulin insensitivity of non–insulin-dependent (type II) diabetes and may increase the insulin requirement of insulin-dependent (type I) diabetes. Remember that hyperglycemia is a normal physiologic response to surgical stress and that the goal of postoperative glucose control is not normal glucose levels but the avoidance of extreme hyperglycemia. In general, maintenance of serum glucose levels of <250 mg/dl is sufficient. It is important to remember that the real risk of diabetic treatment is hypoglycemia resulting from overzealous treatment.

Peripheral insulin resistance will wane as a patient improves. It is useful to treat changes in the diabetic patient's response to insulin with an insulin "sliding scale" or "rainbow" approach. This is a range of insulin doses given in response to the patient's glucose levels. An example of a sliding scale order is given in Table 14–9. It must be emphasized that the sliding scale not only must be initially individualized to the patient's routine insulin needs, but must be frequently monitored and amended to maintain normal to slightly increased glucose levels. When the patient is taking food by mouth well, the preoperative insulin regimen can be reinstated and the sliding scale continued as necessary. Diabetic patients will require insulin despite decreased or suspended oral food intake.

Table 14–9 □ EXAMPLE OF INSULIN SLIDING SCALE ORDER

1. Glucose finger stick every 6 hr and as needed.
2. For glucose

<80 mg/dl	Call house officer, have 1 ampule of 50% dextrose at bedside. If the patient is able to take PO, give 5–10 oz of orange juice. Recheck blood glucose in 30 min.
80–250 mg/dl	No treatment.
251–300 mg/dl	4 U regular insulin SC.
301–350 mg/dl	6 U regular insulin SC.
351–400 mg/dl	8 U regular insulin SC.
>400 mg/dl	10 U regular insulin SC and call house officer.

Table 14–10 □ ONSET AND DURATION OF ACTION OF VARIOUS INSULIN PREPARATIONS DELIVERED SC

Preparation	Onset (hr)	Peak Action (hr)	Duration (hr)
Regular	0.5–1	2–5	5–8
Lente insulin*	1–2.5	7–15	24
NPH†	1–2	6–12	18–24
Ultralente insulin	4–8	10–30	36†

*Lente is a mixture of 30% Semilente Insulin and 70% Ultralente Insulin.
†NPH = neutral protamine Hagedorn.

Insulin requirements of an insulin-dependent diabetic range from 0.5 to 1.2 U/kg/day. This is usually delivered in divided SC doses 2 to 3 times per day in patients who are taking meals. In patients who are on continuous TPN, the insulin may be added to the bag for continuous IV infusion. The times of onset and duration of various insulin preparations are listed in Table 14–10.

Perioperative Insulin Management

Preoperative

The preoperative diabetic patient will usually require insulin on the morning of surgery.
1. Start routine **5% dextrose in water + one-half NS + 20 mEq/L KCl** the evening before surgery at a rate of 75 to 100 ml/hr.
2. Give the patient nothing by mouth after midnight.
3. The morning of surgery, obtain a finger stick glucose reading.
4. For type II patients, administer **5 units of regular insulin SC**.
5. For type I patients, administer about one-half the routine morning dose of regular insulin.
6. Do not administer NPH insulin.

Postoperative

The goal is to maintain blood sugars at <250 mg/dl.
1. Obtain an immediate blood glucose level in the recovery room.
2. Continue **5% dextrose in water + one-half NS + 20 mEq/L KCl at a rate of 75 to 100 ml/hr.**
3. Obtain glucose finger sticks every 6 hours, and administer regular insulin by a sliding scale.

The management of hyperglycemia and hypoglycemia are outlined below. The principles are applicable for diabetic and nondiabetic patients.

Hyperglycemia

Etiology

1. Poor control of diabetes mellitus, or new-onset disease
2. Stress (surgery, infection, and injury)
3. Medications (corticosteroids and thiazide diuretics)
4. TPN administration

Major Threat to Life

- Dehydration
- Diabetic ketoacidosis

Selective Physical Examination

The symptoms of hyperglycemia vary, depending on severity.
Mild hyperglycemia
    Polyuria and polydipsia
Moderate hyperglycemia
    Fluid depletion
    Polyuria and polydipsia
Severe hyperglycemia

VS:	Tachycardia, rapid respiratory rate, and hypotension
MS:	Obtundation, delirium, and coma
HEENT:	"Fruity" breath (ketones)
	Flat neck veins
Resp:	Kussmaul's respiration
Abd:	Anorexia, ileus, and gastric dilation
	Abdominal pain that may mimic an acute abdomen
GU:	Polyuria and polydipsia
Neuro:	Hyporeflexia and hypotonia
ABG:	Acidosis

Management

1. General concepts
   - If a finger stick value is too high or too low, or simply does not make sense, confirm that there are no glucose-containing fluids being administered IV and send a confirmatory serum glucose to the laboratory.
   - A new diagnosis of diabetes should be confirmed with a glucose tolerance test and with serum insulin levels.
        Note: A new diagnosis of diabetes should not be made in settings of severe surgical, infectious, or other hypermetabolic stress.

- The normal control of blood glucose is a balance of the following three elements:
  a. Exercise (which tends to lower blood sugar)
  b. Calorie sources such as food and intravenous fluids (IVFs) (which increase blood sugar)
  c. Insulin (which lowers blood sugar)
  Look for alterations in any of these components when trying to decipher changes in blood sugar trends.

2. Assess the severity.

   This includes a fluid volume status evaluation and laboratory analysis. In addition to finger stick glucose values, frequent blood glucose samples should be sent to the laboratory along with serum electrolytes.

3. Administer fluid resuscitation, if necessary.

   Follow the guidelines listed in Chapter 12 until hemodynamic stability is maintained. The fluid of choice is normal saline (NS). Do not administer glucose-containing fluids initially, as the extra glucose will exacerbate the osmotic diuresis. Care should be used with fluid administration in the elderly and in those patients with a history of congestive heart failure (CHF).

4. Order insulin administration.

   The goal of ongoing insulin administration is the maintenance of serum blood glucose levels of <250 mg/dl. The regimen of delivery depends on the severity of the hyperglycemia and on the severity of the illness. Examine the pattern of blood sugars relative to recent insulin doses and make appropriate adjustments. Use Table 14–10 as a guide to which insulin type to use and when to time its administration.

Mild Hyperglycemia

This condition is often asymptomatic and does not require urgent treatment.

- Confirm an abnormal finger stick reading with a serum glucose level sent to the laboratory.
- Monitor glucose finger sticks every 6 hours and as necessary.
- Monitor serum glucose level and electrolytes every morning.
- Monitor urine by dipstick for reducing sugars and acetate.
- Limit glucose-containing IVFs.
- Administer routine IV insulin doses.

  In the diabetic patient who takes no food orally, administer regular insulin IV as required in doses every 6 hours and cover with a sliding scale. Adjust routine insulin doses as finger stick levels dictate.

- Give SC bolus insulin.

  In the diabetic patient who is able to take regular meals by mouth, administer routine regular and long-acting insulin SC doses and cover with a sliding scale. Adjust routine insulin doses as finger stick levels dictate.

Moderate Hyperglycemia

If the patient is already receiving insulin therapy, an adjustment may be required.

- Confirm an abnormal finger stick reading with a serum glucose level determined by a laboratory.
- Monitor glucose finger sticks every 2 to 4 hours and as necessary.
- Monitor serum glucose level and electrolytes every morning.
- Monitor urine by dipstick for reducing sugars and acetate.
- Give IV bolus insulin.

   5 to 10 units may be given initially. For rapid response, the use of regular insulin, administered IV, is desirable.
- Administer routine IV insulin doses.

   Follow the initial bolus with routine regular insulin IV doses every 6 hours as required, and cover with a sliding scale.
- Advance to SC administration of regular and long-acting insulin as the patient improves and begins to tolerate meals by mouth.
- Determine the cause of poor blood glucose control.

   Change in diet

   Change in infusion rate of glucose-containing IVFs

   Increased metabolic stress

   Inadequate insulin dosages

   Medications

   Pancreatitis

Severe Hyperglycemias

1. Diabetic ketoacidosis

Diabetic ketoacidosis is a severe medical disease. It is seen most commonly in patients with type I diabetes and represents a prolonged lack of insulin. If severe hyperglycemia is present with evidence of acidosis and hypotension, immediate care is required.

- Contact your resident.
- Prepare the patient for transfer to the intensive care unit (ICU).
- Consult the appropriate medical team.
- Give fluid resuscitation.

   Follow the guidelines listed in Chapter 12 until hemodynamic stability is maintained. The fluid of choice is NS. Do not administer glucose-containing fluids initially, as the extra glucose will exacerbate the osmotic diuresis. Care should be used with fluid administration in the elderly and in those patients with a history of CHF.

- Send a baseline serum glucose to the laboratory.

  Also send baseline arterial blood gas (ABG), blood urea nitrogen (BUN), creatinine, serum insulin level, and electrolytes.

- Monitor glucose finger sticks every 1 hour and as necessary.

- Monitor serum glucose, electrolytes, and ABGs every 2 to 4 hours.

- Monitor urine by dipstick for reducing sugars and acetate.

- Give initial insulin bolus.

  Give IV 5 to 10 units regular insulin.

- Give continuous infusion of regular insulin.

  Start with a rate of 0.1 U/kg/hr and adjust as necessary. Continue the infusion until the blood sugars stabilize at 150 to 200 mg/dl. The rate of blood sugar drop should be about 20 to 30 mg/dl/hr (2.0 mmol/L/hr). As the blood sugar falls it will be necessary to slow the insulin infusion to 0.025 to 0.05 U/kg/hr.

- Hold SC insulin doses and oral hypoglycemics.

  When blood sugars have stabilized, SC insulin doses may be added to the regimen. Remember to continue the continuous IV infusion until the SC insulin has taken effect (1–2 hours).

- Add the glucose to IVFs by switching from NS to 5% dextrose in water when the serum glucose level falls below 250 to 300 mg/dl.

- Correct other electrolyte and acid–base abnormalities.

  Common problems include acidemia and hypokalemia. These generally resolve with hydration and insulin therapy. Consider treating a pH of <7.2 with additional $NaHCO_3$ as outlined in Chapter 12. Initial hypokalemia may be treated by addition of KCl to the IVF.

- Determine the cause of poor blood glucose control.

  Dietary indiscretion

  Dehydration

  Increased metabolic stress (infection and illness)

  Inadequate insulin dosages

  Medications

  Pancreatitis

2. **Hyperosmolar nonketotic coma**

   This complication is most commonly seen in patients with poorly controlled type II diabetes. The hyperglycemia may be severe, but ketoacidosis is absent.

   - Contact your resident.
   - Prepare the patient for transfer to the ICU.
   - Consult the appropriate medical team.
   - Give fluid resuscitation.

     Follow the guidelines listed in Chapter 12 until hemodynamic stability is maintained. The fluid of choice is NS. Do not administer glucose-containing fluids initially, as the extra glucose will exacerbate the osmotic diuresis. Care should be used with fluid administration in the elderly and in those patients with a history of CHF. Start with administration of **500 ml of NS over 2 hours**. When the patient is hemodynamically stable, replace fluids as the patient's condition dictates based on a reassessment of fluid status and serum sodium levels. Change to hypotonic fluids, such as one-half NS, at this time.

- Send a baseline serum glucose to the laboratory.

  Also send baseline ABG, BUN, creatinine, serum insulin level, and electrolytes.

- Monitor glucose finger sticks every 1 hour and as necessary.
- Monitor serum glucose, electrolytes, and ABGs every 2 to 4 hours.
- Monitor urine by dipstick for reducing sugars and acetate.
- Give initial insulin bolus.

  Give IV 5 to 10 units regular insulin.

- Give continuous infusion of regular insulin.

  Patients with hyperosmolar nonketotic hyperglycemia require less insulin than those with ketoacidosis. Start in the range of **0.025 to 0.05 U/kg/hr and adjust as necessary**. Continue insulin therapy as described in the discussion of ketoacidosis above.

- Determine the cause of poor blood glucose control.

  Infection

  Dehydration

  Other increased metabolic stress (myocardial infarction and stroke)

Hypoglycemia

Etiology

1. Excessive exogenous insulin or oral hypoglycemics
2. Decreased calorie intake (missed meals or snacks)
3. Increased exercise
4. Medications (alcohol, pentamidine, disopyramide, and monoamine oxidase inhibitors)
5. Hepatic failure (impaired gluconeogenesis)
6. Adrenal insufficiency
7. Too rapid a withdrawal from high-glucose-concentration IV fluids

Major Threat to Life

- Brain hypoglycemia

  The brain is an obligate glucose user, and acute drops in

blood glucose may severely and permanently damage brain functioning.

Selective Physical Examination

The symptoms are divided into two groupings, the more acute **adrenergic** responses, which are due to catecholamine release, and a more indolent **central nervous system** response, which may take 1 to 3 days to develop. Patients treated with oral hypoglycemia medications may not exhibit the adrenergic responses.

VS:	Tachycardia
MS:	Anxiety, confusion, and coma
HEENT:	Diplopia
CVS:	Palpitations
Skin:	Diaphoresis
Neuro:	Headache, perioral and fingertip numbness, focal neurologic abnormalities, tremulousness, seizures, or coma

Management

1. Assess the severity.
   Symptomatic patients require treatment; this may be safely started while the hypoglycemia is being confirmed.
2. Draw blood before treatment for laboratory studies.
   These may include serum glucose, insulin, and C-peptide levels.
3. Give oral glucose.
   If the patient is awake and able to take food by mouth, administer sweetened fruit juice.
4. Give IV glucose.
   If the patient is not able to take food by mouth, administer **50 ml of 50% dextrose in water by slow IV push.**
5. Give **glucagon 0.5 to 1.0 mg SC or IM.**
   This is reserved for patients who have no IV access.
6. Give continuous IV fluids containing glucose.
   This is especially important for the patient who is unable to tolerate food by mouth or for whom hypoglycemia is an expected long-term problem.
7. Recheck finger stick glucose levels in 1 hour and every 2 to 4 hours thereafter until stable.
8. Seek a cause of hypoglycemia.

Nutrition and Wound Healing

A surgical wound has nutritional requirements as does any other tissue. Aberrations in the nutrition status of the patient will have profound effects on the normal progression of wound healing. Collagen synthesis and cross-linking is impaired by protein malnutrition; infiltrating WBCs require adequate tissue levels of glucose; and various vitamins and cofactors should be available or supplemented to effect normal healing. Vitamins A and C and the mineral zinc are of particular importance. A multivitamin is generally enough to supplement these factors.

Patients who are taking high-dose corticosteroids will have delayed wound healing. This is because of decreased inflammatory response, diminished protein synthesis, and inhibition of fibroblast proliferation. This may be reversed in part by administration of a vitamin cocktail outlined in Table 14–5. This should be continued until the wound is well healed.

15

HEADACHE

While on call, you will be asked to evaluate and treat patients with headache. Postsurgical patients may develop headache as a sequela of anesthesia, stress, sleep disturbance, drug reaction, increased intracranial pressure (ICP), and other causes. Other patients may have a history of recurrent, chronic headache. Usually, a slow-onset, chronic headache is associated with a relatively benign process. Rapid-onset headache associated with fever or a change in neurologic status is more concerning as a potentially serious process.

■ PHONE CALL

Questions

1. **How serious is the headache?**

    A serious headache is more likely to represent a concerning problem.

2. **Are there any neurologic changes?**

    When neurologic changes are associated with headache, there is a high likelihood of a serious process. Although some transient neurologic changes can be associated with headache (e.g., migraine headache and visual changes), life-threatening neurologic changes can occur.

3. **Was the headache of sudden onset or gradual onset?**

    Sudden-onset headaches are frequently of vascular origin and include migraine headaches, cluster headaches, subarachnoid hemorrhage, and intracerebral hemorrhage.

4. **What are the vital signs?**

    Hypertension and headache may indicate increased ICP. Make sure you ask about the patient's temperature. Infectious processes of the central nervous system, including bacterial meningitis, may present with fever and headache.

5. **Does the patient have a history of headache? Any medical problems?**

    An easy way to diagnose and treat headache is to know if a patient has a history of chronic, recurrent headache. Ask the RN to ascertain if the headache is a typical chronic headache. If it is a typical headache, find out the medication from which the patient obtains relief.

6. **Did the patient have surgery and is there a ventriculoperitoneal (VP) shunt?**

A severe headache after neurologic surgery may represent cerebral edema or intracranial bleeding. A history of VP shunt and headache may indicate shunt malfunction or infection.

Orders

1. Ask the RN to take a full set of vital signs and to assess the neurologic status if not previously done.

   Although this may seem unnecessary in most patients, it will be useful in the occasional patient who may have an impending serious process.

2. If the patient has a gradual-onset, mild headache without neurologic changes, prescribing an analgesic agent such as acetaminophen 650 mg orally (PO) (for adults) is appropriate. The pediatric dose of **acetaminophen** is **10 mg/kg/ dose PO**.

   Instruct the RN to call you back if the headache does not improve in 1 to 2 hours.

3. If the headache is associated with a deteriorating level of consciousness, ask the nurse to insert an intravenous (IV) line and place the patient on O_2.

Inform RN

"Will arrive at the bedside in . . . minutes."

Headaches associated with altered mental status, change in level of consciousness, fever, or vomiting require you to assess the patient immediately. These signs frequently represent serious intracranial processes such as bleeding, swelling, or infection. Failure to recognize and treat serious intracranial problems may result in permanent neurologic dysfunction or death. If a patient who was treated for a mild headache obtains no relief or develops worsening pain, a bedside evaluation is appropriate.

■ ELEVATOR THOUGHTS

What causes headaches?

Slow-Onset or Chronic Headache

1. Migraine headache
2. Cluster headache
3. Temporomandibular joint (TMJ) disorder
4. Drugs (e.g., nitrates and calcium channel blockers)
5. Tension headache
6. Cervical osteoarthritis
7. Referred pain

Acute Headache

- Infectious causes
  1. Meningitis
  2. Encephalitis
  3. VP shunt infection
  4. Subdural abscess
  5. Brain abscess
  6. Craniotomy wound infection
  7. Headache associated with viral syndrome or flu
- Vascular causes
  1. Arteriovenous malformation (AVM)
  2. Subarachnoid hemorrhage
  3. Intracerebral hemorrhage
  4. Intracranial aneurysm
  5. Malignant hypertension
- Increased intracranial pressure causes
  1. Cerebral edema
  2. Hydrocephalus
  3. Tumors
  4. Space-occupying fluid collections (blood and abscess)
- Local causes
  1. Postcraniotomy or postsurgical pain
  2. Temporal arteritis
  3. Visual process (acute-angle glaucoma)

■ MAJOR THREAT TO LIFE

- Herniation syndromes
- Meningitis
- Subarachnoid hemorrhage

Brain herniation refers to a process in which increased ICP forces a vital portion of the brain to be displaced under a rigid intracranial supporting structure. This leads to compression and loss of function of the displaced area of brain. The three rigid areas that tend to entrap brain tissue are the foramen magnum, tentorial edge, and falx cerebri. Patients with increased ICP and impending brain herniation are usually unconscious. They demonstrate a deteriorating neurologic examination and are at high risk for death. Tables 15–1 and 15–2 give the main types of herniation syndromes and the classic signs. Meningitis may be caused by a range of factors including bacterial, fungal, or viral infection. Patients with bacterial meningitis often present with a rapidly deteriorating course and must be treated with intravenous antibiotics early. Subarachnoid hemorrhage, most frequently caused by trauma, ruptured berry aneurysms, and AVMs, must be recognized and treated rapidly.

Table 15–1 ▫ **MAJOR HERNIATION SYNDROMES**

Type	Regions Involved
Uncal herniation	Lateral mass displaces uncus of temporal lobe medially over tentorial edge
Central herniation	Downward displacement of brainstem through foramen magnum
Cerebellar herniation	Cerebellum herniates downward through foramen magnum
Subfulcine herniation	Cingulate gyrus is displaced below falx cerebri

■ BEDSIDE

Quick Look Test

Does the patient look well (only mildly uncomfortable), sick (very uncomfortable or distressed), or critical (about to die)?

Patients with processes causing increased ICP look sick. They frequently have either an altered mental status or a deteriorating neurologic examination. On the other hand, patients with chronic headaches are often mildly uncomfortable but do not appear sick.

Airway and Vital Signs

What is the patient's blood pressure (BP) and heart rate (HR)?

Headache may be caused by severe hypertension with systolic blood pressure (SBP) of >190 mm Hg or diastolic blood pressure (DBP) or >110 mm Hg. Hypertension in comatose

Table 15–2 ▫ **TYPICAL PRESENTING SIGNS OF MAJOR HERNIATION SYNDROMES**

Stage of Herniation	Sign
Early	Ipsilateral pupillary dilation
	Progressive decrease in mental status
	Respiratory pattern changes (Cheyne-Stokes)
Progressing	Decreasing level of consciousness
	Hyperventilation
	Contralateral hemiplegia
	Decerebrate posturing
	Pupillary constriction
Advanced	Bilateral decerebrate rigidity (uncal herniation)
	Irregular respiration
	Flaccidity (central herniation)
	Death

patients with head injury or increased ICP may be due to herniation. In the advanced stages of herniation or near death, hypotension may occur. Bradycardia associated with hypertension may occur with increased ICP.

What is the patient's temperature?

Fever and headache may indicate meningitis, subdural empyema, brain abscess, or shunt infection.

Selective Physical Examination I

Does the patient have increased ICP or meningitis?

VS: Assess BP, HR, respiratory rate, and temperature
HEENT: Look for signs of head injury
        Nuchal rigidity (most common with subarachnoid
           hemorrhage or meningitis)

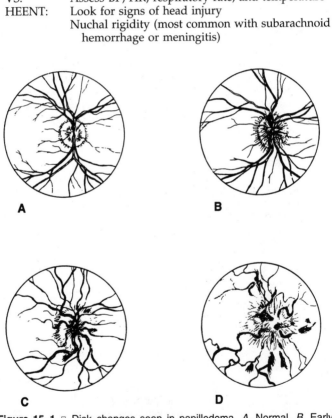

Figure 15–1 □ Disk changes seen in papilledema. *A*, Normal. *B*, Early papilledema. *C*, Moderate papilledema with early hemorrhage. *D*, Severe papilledema with extensive hemorrhage. (From Marshall SA, Ruedy J: On Call: Principles and Protocols, 2nd ed. Philadelphia, WB Saunders Co, 1993, p 107.)

Papilledema (sign of increased ICP) (Fig. 15–1)
Check for presence of a VP shunt.
Check for craniotomy wound infection.

Neuro: Mental status examination: evaluate for acute changes (Table 15–3)
Pupillary examination: note size, reactivity, and symmetry of the pupils
Brudzinski's sign and Kernig's sign (Fig. 15–2)
Brief motor examination (Table 15–4)

If there are signs of nuchal rigidity, acute mental status changes, motor changes, or papilledema, a full and detailed neurologic examination is indicated.

Initial Management

Headache Associated with Increased Intracranial Pressure

1. Elevate head of the bed.
2. Order computed tomography (CT) scan immediately.
3. Obtain neurosurgical consultation.
4. If the ICP is greatly elevated, hyperventilate the patient if intubated (e.g., trauma patient); lower the arterial partial pressure of carbon dioxide ($PaCO_2$) to 25 to 30 mm Hg.

   Most patients with greatly elevated ICP are unconscious, are unstable, and require intubation. Those patients who are

---

Table 15–3 □ THE MENTAL STATUS EXAMINATION

Response to External Stimuli

Assess if patient is awake and alert
Assess response to verbal commands
If patient does not respond to verbal commands, evaluate response to pain (localization, withdrawing to painful stimuli, and posturing in response to pain)

Response to Cognitive Testing

Test orientation to person, place, and time
Memory testing
    Serial 7s
    Naming three objects in 5 minutes (short-term memory)
    Naming of past presidents and major past events
    Simple calculations
Evaluate speech
    Fluency
    Rate

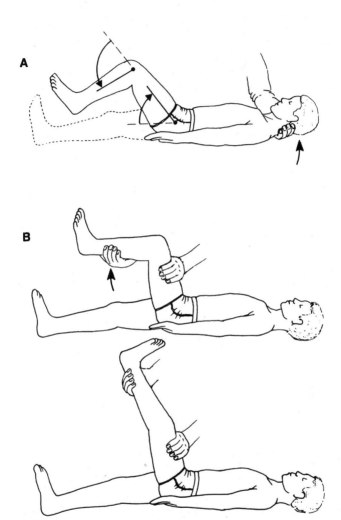

Figure 15–2 □ *A*, Brudzinski's sign. The test result is positive when the patient flexes his or her hips and knees in response to passive neck flexion by the examiner. *B*, Kernig's sign. The test result is positive when pain or resistance is elicited by passive knee extension, from the 90-degree hip/knee flexion position. (From Marshall SA, Ruedy J: On Call: Principles and Protocols, 2nd ed. Philadelphia, WB Saunders Co, 1993, p 109.)

Table 15–4 □ BRIEF MOTOR EXAMINATION

Muscle tone and bulk (fasciculation and atrophy indicate lower motor neuron disorder, increased tone and spasticity indicate upper motor neuron disorder)
Muscle strength (grades 0–5)
Muscle symmetry (look for unilateral weakness)
Reflex testing (hyporeflexia, upper motor neuron; hyperreflexia, lower motor neuron)
Gait (if possible)

still conscious may need elective intubation if the need to lower the ICP is emergent.

5. Consider the use of diuretics.

Mannitol is a good osmotic diuretic and may be given up to **1 g/kg IV every 3 hours**. Hold for serum osmolarity of >305.

6. Steroids are useful stabilizers of the blood–brain barrier.

Consider **dexamethasone (Decadron) 10 to 50 mg IV once, then 2 to 5 mg IV/IM every 6 hours**. Place the patient on a histamine H_2 blocker to decrease the risk of a peptic ulcer.

7. Consider loading with **phenytoin (Dilantin)** to reduce the risk of seizure.

Load with **18 mg/kg IV at a maximum rate of 25 mg/ min. Maintain at 100 mg IV every 8 hours**. Check serum phenytoin levels.

Headache Associated with Nuchal Rigidity and No Sign of Increased Intracranial Pressure

1. If bacterial meningitis is suspected (by history or presence of fever), establish IV access.
2. Order CT scan of the head immediately if possible.
3. Order lumbar puncture (LP) immediately.
   - Note: Do not perform LP if there is evidence of increased ICP (risk of herniation). Obtain a CT scan first.

   Measure the opening pressure and note the appearance of the cerebrospinal fluid (CSF). Also obtain cell counts, bacterial and fungal cultures, Gram stain, and India ink stain. Bacterial meningitis is most often associated with cloudy CSF, increased white blood cell (WBC) count and protein, and decreased glucose. Viral meningitis may be associated with turbid fluid, increased WBCs, slightly elevated protein, and normal glucose. A subarachnoid hemorrhage usually presents with bloody CSF, about 1 WBC for every 100 red blood cells, increased protein, and normal glucose.
4. Start IV antibiotics immediately if LP suggests meningitis.

   See Table 15–4 for guidelines.
5. Consider phenytoin prophylaxis.

Headache with Nuchal Rigidity and Signs of Increased Intracranial Pressure

1. **Do not perform LP (risk of herniation).**
2. Order CT scan immediately.
3. Start empirical IV antibiotics.
4. Consider brain abscess of subdural empyema.
5. Obtain neurosurgical consultation for mass lesions.
6. Consider phenytoin prophylaxis.

Selective History and Chart Review

Once emergent management is taken for life-threatening processes associated with headache, a more detailed evaluation may be performed. If the patient has an isolated headache and has not required aggressive initial management, a carefully taken history will often clarify the best management.

Does the patient have a history of headaches?

Frequently, patients suffer from recurrent headaches and can describe the form of treatment that best relieves the symptoms. Patients with a history of migraine or cluster headaches may also describe the form of drug therapy that is effective for relief of the symptoms.

Does head position affect headache severity?

Patients with headaches sensitive to vertical positioning of the head may have an increased ICP.

Does the patient have TMJ syndrome or referred headache pain?

Patients with TMJ syndrome frequently develop headaches as a result of muscle spasm. These patients clench and grind their teeth while asleep and then awaken with a headache. They may be helped with nonnarcotic analgesics such as nonsteroidal anti-inflammatory drugs (NSAIDs) and muscle relaxants (e.g., Flexeril). Ask the patient what type of therapy has worked best in the past. Ultimately, many of these patients will need dental treatment and a mouth guard to wear while sleeping, to prevent clenching and grinding.

Is there a history of head trauma in the recent or remote past?

Epidural hematomas are caused by a collection of blood between the calvaria and the dura and are usually seen associated with a skull fracture. Subdural hematomas are usually caused by brain surface bleeding or bleeding from venous structures near the brain surface. Subdural hematomas may be acute (symptoms within 72 hours of injury), subacute (3–20 days after injury), or chronic (3 weeks or longer after injury). Mass effect and an abnormal neurologic examination usually require craniotomy and removal of the clot.

Are there any prodromal or visual changes?

Visual auras may occur before migraine headaches and include blurred vision and scintillations. Remember that visual changes may be associated with transient ischemic attacks.

Does the patient have a fever and a VP shunt?

VP shunts have a 5 to 10% infection rate; organisms causing infection include *Staphylococcus aureus, S. epidermidis*, and Gram-negative rods. Shunt culture (sterilely obtaining fluid from the reservoir) is indicated. IV and intrathecal antibiotics are indicated for shunt infections; infected shunts may ultimately need to be removed and replaced at a different site. Consult with a neurosurgeon for shunt problems.

What drugs is the patient receiving?

Nitrates, calcium channel blockers, and other drugs may cause headaches.

Has the patient had a recent lumbar puncture or spinal anesthesia?

Removal of small amounts of CSF can cause headache, especially when the patient is upright. Treatment is bedrest.

Selective Physical Examination II

VS: Repeat now
HEENT: Scalp lacerations and depressed skull fractures
           Hemotympanum (blood medial to tympanic membrane) or raccoon eyes (basilar skull fracture)
           CSF otorrhea or rhinorrhea (dural tear and possible basilar skull fracture)
           Red eye (narrow-angle glaucoma)
           Eyelid ptosis (cranial nerve 3 dysfunction or levator disinsertion)
           Retinal hemorrhages (hypertension or trauma)
           Tender, enlarged temporal arteries (temporal arteritis)
           Tenderness over the frontal or maxillary sinuses (sinusitis)
           Crepitus and tenderness over the TMJ; possible restricted mouth opening (TMJ syndrome)
Neuro: Perform a complete neurologic examination
           Mental status (if not already tested): evaluate the level of consciousness and look for new-onset somnolence
           Cranial nerves: look for asymmetries
           Motor examination including gait and reflexes: look for asymmetries, weakness, and abnormal reflexes
           Sensory examination

■ **DEFINITIVE MANAGEMENT**

Evidence of Head Trauma

A patient who has had head trauma with a loss of consciousness should have a head CT scan. The other alternative is to admit the patient for close neurologic observation. The head CT scan is advantageous because it may be a less costly and a more efficient way to screen for head injury. Any significant intracranial mass or brain injury discovered on head CT scanning requires evaluation by neurosurgery.

Posttraumatic Headache

If a patient has suffered head trauma without a loss of consciousness, it is important to be able to follow this patient's neurologic examination in the immediate posttraumatic period. Care must be used to not sedate the patient with an analgesic. It is best to use acetaminophen for mild headache. For more severe pain, use **codeine 30 mg intramuscularly (IM)**. Do not use drugs that inhibit platelet function (NSAIDs).

Pseudotumor Cerebri

This condition, also known as benign intracranial hypertension, presents as headache and increased ICP (papilledema), without obvious intracranial mass on CT scanning. This condition does not require emergent management at night, and referral to a neurologist may be made during normal working hours.

Migraine Headache

Migraines may present in a variety of ways, although they are often lateralized and throbbing. Many patients have a short prodromal period, or "aura," before the severe migraine pain begins. Migraine headaches may be associated with blurring of vision, visual field defects, visual hallucinations, aphasia, numbness, paresthesias, or transient focal weakness. Triggering factors include sleep deprivation, emotional distress, reactions to food, and certain drugs (e.g., oral contraceptives). Treatment for mild pain includes aspirin or acetaminophen. If a more severe migraine begins and is still in its prodromal stage, **Cafergot**, a combination of ergotamine tartrate and caffeine, may be helpful. The patient should take **2 tablets** (1 tablet = 1 mg ergotamine + 100 mg caffeine) **at the onset of the headache or the prodrome**. If the symptoms have not subsided **at 20 minutes**, the patient should be given **1 more tablet every 30 minutes, up to 6 tablets/24 hours**. If the patient vomits during the migraine headache, **ergotamine IM (0.25–0.5 mg)** can be given. Frequently, a narcotic analgesic such as **meperidine (Demerol) 75 to 100 mg IM** is required for adequate analgesia. Avoid the use of ergotamine-containing preparations in patients who are pregnant or who have a history of unstable angina or poorly controlled hypertension.

Cluster Headache

These headaches are most common in middle-aged men. Pain begins as an episode of unilateral periorbital pain that lasts about 1 hour. Pain generally occurs daily for several weeks. Pain is accompanied by eye tearing, rhinorrhea or nasal congestion, or Horner's syndrome. Adequate treatment is difficult. Ergotamine tartrate aerosol or **inhalation of 100% oxygen for 15 to 20 minutes** is usually helpful. The use of narcotic analgesics, such as meperidine, is also useful.

Tension Headache

These headaches are extremely common. They usually present as vise-like, generalized pain. The posterior neck muscles are frequently involved and are often tender. Headache may be exacerbated by stress, noise, or fatigue. Treatment involves aspirin or acetaminophen, and relaxation techniques. Hot baths and massage are also useful. Avoid the use of benzodiazepines chronically in these patients.

Temporal Arteritis

This condition involves inflammation of the temporal arteries, which may become thrombosed. In addition to temporal arteries, vertebral and ophthalmic arteries may also be involved. Clinical examination reveals tenderness of the superficial temporal artery over the scalp. Temporal arteritis must be treated immediately, because untreated disease can lead to blindness. If the diagnosis is suspected, start the patient on **prednisone 60 mg PO every day**, obtain an erythrocyte sedimentation rate (ESR) (look for ESR of >60 mm/hr), and arrange for the surgical service to perform a temporal artery biopsy.

Malignant Hypertension

Uncontrolled sustained hypertension, with diastolic pressures of >130 mm Hg, leads to widespread arteriolar damage. This is manifested by headache, retinal hemorrhages, papilledema, renal failure, myocardial infarction, and stroke. Refer to Chapter 16 for the treatment of malignant hypertension.

16

HYPERTENSION

The goal on call is to treat hypertensive episodes that are symptomatic or that put the patient at risk for myocardial infarction (MI), stroke, or bleeding. As the on-call physician, it is best to leave the fine-tuning of a patient's blood pressure (BP) to the primary team caring for the patient.

■ PHONE CALL

Questions

1. **What is the BP?**

   Always evaluate the magnitude of the BP elevation. A mild BP elevation is not serious. However, an episode of malignant hypertension may result in sudden death.

2. **Why is the patient in the hospital? Did the patient have surgery? If so, what was the operation and when was it performed?**

   It is important to ascertain why the patient is in the hospital and whether the patient is postoperative. For example, a diagnosis of pheochromocytoma would explain elevated BP.

3. **Is the patient in pain or anxious?**

   Pain and anxiety result in sympathetic stimulation and elevation of BP.

4. **Is there a history of hypertension? If so, is the patient taking any antihypertensive medications?**

   Patients with a history of hypertension are likely to have BP control problems while in the hospital. Patients taking antihypertensive medications frequently miss doses of medication just before admission. Sometimes, hypertensive patients are not placed on their BP medications on admission.

5. **Are there any symptoms of a hypertensive emergency, such as chest pain, back pain, shortness of breath (SOB), headache, neck stiffness, vomiting, or seizures?**

   MI or aortic dissection may cause chest pain or back pain. SOB may be caused by MI or pulmonary edema secondary to severe hypertension. Headache, neck stiffness, vomiting, and seizures may be related to subarachnoid hemorrhage or stroke.

Orders

If asked to treat a patient with mildly symptomatic elevation in BP, ask the RN if the patient is currently taking antihypertensive drugs. If the patient is not currently on drug therapy for hypertension and is otherwise healthy and not pregnant, consider ordering **nifedipine 10 mg orally (PO) or sublingually (SL)**. A patient currently on antihypertensive therapy may benefit from an additional incremental dose of the current medication.

In the event of a hypertensive emergency (diastolic BP >120 mm Hg), a functional intravenous (IV) line should be available. If an IV is not in place, order an IV placed immediately. Run crystalloid to keep the vein open.

Inform RN

"Will be at the bedside in . . . minutes."

Mild BP elevation is not an emergency, and it can usually be handled over the phone. However, hypertensive emergencies require your immediate evaluation and treatment of the patient.

These hypertensive emergencies include the following conditions:

1. Preeclampsia and eclampsia
2. Aortic dissection
3. Hypertensive crisis
4. Hypertensive withdrawal syndromes (e.g., cocaine and alcohol)
5. Coronary ischemia or infarction
6. Catecholamine crisis
7. Hypertensive encephalopathy
8. Pulmonary edema

■ ELEVATOR THOUGHTS

What causes hypertension?
- Essential hypertension
- Renal disease
- Preeclampsia and eclampsia
- Pain
- Fear or emotional stress
- Fluid overload
- Increased intracranial pressure (ICP) (e.g., intracranial tumor or bleed)
- Cushing's syndrome
- Pheochromocytoma
- Coarctation of the aorta
- Hypoxia
- Drugs of abuse (e.g., cocaine or amphetamine toxicity)
- Drug interactions (e.g., monoamine oxidase [MAO] inhibitors and tricyclics)
- Drug withdrawal

There are many causes of hypertension. Essential hypertension is the most common form of high BP and accounts for >90% of chronic hypertension cases. The cause of essential hypertension is not known.

Preeclampsia is a condition associated with pregnancy and is manifest by hypertension, proteinuria, generalized edema, and sporadic liver function abnormalities (including coagulopathy). Eclampsia includes the findings of preeclampsia but also includes generalized seizures. Hypertension in the setting of pregnancy is dangerous for both the fetus and the mother. Special care must be used in treating these conditions, because some antihypertensive agents have adverse effects on fetal development.

Pain is a common cause of hypertension in postsurgical and trauma patients. Ascertain that postoperative patients have appropriate pain control. Inadequate sedation of intubated patients may lead to hypertension. Emotional states such as anxiety and fear also contribute to elevated BPs.

Increased ICP may be a cause of hypertension in neurosurgical and trauma patients. Tumors, subdural or epidural hematomas, or diffuse brain swelling may all cause increased ICP.

Endocrine disorders may be associated with hypertension. Cushing's disease associated with adenoma or exogenous steroid use may cause significant hypertension. Pheochromocytoma may cause a malignant hypertensive crisis through overproduction and release of large quantities of epinephrine and norepinephrine.

Cocaine and amphetamines block reuptake of norepinephrine in nerve synapses. These drugs may cause severe hypertension when taken in overdose amounts. MAO inhibitors and tricyclic antidepressants may also cause hypertension and toxicity when taken in overdose amounts. These drugs may cause serious interactions when taken with indirect-acting (tyramine) or direct-acting (epinephrine) catecholamines.

Withdrawal from alcohol and drugs can lead to hypertension and severe sympathetic overactivity. Alcohol withdrawal is associated with significant morbidity and mortality. Withdrawal of cocaine or other sympathomimetic drugs can produce hypertension after chronic use. Narcotic withdrawal may cause tremulousness, hypertension, and tachycardia.

■ MAJOR THREAT TO LIFE

The following conditions, secondary to hypertension, are either directly life threatening or may lead to complications that are life threatening:

1. Malignant hypertension
2. Cerebrovascular accident (CVA) (stroke)
3. MI

4. Pulmonary edema
5. Aortic dissection
6. Eclampsia
7. Drug withdrawal
8. Hypertensive encephalopathy

■ BEDSIDE

Quick Look Test

Does the patient look well (comfortable), sick (uncomfortable or distressed), or critical (about to die)?

Most patients with mild elevations in BP are asymptomatic and look comfortable. Most patients with signs and symptoms of chest pain, SOB, or pain in the chest or back associated with hypertension will look distressed.

Airway and Vital Signs

Is the airway adequate?

Hypertension may be seen in a patient with airway obstruction or hypoxia. In both intubated and nonintubated patients, assess that ventilation and oxygenation are adequate.

What is the BP?

Take the BP in both arms. If the readings are not within 5 mm Hg of each other, repeat both pressures. Recall that coarctation of the aorta and aortic dissection may produce different BP readings in the two extremities.

What is the heart rate?

Hypertension and tachycardia are seen in states of catecholamine excess. This is commonly found in hypertensive crisis, drug overdose, and drug withdrawal. If the patient is hypertensive and bradycardic, look for signs of increased ICP. Beware that beta blockers may produce bradycardia in a patient with hypertension.

Selective History and Chart Review

Does the patient have a history of hypertension?

Was the patient taking any medications outside the hospital?

Is the patient being continued on antihypertensive medications while in the hospital?

Patients who take antihypertensive medications frequently do not have these medications continued on admission to the hospital. This is usually an oversight at the time of admission.

Discontinuation of antihypertensive therapy may be responsible for poor BP control.

Does the patient have any symptoms suggestive of a hypertensive emergency?

Ask the patient about the following symptoms:

1. Chest pain (MI or aortic dissection)
2. Back pain (aortic dissection)
3. SOB (pulmonary edema)
4. Headache (increased ICP or hypertensive encephalopathy)
5. Unilateral weakness or paresis (CVA)

Selective Physical Examination

The physical examination should be directed at looking for evidence of hypertensive crisis.

VS: Repeat now; be sure to perform BP readings on both arms if not already done.

HEENT: Fundoscopy: first look for papilledema, which is evidence of malignant hypertension; evidence of more chronic hypertensive changes, such as arteriolar narrowing, hemorrhages, or exudates, should also be noted.

Resp: Note crackles or rales (pulmonary edema) and evidence of pleural effusions (congestive heart failure [CHF]).

CVS: Listen for S_3 (CHF); look for evidence of elevated jugular venous distention.

Neuro: Look for focal weakness or paresis (CVA); also note changes in mental status, including level of agitation, and confusion (increased ICP or hypertensive encephalopathy).

■ MANAGEMENT

Hypertensive Crisis

This state is defined when the diastolic BP is >120 mm Hg. The severity of the crisis depends on both the absolute BP and the rapidity with which the BP elevation occurs. Hypertension associated with target organ damage (TOD) is an emergency, and it must be treated immediately. Common examples of TOD are shown in Table 16–1.

Hypertensive crisis with associated TOD changes should be treated with IV drug therapy. For patients in an intensive care unit (ICU) environment and with an arterial line, sodium nitroprusside is the first-line drug to reduce severe hypertension.

Table 16–1 ▫ **TARGET ORGAN DAMAGE ASSOCIATED WITH HYPERTENSIVE CRISIS**

Target Organ/System	Associated Changes
Cardiac/respiratory	Myocardial ischemia
	Infarction
	Pulmonary edema
Renal	Hematuria
	Azotemia
Central nervous system	Mental status changes
	Seizures
	Coma
Central nervous system (retina)	Papilledema
	Hemorrhages
	Exudates

Sodium nitroprusside is rapid acting and is easily titratable. Its action is short lived when infusion is discontinued. Start therapy with a **0.5 µg/kg/min IV drip and titrate the dosing as tolerated.** Patients with renal failure should be started at **0.25 µg/kg/min.** Most patients will respond to doses of <2 µg/kg/min. Dosing should never be >10 µg/kg/min. Sodium nitroprusside is light sensitive and is associated with thiocyanate toxicity and methemoglobinemia when given in high doses (>2–3 µg/kg/min) or for prolonged duration. Patients with renal dysfunction are also at increased risk for thiocyanate toxicity. Toxicity is associated with acidosis, dyspnea, vomiting, and dizziness. Thiocyanate levels should be checked every 2 to 3 days.

If sodium nitroprusside is not readily available or if intra-arterial monitoring has not been established, other IV agents may be useful. IV bolus therapy may be initiated with labetalol, diazoxide, and hydralazine. These drugs allow rapid BP reduction. Continuous IV infusion can be continued with labetalol and diazoxide. The effects of these drugs are not as easy to control as those of sodium nitroprusside, due to longer duration of action. Table 16–2 provides a list of common IV antihypertensive agents and their onsets, durations, dosages, and commonly occurring adverse effects.

Aortic Dissection

Patients with aortic dissection will often present with a history of sudden, severe chest pain with radiation to the back, the abdomen, and the extremities. Shock usually occurs with the later stages of the process. More than 60% of dissections occur in the ascending aorta, whereas 20% occur in the distal arch and 20% in the descending thoracic or abdominal aorta. Mediastinal widen-

Table 16-2 □ AN OVERVIEW OF COMMON INTRAVENOUS ANTIHYPERTENSIVE AGENTS

Drug	Route Available	Onset	Mechanism and Duration	Dosage	Considerations
Sodium nitroprusside	IV infusion	Immediate	Smooth muscle relaxant, 3 min	0.5 μg/kg/min starting dose, then titrate to achieve desired effect, up to 10 μg/kg/min as tolerated; consider 0.25 μg/kg/min in renal failure	Hypotension, nausea, vomiting, thiocyanate toxicity; check thiocyanate levels
Nitroglycerin	IV infusion	Immediate	Preload and afterload reduction, venous dilatation, 15 min	5–20 μg/min, titrate to achieve desired effect	Useful for moderate hypertension in patients with myocardial ischemia; watch for excessive preload reduction in patients with right-sided heart failure
Labetalol	IV bolus	5 min	Alpha and beta blockade, 3–5 hr	10–80 mg every 5 min, to 300 mg	Beware of inducing heart failure and hypotension; very effective agent
Diazoxide	IV infusion IV bolus	1–3 min	Direct arterial dilatation, 6–10 hr	5–100 μg/min 50–100 mg every 5 min to 500 mg	Causes reflex tachycardia; avoid use in acute MI or in dissecting aortic aneurysm
Hydralazine	IV infusion IV bolus	10 min	Vasodilation, 3–5 hr	10–30 mg/min 5–10 mg every 10 min	Tachycardia, hypotension; consider different agent if no significant effect after 20–30 mg
Esmolol	IV infusion	1–3 min	Selective beta blocker, 10 min	200–400 μg/kg/min for first 1–3 min, then 50–200 μg/kg/min	Watch for heart block, hypotension, and bronchospasm

IV = intravenous; MI = myocardial infarction.

ing may be visible on chest x-ray. Computed tomographic scanning with contrast provides a noninvasive diagnostic tool. Aortography is diagnostic.

Aortic dissections that involve the ascending aorta are known as type A. These dissections mandate emergent surgery due to the high likelihood of aortic rupture and cardiac tamponade. Type B dissections begin at the subclavian artery, and surgical therapy is often deferred. Control of the process is attempted with antihypertensive therapy. Severe pain, inability to control BP, compromise of blood flow to end-organs, or high risk of rupture are complications of type B dissections that mandate surgery.

The mainstay of treatment includes bed rest and antihypertensive therapy. The goal of antihypertensive therapy is to achieve a systolic BP of 100 to 120 mm Hg or the lowest possible BP that allows adequate organ perfusion. For BP control, a sodium nitroprusside drip is the treatment of choice because of the ability to titrate the BP finely without tachyphylaxis. A beta blocker must be used concurrently with sodium nitroprusside, because sodium nitroprusside alone causes an increase in left ventricular dv/dt and subsequent arterial shearing forces. **Propranolol** may be used at **0.5 mg IV followed by 1 mg IV every 5 minutes until the pulse pressure is reduced to 60 mm Hg or to a total dose of 0.15 mg/kg in any 4-hour period**. Esmolol may be more convenient to use, since it is a cardioselective beta blocker and is less likely to cause problems in asthmatics or patients with chronic obstructive pulmonary disease. Consider **200 to 400 μg/kg/min esmolol for the first 1 to 3 minutes followed by 50 to 200 μg/kg/min**. When using beta blockers concurrently with sodium nitroprusside, be careful to avoid hypotension and heart block.

Second-choice therapy in treating aortic dissection is labetalol. It can be used successfully as a single agent, but it should be reserved for situations in which sodium nitroprusside cannot be tolerated or when it is not available. Start with **labetalol 20 to 80 mg IV bolus, up to 250 mg. Begin continuous infusion at 0.5 to 2.0 mg/min**.

Preeclampsia and Eclampsia

Managing hypertensive pregnant patients is difficult and should be done only with the consultation of an obstetrician. Attempt to contact the patient's obstetrician if possible. Treatment for hypertension in pregnant patients should be considered when the diastolic BP is >100 mm Hg. The treatment of choice when the mother is near term is magnesium sulfate given as an IV infusion. Magnesium sulfate does not decrease BP, but it decreases fetal and maternal morbidity until delivery can be induced or cesarean section is performed. Ask the obstetrician to order and manage the magnesium sulfate drip.

If antihypertensive therapy is required for a pregnant patient, **methyldopa 250 to 500 mg IV bolus** is the recommended first-line therapy. An alternative drug is **hydralazine 5 to 10 mg IV every 10 minutes**, followed by oral maintenance therapy (Table 16–3). Some antihypertensive agents have been associated with perinatal morbidity and mortality. Angiotensin-converting enzyme inhibitors are toxic to the fetus. Beta blockers such as propranolol have been shown to alter uterine contractility; calcium channel blockers also alter uterine contractility. Diuretic use in pregnant patients has been shown to cause neonatal toxicity and maternal dehydration.

Hypertensive Encephalopathy

In this condition, severe hypertension is accompanied by drowsiness, confusion, headache, nausea, and deteriorating mental status. A greatly elevated BP, often >250/150 mm Hg, is characteristic. Common findings include papilledema, retinal hemorrhages, and exudates. There are usually no focal neurologic deficits found early in the progression of the disease. However, if focal neurologic deficits are present, a concurrent CVA may have occurred.

Treatment requires transfer to an ICU for electrocardiographic (ECG) and BP monitoring. A single **5- to 10-mg PO dose of nifedipine** can gently bring down BP while ICU transfer is taking place. Once the patient is in the ICU, an arterial line should be placed. First-line drug therapy is sodium nitroprusside, as outlined in Table 16–2. In patients with known or suspected atherothrombotic cerebrovascular disease, remember to bring down the BP slowly. These patients are at increased risk of CVA if blood pressure is reduced too quickly. It is reasonable to attempt to reduce the mean arterial BP by about 25% over the first several hours of therapy. Slowly titrate the infusion of nitroprusside to gradually decrease the BP.

There are other options for treating the hypertension associated with hypertensive encephalopathy. Diazoxide and labetalol may be used as outlined in Table 16–2. Once BP control is achieved through parenteral means, an appropriate oral regimen can be selected for maintenance (see Table 16–3).

Hypertension Associated with Myocardial Ischemia or Pulmonary Edema

Patients with hypertension and myocardial ischemia/infarction or pulmonary edema should be transferred to the ICU immediately. Consider **SL nitroglycerin 0.3 mg** to control chest pain during the transfer. Once in the ICU, begin **nitroglycerin infusion at 5 μg/min**, and **titrate** the dose **to 20 μg/min** to attempt to

Table 16–3 □ AN OVERVIEW OF COMMON ANTIHYPERTENSIVE AGENTS AVAILABLE BY ORAL, SUBLINGUAL, AND TRANSCUTANEOUS ROUTES

Drug	Route Available	Mechanism	Initial Dosage
Nifedipine	PO/sublingual	Calcium channel blocker	10 mg 3 times per day, may repeat sublingual dosing once
Nifedipine XL	PO	Calcium channel blocker	30 mg every day
Verapamil	PO	Calcium channel blocker	80 mg 3 times
Verapamil XL	PO	Calcium channel blocker	120 mg PO every day
Atenolol	PO	Selective beta antagonist	50 mg PO every day
Metoprolol	PO	Selective beta antagonist	50 mg PO 2 times per day
Propranolol	PO	Nonselective beta antagonist	40 mg PO 2 times per day
Labetalol	PO	Alpha and beta antagonist	100 mg PO 2 times per day
Captopril	PO	ACE inhibitor	10 mg PO every day
Enalapril	PO	ACE inhibitor	5 mg PO every day
Lisinopril	PO	ACE inhibitor	10 mg PO every day
Clonidine	PO	Centrally acting agent	0.1 mg PO 2 times per day
Clonidine patch	Transcutaneous	Centrally acting agent	TTS 1/weekly
Chlorothiazide	PO	Thiazide diuretic	500 mg PO every day
HCTZ	PO	Thiazide diuretic	25 mg PO every day
Furosemide	PO (or IV)	Loop diuretic	20 mg PO every day
Spironolactone	PO	Potassium-sparing diuretic	50 mg PO every day

PO = by mouth; HCTZ = hydrochlorothiazide; IV = intravenous; ACE = angiotensin-converting enzyme; TTS = transdermal therapeutic system.

control both the hypertension and the chest pain. Nitroglycerin reduces the myocardial demand for oxygen while reducing both preload and afterload. Nitroprusside is not the first-line drug therapy in hypertensive patients with myocardial ischemia because nitroprusside may cause a coronary steal phenomenon and increase the area of myocardial ischemia. Treat pulmonary edema as outlined in Chapter 28.

Catecholamine Crisis

There are many conditions that greatly increase catecholamine or catecholamine-like activity. Cocaine and amphetamine toxicity, antihypertensive drug withdrawal, alcohol withdrawal, and food or drug interactions with MAO inhibitors can lead to hypertensive crisis. Taking a good history is important in delineating what substances may be involved.

Pheochromocytomas may release dopamine, epinephrine, norepinephrine, and vasoactive peptides, resulting in severe hypertension. Classic symptoms include episodic hypertension associated with pallor and subsequent flushing, palpitations, headache, nervousness, excessive perspiration, and anxiety. In about one-half the cases, hypertension is sustained. Elevated levels of urinary vanillylmandelic acid and metanephrine are suggestive; direct measurement of elevated urinary or serum epinephrine or norepinephrine is diagnostic.

A patient with malignant hypertension and catecholamine crisis should be transferred to the ICU. ECG and intra-arterial BP monitoring is appropriate. Drug therapy is as follows:

1. Cocaine and amphetamine toxicity
   Propranolol 1 to 3 mg every 2 to 5 minutes IV to a maximum of 8 mg. Attempt to control both BP and tachycardia. Sedation may be helpful to reduce anxiety.
2. Pheochromocytoma
   The alpha-adrenergic blocking drugs are the treatment of choice. **Phenoxybenzamine hydrochloride** may be given **at an initial dose of 10 mg IV every 8 hours.** Phenoxybenzamine is a selective alpha blocker with a long duration of action. The dosage may be increased until all signs of catecholamine toxicity have resolved. Watch for postural hypotension with use of alpha-blocking drugs. Propranolol may be useful when cardiac dysrhythmias and severe tachycardia present. However, use propranolol only after alpha blockade has been performed (hypertensive crisis can ensue if alpha blockade is not performed and beta blockade is given).

17

HYPOTENSION AND SHOCK

Hypotension is a common and serious complication of a patient's hospital course. In mild and early stages there are many compensatory responses that can support tissue perfusion. If it worsens, circulatory collapse can ensue, resulting in shock. Shock is the extreme form of hypotension and refers to the condition of inadequate end-organ tissue perfusion. With a small amount of information and knowledge of a patient's trends over time, the early warning signs of hypotension may be detected and appropriately treated. Shock may not always be avoided, but the patient can receive the benefits of adequate circulation throughout the hypotensive episode.

The phone call will usually deal with a blood pressure (BP) number. Although this is of value, it is important to remember that there is no absolute systolic or diastolic number that defines hypotension. It is different in each patient. Look at the body's response, i.e., the pulse relative to the BP, orthostatic BPs, and tissue perfusion (especially skin, kidneys, and brain) before assuming that a particular BP is inadequate.

■ PHONE CALL

Questions

1. **What is the BP, and is this number a change in the BP trends?**
2. **How was the BP measured?**
   Consistency is the key. BPs will vary somewhat depending on the size of the BP cuff used, the limb used, and whether the value was derived from a normally functioning arterial line.
3. **What is the pulse?**
   Be especially mindful of orthostatic BPs with pulses. Is this a change in pulse trends?
4. **Are there changes in end-organ perfusion?**
   Is the patient conscious (brain)? What is the urine output (UO) (kidney)? Are the distal extremities warm (skin)?
5. **Has the patient undergone a surgical procedure, and if so, how long ago?**
   Is the patient having a surgically related loss of fluid such as postoperative bleeding or sequestration into a third space?

6. **Are there any other symptoms such as chest pain, respiratory distress, or rash?**
7. **Are there any changes in vital signs?**

   Be especially mindful of fever. Fever with hypotension is evidence of impending septic shock.

Orders

1. Order intravenous (IV) access.

   For rapid fluid replacement, a large-bore (16 gauge) peripheral IV is best. This will allow more rapid vascular space volume expansion than will central venous access. Begin fluid resuscitation through any existing line while another appropriate line is started. More than one line may be used and may be desirable.

2. Begin volume expansion.

   Rapid fluid replacement begins with crystalloid. This is the cheapest and most readily available fluid. Start with a **bolus of normal saline (NS) 500 ml IV** and repeat as necessary until the BP improves. If massive blood loss is the cause of the hypotension, consider replacement with O type, Rh negative uncrossmatched blood and NS.

3. Support cerebral perfusion.

   Place the patient in Trendelenburg's position with the feet elevated.

4. Support oxygenation.

   Have a pulse oximeter placed on the patient, and deliver O_2 by mask to keep the saturation at >90%. If tissue perfusion is poor, the pulse oximeter may not be effective. Deliver O_2 at 4 to 10 L/min by mask.

5. If the patient is anaphylactic (hives, hypotension, and respiratory distress), have epinephrine available for administration, as follows:

   Epinephrine (1:1000) 0.5 ml (0.5 mg) subcutaneously (SC) and

   Epinephrine (1:10,000) 5 ml (0.5 mg) IV.

   (Label these carefully by their route of administration, so no mistake is made. Either may be necessary, depending on the severity of the reaction.)

6. Send laboratory studies. The following should be sent immediately:

   - Complete blood count (CBC)

     Remember that the hemoglobin may be initially normal (or unchanged) in settings of acute hemorrhage.

   - Arterial blood gas (ABG)

     This will give information on acid–base status and oxygenation. Pay special attention to the base deficit. This is a good initial indication of the severity of the hypoperfu-

sion and may be followed sequentially to assess the efficacy of the resuscitation.
- Baseline serum chemistries

    Rapid fluid expansion will require frequent assessment of serum Na^+, K^+, Cl^-, blood urea nitrogen, and creatinine.
- Baseline urine chemistries

    End points of fluid resuscitation include normal urine output (UO) and normal specific gravity (1.010).
- Consider an immediate type and crossmatch for blood if acute hemorrhage is the cause of hypotension.
7. Consider other studies, as follows:
    - Portable chest x-ray immediately to assess for pneumothorax or pulmonary infection
    - 12-lead electrocardiogram (ECG)

Degree of Urgency

The patient must be evaluated immediately.

■ ELEVATOR THOUGHTS

What causes shock?

Remember that shock is inadequate for end-organ perfusion. Perfusion is based on appropriate cardiac function, blood volume, and peripheral vascular tone in relationships described by the following formulas:

$$\text{Cardiac output (CO)} = \text{heart rate (HR)} \times \text{stroke volume (SV)}$$

$$\text{BP} = \text{CO} \times \text{systemic vascular resistance (SVR)}$$

Factors that cause shock act at one or more of the elements that contribute to BP (CO or SVR).
1. Cardiogenic
    - Pump malfunction (inadequate HR or SV)
    - Occlusion of the outflow tract (inadequate CO)
2. Hypovolemic (inadequate SV)
3. Septic (inadequate SVR)
4. Anaphylactic (inadequate SVR)

■ MAJOR THREAT TO LIFE

- Shock
- Complications of inadequate perfusion
    1. Myocardial infarction (MI)
    2. Stroke
    3. Multiple organ failure

■ BEDSIDE

Quick Look Test

A hypotensive patient who is not yet in shock will appear well to mildly ill. A patient who is in shock will appear ill or moribund.

Airway and Vital Signs

1. Maintain the airway.

   If the patient is unconscious, place the patient in a supine position. Remove dentures and other foreign objects. Make sure the airway is patent and clear. An oral airway may be necessary. If the patient is very ill, consider endotracheal (ET) intubation. If patients cannot protect their own airways (aspiration or absent gag reflex), intubation is required to decrease the risk of aspiration pneumonia. Place the patient in the left lateral decubitus position until intubation is performed. Contact the intensive care unit (ICU)/cardiac care unit (CCU) for immediate transfer of the patient. Contact your resident.

2. Maintain respirations.

   If the patient is breathing spontaneously, maintaining the airway may be sufficient. Note the respirations, however; rapid, sonorous respirations are indicative of acidosis, which will require treatment. In addition, the work of breathing may be more effort than the patient can maintain, and ET intubation will be required to save the patient's energy.

3. Maximize oxygenation.

   The definition of shock is poor delivery of oxygen to the tissues. Oxygen delivery to the patient should be optimized to take advantage of what little perfusion is available.

4. Assess blood pressure.

   This should be done continuously during fluid resuscitation. In the ICU/CCU this may be done by continuous arterial line monitoring (see Chapter 19 for placement information). On the ward, serial BPs may be taken, or a mechanical BP device may be left on the patient during the resuscitative effort.

   Orthostatic BPs can help determine the intravascular volume status (see Chapter 12). Orthostatics are HR and BP taken while the patient is lying flat, while the patient is sitting, and while the patient is standing. If possible, allow 1 or 2 minutes to pass between each change in position so the patient may equilibrate. A rise in HR of 15 beats/min or a drop in systolic blood pressure of 15 mm Hg or any drop in diastolic blood pressure with a change in position is evidence of a significant intravascular deficit.

The absolute number of systolic pressure must be considered with the state of tissue perfusion. The three organs that give the most readily available information are the skin, the kidney, and the brain. Confirm the following:

- The skin is warm and moist

    One response to hypotension is to decrease perfusion of the peripheral vascular beds. Skin that is poorly perfused is cool, blue, and dry.

- The UO is adequate

    Normal UO is usually considered >20 ml/hr. A smaller urine volume is considered oliguria and may be due to hypotension.

- The patient is mentating well or at least at the baseline level

    Decreased tissue perfusion causes delirium, lethargy, and confusion. Extreme cases cause coma.

    If the patient has evidence of decreased tissue perfusion, this is the clinical definition of shock.

5. Assess the HR.

    Hypotension can have primary cardiac causes. Noting the timing and the quality of the pulse and analyzing the ECG can give vital information, as follows:

- Bradycardia

    Defined as <50 beats/min, bradycardia has many etiologies including the following:

    a. Autonomic dysfunction: The most common dysfunction is iatrogenic; beta blockade, or calcium channel blockers at normal or overdose levels, can cause an inability of the body to adequately respond to a hypotensive challenge; remember that the normal response to hypotension is a compensatory tachycardia; without the compensatory increase in HR, tissue perfusion can be in peril; other causes include sick sinus syndrome or primary autonomic neuropathy.

    b. Heart block: Usually as the result of acute MI, complete block is readily apparent on ECG (Fig. 17–1); see Chapter 9 for a complete discussion of the diagnosis and treatment of arrhythmias.

    c. Vasovagal reaction: This is generally a response to pain, change in position, or straining; if present, the hypotension is generally short lived.

- Tachycardia

    Sinus tachycardia is the expected response to hypotension. This includes HRs from 80 to 150 beats/min. Greater than this number is indicative of a tachyarrhythmia, which may require treatment. A rapid HR is not always associated with adequate stroke volume, as the

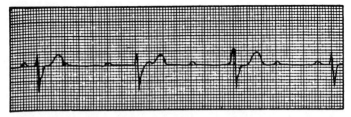

Figure 17–1 □ Bradycardia; third-degree atrioventricular block. (From Marshall SA, Ruedy J: On Call: Principles and Protocols, 2nd ed. Philadelphia, WB Saunders Co, 1993, p 131.)

heart may not have sufficient time for filling after each beat. Significant tachyarrhythmias include the following:

    a. Atrial fibrillation: The ventricular response rate varies but may be as rapid as 240 beats/min (Fig. 17–2). Note the absence of p waves.

    b. Supraventricular tachycardia (Fig. 17–3): The QRS complex may be narrow or wide.

    c. Ventricular tachycardia (Fig. 17–4): Note the wide QRS complex.

Any of these tachyarrhythmias are life threatening. Notify your resident immediately and institute cardiac life support (ACLS) protocols as necessary.

- Asystole

  This lack of rhythm would obviously result in hypotension. ACLS protocols should be instituted immediately.

- Electromechanical dissociation

  Electromechanical dissociation (EMD) is an uncoupling of the electrical stimulation of the heart as seen on ECG from the mechanical action of pumping. Whenever a rhythm is noted on cardiac monitoring, confirm that the rhythm actually corresponds to a palpable pulse.

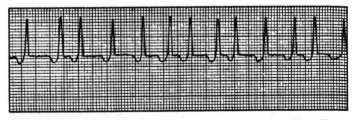

Figure 17–2 □ Atrial fibrillation with rapid ventricular response. (From Marshall SA, Ruedy J: On Call: Principles and Protocols, 2nd ed. Philadelphia, WB Saunders Co, 1993, p 154.)

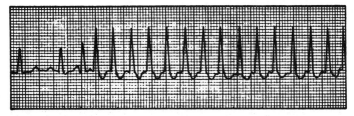

Figure 17–3 □ Supraventricular tachycardia. (From Marshall SA, Ruedy J: On Call: Principles and Protocols, 2nd ed. Philadelphia, WB Saunders Co, 1993, p 154.)

EMD is also a medical emergency and requires institution of ACLS protocols.

Initial Management

In addition to the measures started in the orders section above,

1. If the patient is bradycardic, give **atropine 0.5 mg IV; may repeat every 15 minutes to a total dose of 2 mg**.
2. If the patient has a tachyarrhythmia, refer to Chapter 9 for a complete discussion on treatment.

Selective Physical Examination

Look for clues as to the cause of the hypotension. This may be done while resuscitative efforts are under way. Examination of the patient does not preclude initiation of fluid replacement.

Fluid status: Perform a rapid fluid status assessment (see Chapter 12)

VS: Repeat frequently during the resuscitative effort

MS: Declining mental status, delirium, confusion, or coma (decreased tissue perfusion)

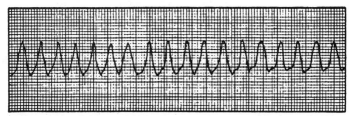

Figure 17–4 □ Ventricular tachycardia. (From Marshall SA, Ruedy J: On Call: Principles and Protocols, 2nd ed. Philadelphia, WB Saunders Co, 1993, p 155.)

HEENT:	Elevated jugular venous distention (JVD) (congestive heart failure [CHF]); flat neck veins (hypovolemia)
CVS:	S_3 (CHF); arrhythmia
Resp:	Wheezes (anaphylaxis and CHF); crackles (CHF)
GU:	Oliguria (decreased tissue perfusion)
Skin:	Cyanosis, cool, and clammy (decreased tissue perfusion); hives with urticaria (anaphylaxis)
Extrem:	Ankle or presacral edema (CHF)
Additional tests:	As outlined above in the orders

■ MANAGEMENT

- **Normalize intravascular volume**.

    The goal of this treatment is to optimize cardiac preload. Look quickly at the neck veins of the patient. If the veins are distended, then preload may be high, and it is the pump that is not working well. The finding of rales and peripheral edema will also support the diagnosis of CHF. This is cardiogenic shock and is treated with fluid restriction and preload reduction (see Chapter 28 for the treatment of CHF).

    If the neck veins are flat, then preload may be inadequate. All forms of shock other than cardiogenic are treated initially with fluid. The fluid of choice is crystalloid. The absolute volume required is patient dependent and may be large. Repeat boluses of NS or lactated Ringer's in volumes of 200 to 500 ml are sufficient. These are given until tissue perfusion returns.

    Fluid resuscitation will require frequent monitoring of fluid and electrolyte status for safety.

    1. Send baseline electrolytes, urinalysis, and CBC.

        Repeat electrolytes every 6 to 8 hours during rapid fluid replacement until the patient stabilizes, then reduce as is reasonable.

    2. Send baseline ABG for a base deficit.

        Base deficit is a reasonable reflection of serum lactate levels. This is a good screening test of the severity of the initial hypoperfusion and may be followed hourly to assess the resuscitation. As perfusion improves, base deficit will return to normal.

    3. Place a Foley catheter to monitor UO.

        Adequate UO (>20 ml/hr) is a good end point to use to judge hydration.

    4. Place the patient on cardiac monitoring, especially if the patient is at risk for MI or CHF.

5. If necessary, gain central venous access to monitor central venous pressure (CVP) (see Chapter 19 for techniques to gain access to the central venous system).

Normal CVP is 0 to 6 cm H_2O (this corresponds to a JVD of 2–3 cm). For some patients it may be necessary to maintain a CVP in the 7 to 10 cm H_2O range to ensure adequate preload. A CVP of >15 cm H_2O is indication of left ventricular dysfunction. For patients with a history of cardiac events or for very ill patients, a Swan-Ganz catheter may be necessary to give adequate cardiac data. Swan-Ganz catheterization is best left for ICU/CCU management and is not frequently used in patients on the ward.

- **Give inotropic agents**.

Further support cardiac output and perfusion with vasopressor agents as necessary. Inotropic support should not be given without first optimizing the intravascular fluid volume. The action of these agents results from interaction at the various adrenergic receptors:

1. Alpha: Located on vascular smooth muscle; effects include vasoconstriction, resulting in increased SVR.
2. Beta$_1$: Effects are inotropic and chronotropic, resulting in increased CO.
3. Beta$_2$: Effects include dilation of smooth muscles, resulting in decreased SVR.

These agents generally require central venous access and ICU/CCU transfer. Commonly used drip preparations are summarized in Table 17–1. The physiologic effects are summarized in Table 17–2. Because increasing SVR will ultimately diminish the blood flow to some organs, watch carefully for changes in UO or other end-organ dysfunction when administering alpha-adrenergic agents.

- **Correct hypoxia**.

Part of maintaining adequate tissue perfusion is optimizing the oxygen delivered to the end-organs. If the patient is in shock, distal extremity perfusion may not be adequate for a pulse oximeter to give reliable data. Rely on ABG data. Deliver O_2 by mask to maintain arterial partial pressure of O_2 (PaO_2) of >60 mm Hg. Monitor ABG data as needed. Consider transfusions of packed red blood cells for a hematocrit of $<25\%$.

- **Correct acidosis**.

Poor tissue perfusion results in tissue hypoxia. The conversion to anaerobic metabolism is associated with the buildup of lactic acid and metabolic acidosis. Monitor this with ABGs and base deficits. Acidosis secondary to hypoperfusion is generally treated by improving the peripheral circulation. The administration of sodium bicarbonate is reserved for code situations. In some cases, correction of pH of <7.2 with bicar-

Table 17-1 □ COMMON INTRAVENOUS DRIP INOTROPIC AGENTS

Name	Action	Indication	Dose Range	Comments
Amrinone	Nonadrenergic	Cardiogenic shock	5–20 μg/kg/min	Long half-life (6 hr)
Dobutamine	β₁-adrenergic	Cardiogenic shock	2.5–10 μg/kg/min	Titrate to desired BP
Dopamine	Dopaminergic	Renal perfusion	1–2 μg/kg/min	
	α, β₁-adrenergic	Cardiogenic shock	2–10 μg/kg/min	Titrate to desired BP
	α-adrenergic	Hypotension	10–20 μg/kg/min	Titrate to desired BP
Epinephrine	α, β-adrenergic	Hypotension, low SVR	0.025–0.1 μg/kg/min	Titrate to desired BP, increased myocardial O₂ use
Isoproterenol	β-adrenergic	Bradycardia, septic shock	0.05–0.5 μg/kg/min	Titrate to desired BP, increased myocardial O₂ use
Norepinephrine	α, β-adrenergic	Hypotension, low SVR	0.05–0.5 μg/kg/min	Titrate to desired BP, increased myocardial O₂ use

BP = blood pressure; SVR = systemic vascular resistance.

Table 17–2 □ PHYSIOLOGIC EFFECTS OF INOTROPIC AGENTS

Name	CO	PCWP	SVR	MAP	HR	CVP	PVR
Amrinone	↑	↓	↓	↔	↑	↓	↓
Dobutamine	↑	↓	↓	↑	↑	↓	↓
Dopamine							
1–6 µg/kg/min	↑	↑↓	↑↓	↑↓	↑	↑↓	↔
7–20 µg/kg/min	↑	↑	↑	↑	↑	↑	↑
Epinephrine	↑	↔	↑↓	↑	↑	↔	↑
Isoproterenol	↑	↓	↓	↓	↑	↓	↓
Norepinephrine	↑	↑	↑	↑	↔	↑	↑

CO = cardiac output; PCWP = pulmonary capillary wedge pressure; SVR = systemic vascular resistance; MAP = mean arterial pressure; HR = heart rate; CVP = central venous pressure; PVR = pulmonary vascular resistance; ↑ = increased; ↓ = decreased; ↔ = unchanged.

bonate is desirable. See Chapter 12 for a complete discussion of acidosis.

- **Give additional treatment** based on underlying etiology, as follows:

Cardiogenic Shock
Hypotension and Elevated JVD

The causes of cardiogenic shock are essentially the causes of CHF. MI heads the list. The treatment for CHF is described in Chapter 28. It is important to confirm that the patient is in CHF. Other causes of hypotension associated with elevated JVD include the following (each is an emergent situation and necessitates contacting the resident):

1. Tamponade
   Look for Beck's triad of hypotension, elevated JVD, and muffled heart tones. Pulsus paradoxus of >10 mm Hg also suggests this diagnosis. It is treated by emergent pericardiocentesis as described in Chapter 28.
2. Pulmonary embolus
   Cyanosis and marked hypoxia may suggest this diagnosis. Look also for evidence of right-sided heart failure, i.e., enlarged liver, peripheral edema, right ventricular heave, tricuspid murmur, and increased pulmonary heart sound.
3. Superior vena cava obstruction
   Look for swelling that is limited to the face and upper extremities. Also, collateral venous return may be prominent.
4. Tension pneumothorax
   Respiratory distress and hypoxia associated with hyper-resonance of a hemithorax. The trachea may be deviated away from the side of the pneumothorax. It is initially treated with placement of a 16-gauge angiocatheter into the thorax at the midclavicular line between the first and second ribs. This will confirm the diagnosis and allow a venting of built-up pressure. A tube thoracostomy must then be placed (see Chapter 28).

Hypovolemic Shock
Hypotension with Fluid Loss or Redistribution

The source of intravascular fluid loss may not be readily apparent.

1. Postoperative or acute gastrointestinal blood loss should be evaluated and treated as described in Chapters 26 and 13, respectively.
2. Excess fluid loss or sequestration should be treated with NS replacement; sequestration, as with acute pancreatitis, may require massive fluid replacement.
3. Inotropic agents are used to maintain perfusion unresponsive to fluid resuscitation alone.

Use of most vasopressor agents requires placement of central venous access and ICU/CCU transfer. Occasionally, **dopamine** administration in doses of **2–5 µg/kg/min** are used in patients to facilitate renal perfusion.

4. Certain medications may contribute to poor perfusion by their effects on the heart or the circulatory system. Among the more common offenders are
   - Opiates
   - Nitroglycerin
   - Beta blockers
   - Calcium channel blockers
   - Other antihypertensives
   - Sedative medications

   The treatment of medication-associated hypovolemia is often fluid support, Trendelenburg's position, and time.

5. Some medications have specific antidotes.
   - Opiates can be reversed with **naloxone (Narcan) 0.2 to 2.0 mg IV, intramuscularly (IM), SC,** or **endotracheal tube (ET) with repetition of the dose every 5 minutes to a total dose of 10 mg**.
   - Some benzodiazepines can be reversed with **flumazenil (Romazicon) 0.2 mg IV over 30 seconds. A dose of 0.3 mg may be given** if there is no response in 5 minutes, **followed by subsequent doses of 0.5 mg every 5 minutes to a total dose of 3 to 5 mg. The effective dose may be repeated every 20 minutes, delivered at a rate of 0.2 mg/min to a total of 3 mg/hr.**

Septic Shock

Hypotension and Fever

Note that the onset of septic shock may be increased tissue warmth associated with tachycardia, as the peripheral beds initially dilate. During the early stages of sepsis, respiratory alkalosis is the rule. As hypoperfusion worsens, acidosis becomes apparent. In addition to supportive measures, the treatment of septic shock is based on identification of the offending microorganism, correction of the source, and administration of appropriate IV antibiotics. This usually starts off as empirical wide-spectrum therapy, which is subsequently narrowed as the organism is identified. Fluid resuscitation is usually supported with vasopressor administration. Prolonged hypotension requires transfer to the ICU/CCU.

Anaphylactic Shock

Hypotension, Hives, and Wheezing

The onset of anaphylactic shock is usually associated with an identifiable source (e.g., penicillin and contrast dye). Treatment of anaphylactic shock is outlined in Chapter 8.

Irreversible Shock and Multiple Organ Failure Syndrome

Prolonged or refractory shock will lead to the complications of hypoperfusion. This affects most organ systems and is termed multiple organ failure syndrome (MOFS). The etiology of MOFS is unclear. There is not specific treatment other than ICU/CCU level support. Despite aggressive treatment of injuries and infections and adequate delivery of oxygen to the tissues, the mortality of patients with MOFS remains quite high.

■ SPECIAL SURGICAL CONSIDERATIONS

Preoperative Considerations

1. Shock may be the reason to operate.
   If a septic source cannot be found in a patient with abdominal pain, consider necrotic bowel as a source.
2. Shock is an indication to cancel an elective case.
   Contact your resident or attending physician.

Postoperative Considerations

1. Sequestration of fluids may result in hypovolemic shock.
   This is common after major abdominal procedures. Adequate preoperative and intraoperative hydration may not be sufficient to maintain hydration in a postoperative patient.
2. In a recent postoperative patient who develops hypotension, always consider postoperative bleeding as a possible source.
   Remember that the initial hemoglobin may be normal despite significant blood loss. A change may not be noted until after rehydration has occurred.

Remember

1. Prolonged hypotension with decreased tissue perfusion will have late complications such as MI, acute tubular necrosis, and stroke. These usually happen 2 to 3 days after a significant hypotensive event.
2. Though toxic shock syndrome is most common in premenopausal women, it can occur in any patient, regardless of sex or age.
3. Nearly all forms of shock will require ICU/CCU care and monitoring. Do not hesitate to discuss transfer of the patient with your resident.

18

INSOMNIA

The hospital is unfamiliar to many patients. The late-night "sleeping hours" in hospitals are interrupted with disruptions from other patients, nursing checks, and noisy monitoring equipment. Many patients become very fatigued, yet are unable to sleep. Calls requesting "sleepers" for patients will be common. For this type of call, it is generally not necessary to examine the patient at the bedside. Ordering a safe, effective sleep-inducing medication is appropriate.

■ PHONE CALL

Questions

1. **What is the patient's reason for hospitalization, and is the patient preoperative or postoperative?**

    Learn why the patient is in the hospital. If the patient is postoperative, is he or she in pain? If so, order an appropriate analgesic. If the patient is preoperative, is he or she anxious? A preoperative patient may benefit from a sleeping medication.

2. **Does the patient have any medical problems?**

    Ask the RN about the patient's pertinent medical history. Benzodiazepines are among the most commonly prescribed sedative/hypnotics. These drugs are oxidized in the liver. Care must be used when administering these drugs in patients with liver disease. Also be careful when using benzodiazepines in patients who have recently consumed alcohol, because alcohol increases the toxicity of benzodiazepines.

3. **What is the patient's age?**

    Beware of using benzodiazepines for elderly or frail patients. The half-life of these drugs may be increased up to fourfold in elderly patients. Think about using a sleeping medication with a short half-life. Some elderly patients do best with a nonbenzodiazepine drug.

4. **Does the patient have any drug allergies or a history of adverse reactions to drugs?**

    Obviously, avoid using a drug to which a patient has had an allergic or adverse reaction. Common adverse reactions to sedative/hypnotic drugs include excessive sedation, prolonged drowsiness, and nightmares.

5. **Has the patient been provided a sleeping medication recently that was effective?**

There is no reason to change a medication that has been effective previously.

Orders

The key to selecting an appropriate sleeper is to choose a drug that causes the least long-term sedation and the fewest side effects. The following are important suggestions:

- **Diphenhydramine hydrochloride (Benadryl)** is a safe drug to use in elderly or frail patients.

  It has both an antihistamine and a sedative effect. It is metabolized in the liver, so the drug will have a prolonged half-life in patients with cirrhosis. In frail or elderly patients, consider a dose of **25 mg orally (PO) just before sleep**. If this is not effective, the dose can be repeated.

- Chloral hydrate is especially safe and effective in children.

  This drug is metabolized in the liver and has an active metabolite that determines the half-life of action.

- A relatively new nonbenzodiazepine sleeper, Ambien, acts at the gamma-aminobutyric acid receptor. It has relatively few side effects and a short half-life and is a safe drug.

- The benzodiazepines are the most commonly prescribed

Table 18–1 □ **DRUGS USEFUL FOR INSOMNIA: SEDATIVE/ HYPNOTICS**

Drug	Dose	Half-life
Common benzodiazepines		
Triazolam (Halcion)*	0.125–0.5 mg PO just before sleep	2–3 hr
Flurazepam HCl (Dalmane)	15–30 mg PO just before sleep	50–100 hr
Temazepam (Restoril)*	15–30 mg PO just before sleep	9–12 hr
Nonbenzodiazepine agents		
Diphenhydramine HCl (Benadryl)	25–50 mg PO just before sleep	2.4–9 hr
Zolpidem tartrate (Ambien)	10 mg PO just before sleep	2.5 hr
Chloral hydrate	25–50 mg/kg, to 1000 mg maximum, PO or PR just before sleep	8–11 hr

*Benzodiazepine drugs with inactive metabolites. Benzodiazepines with inactive metabolites are useful in patients with liver disease.
PO = orally; PR = rectally.

sleeping medications and are useful in many adult patients with normal liver function.

The benzodiazepines combine sedation with an anxiolytic effect. Beware that the benzodiazepines may be habit forming with long-term use and have the potential for abuse. In addition, some benzodiazepines are more useful for anxiolytic purposes than for insomnia (e.g., diazepam [Valium] and lorazepam [Ativan]).

Table 18–1 gives common drugs useful for insomnia.

19

INTRAVASCULAR ACCESS

Intravascular access is a means to administer fluids and medications, and it is a valuable tool for gathering hemodynamic information. The loss of "access" is a common reason for a phone call. This chapter will provide orientation to various types of intravascular access, procedures to attain them, and common complications and problems. Some hospitals require informed consent before some of these procedures are performed; find out what the specific regulations are at your institution. Proprietary kits for intravascular line placement have specific instructions to follow for safe placement. The suggestions below do not attempt to supersede the written instructions supplied with each kit. Read the kit instructions, and follow the steps carefully. Perform procedures only if you are comfortable with them; enlist the help of more experienced personnel if you are unsure.

Loss of Line Function

■ PHONE CALL

Questions

1. **Why does a patient need intravascular access?**
   Reasons may range from hemodynamic monitoring by arterial or central venous lines, nutrition or medication delivery through central access, need for hemodialysis, or administration of medication or fluids through peripheral lines.

2. **Is the access still necessary?**
   Often lines remain in place long after their usefulness is gone. There may be enteral routes or other options available for use. Even if you determine continued need for intravascular access, the patient may be stable enough to wait for intravenous (IV) line placement in the morning by the regular care team.

3. **Are there immediate problems with the access?**
   These are discussed in the sections for the individual lines, but the question should be asked, because some problems such as severe bleeding or shortness of breath (SOB) may be life threatening.

4. **How long has the existing line been in place?**
   Long-term access lines such as long-arm or PICC (periph-

erally inserted central venous catheter) lines or Hickman-type catheters are designed to remain in for weeks to months but may have thrombotic or infectious complications. Other "medium-term" lines such as multilumen central venous access catheters or arterial lines may require removal and reinsertion with a clean line every 3 to 5 days to minimize infectious risk.

5. **Are there any other symptoms?**
6. **Are there any changes in vital signs?**

Orders

1. Have the means available to restart the access, if necessary, which may include peripheral IV trays or specific kits for arterial line or central venous access.
2. Respond to any immediate problem such as bleeding or SOB as necessary.

Degree of Urgency

Loss of peripheral access is not an emergency unless a specific, important medication such as heparin is interrupted. If there is a significant change in vital signs or symptoms, the patient must be evaluated immediately.

■ ELEVATOR THOUGHTS

What causes loss of IV access?
1. Reevaluate the need for intravascular access.
2. Think about the various options for vascular access.
    There may be more than one approach that is appropriate in an individual patient.
3. Causes of loss of function of a line are as follows:
    - Kinking of the line
    - Loose or disconnected line
    - IV pump failure
    - Intraluminal blockage
    - Thrombosis of the vessel
    - Thrombophlebitis
    - Misplacement of the line by initial insertion or migration

■ MAJOR THREAT TO LIFE

- Loss of vital hemodynamic information
- Interruption of important medication

■ Life-threatening complication, such as pneumothorax after central venous line placement, or arterial thrombosis of a peripheral limb associated with an arterial line.

■ BEDSIDE

Quick Look Test

If there is a specific complaint related to the line, such as SOB or pain, the patient may look distressed. A malfunctioning line usually produces no symptoms. The patient may be distressed by the IV infusion pump alarms or by a leak in the IV tubing.

Airway and Vital Signs

There is generally no derangement in vital signs due to the nonfunction of the line, unless the medications delivered are responsible for altering cardiopulmonary physiology (such as inotropic agents). If thrombophlebitis is present, fever may be apparent.

Selective Physical Examination

VS:	Repeat as necessary.
Line site:	Inspect the line: look for kinks and loose connections. Inspect the IV pump: is it on and functioning correctly? Inspect the fluid: is there fluid remaining in the IV bottle?
Skin:	Is there redness, swelling, purulence, or clear fluid collection under the dressing?
Extrem:	If the IV is in a peripheral site, look for swelling or discoloration of the limb; feel for distal pulses.
Additional tests:	
1. CXR:	This is for evaluation of inferior jugular (IJ) and subclavian central line tip placement. The tip should be at the superior vena cava (SVC). Occasionally, after placement of a subclavian line, the tip can be found in the IJ vein. If out of place, the line must be repositioned. The CXR is also diagnostic when evaluating for pneumothorax following central line placement.
2. Aspiration:	Aspiration should be done in a sterile fashion. Wipe the connection with a

small amount of iodine. Disconnect the IV tubing from the hub of the line, and immediately attach a 5- to 10-ml syringe to the hub. For a central line, wait for exhalation before detaching the IV tubing. Gently aspirate. Removal of a small-tip thrombus is usually sufficient to clear the line. Continue to aspirate until 3 to 5 ml of blood have been collected. Discard the blood and reconnect the line to the IV tubing. Replace a sterile dressing. Never flush the line, because this might dislodge a larger clot propagating from the tip of the catheter into the vena cava and result in a pulmonary embolus.

■ MANAGEMENT

1. If repositioning or aspiration of the line is unsuccessful in restoring function, another way of delivering medication is required. Ask a few basic questions:
   - Does the patient still need intravascular access?
     Is the patient taking food or medication orally (PO)? Can current medication be switched to PO or intramuscular (IM) administration?
   - Must the access be central access?
     Is the patient on medication that requires central access, such as total parenteral nutrition (TPN), chemotherapy, inotropic drugs, or irritating medication such as amphotericin?
   - Are there other ports on an existing central catheter that are usable? If the site is clean, the line may be changed to a new one over a wire (Seldinger technique).
     If there is a problem with the site, such as erythema, the existing line must be removed regardless of the patency of the other lumens.
2. A new site is required if
   - The current skin site is red or purulent
   - The patient is febrile
   - The line is clogged through the distal port (as this also may dislodge a clot propagating from the tip of the catheter)
3. Restart IV access if required.
4. If removal of the existing central line is required, remember to send the catheter tip for culture, if required; also hold pressure at the skin site after removal for 10 minutes (by the clock) to ensure adequate hemostasis.

■ SPECIAL SURGICAL CONSIDERATIONS

Occasionally, a surgical house staff member is called to remove a longer-term line such as a Hickman catheter. These differ from temporary central venous access in that a Dacron fiber cuff is present under the skin a short distance from the insertion site. The toughness of the adherence of the subcutaneous tissue to this cuff depends on the length of time during which the catheter has been in and on the healing properties of the patient. The removal of these lines is discussed below.

Bleeding from the Site

■ PHONE CALL

Questions

1. **Is this the only site of bleeding?**
   Blood oozing from more than one site may be evidence of coagulopathy.
2. **Is the line functional?**
3. **Did the patient undergo a surgical procedure, and if so, how long ago?**
4. **Are there any other symptoms?**
5. **Are there any changes in vital signs?**

Orders

1. Have the means available to restart the access, if necessary; this may include peripheral IV trays or specific kits for arterial line or central venous access.
2. Respond to any immediate problems.

Degree of Urgency

If there is a significant change in vital signs or symptoms, the patient must be evaluated immediately.

■ ELEVATOR THOUGHTS

What causes bleeding from an IV site?
1. A new site will ooze slightly, which should stop within several hours.
2. Coagulopathy, causing bleeding, may result from the following:

- Medications including heparin, warfarin, streptokinase, and tissue plasminogen activator (t-PA).
- Platelet dysfunction from thrombocytopenia or nonsteroidal anti-inflammatory drugs (NSAIDs).
- Clotting factor deficiency
- Dilutional coagulopathy
- Disseminated intravascular coagulation (DIC)

■ MAJOR THREAT TO LIFE

- Soft-tissue swelling; subcutaneous blood can exert pressure on surrounding structures; depending on the site of the line, the hematoma can displace lung (with a subclavian line) or trachea (with an IJ line)
- Loss of vital hemodynamic information
- Interruption of important medication
- Life-threatening complication, such as pneumothorax after central venous line placement, or arterial thrombosis of a peripheral limb associated with an arterial line

■ BEDSIDE

Quick Look Test

Minor bleeding is not associated with discomfort. If the bleeding is due to impending sepsis, the patient may appear ill.

Airway and Vital Signs

If the line is in the IJ site, pay special attention to the patient's airway. Is the patient breathing well? If a significant amount of blood is lost, pulse rate may be elevated and blood pressure (BP) may drop.

■ MANAGEMENT

1. Inspect the wound.
   Remove the dressing and clean around the site. Try to identify a specific site of oozing, which is often not possible.
2. If no specific site can be identified, apply pressure (with a gloved hand) at the site for 20 minutes (by the clock).
3. Recheck the site, being careful not to dislodge any clot that may have formed; if bleeding continues, hold pressure for another 20 minutes.

4. If bleeding continues, consider evaluation of the patient for coagulopathy.

See Chapter 26 for evaluation and treatment of bleeding disorders.

5. Bleeding may compromise the function of the line, and if this is the case, consider replacement of the line but at another site.

Purulence at the Site

■ PHONE CALL

Questions

1. **Is the patient febrile?**
2. **Are there other signs of infection?**
3. **Is the line functional?**
4. **Did the patient undergo a surgical procedure, and if so, how long ago?**
5. **Are there any other symptoms?**
6. **Are there any changes in vital signs?**

Orders

1. Have the means available to restart the access, if necessary.
   This may include peripheral IV trays or specific kits for arterial line or central venous access.
2. Respond to any immediate problems.

Degree of Urgency

If there is a significant change in vital signs or symptoms, the patient must be evaluated immediately.

■ ELEVATOR THOUGHTS

What causes purulence at an IV site?
1. Local site infection
2. Suppurative thrombophlebitis
3. Line sepsis

■ MAJOR THREAT TO LIFE

- Sepsis

■ BEDSIDE

Quick Look Test

A local wound infection may cause only minor discomfort at the site. If the patient has suppurative thrombophlebitis or impending sepsis, he or she will appear ill.

Airway and Vital Signs

Evaluate the patient as if sepsis is impending. Look at fluid status, pulse rate, and BP, including orthostatics. Fever is the hallmark of severe infection and usually indicates that the line must be removed.

■ MANAGEMENT

1. Evaluate the site.
   If there is redness of the skin or any purulence from the wound site, the line must be removed. Clean the site carefully before removal. Do this sterilely so that the tip of the line may be sent for culture.
2. Express pus from the skin site if possible; this may also be sent for Gram stain and culture.
3. If the patient is febrile, blood cultures should be sent.
   It is possible to draw one sample through the existing line, but be sure to draw one elsewhere from a new skin puncture.
4. Appropriate antibiotics must be started.
   Most site infections are staphylococcal; these respond best to synthetic penicillins, first-generation cephalosporins, or vancomycin. Focus the antibiotic therapy based on culture and Gram stain results.
5. If IV access is still required, the line must be replaced.
   Try not to do this while the patient is febrile and is at risk for exhibiting bacteremia. Avoid skin sites that are red, macerated, or breaking down.
6. Suppurative thrombophlebitis must be suspected if the white blood cell (WBC) count is elevated or if the patient is septic.
   Do not be fooled by the absence of skin findings. The hallmarks include tenderness at an existing or previous IV insertion site in the setting of fever and elevated WBC count.

Vein sites must be explored surgically in the patient who has no other source of fever. Recovery of normal vein is a negative result. Vein occluded with clot or pus is evidence of thrombophlebitis, and the entire infected vein must be excised. The skin is left open to drain. Send a portion of the excised vein to pathology for histology and a portion to microbiology for culture and sensitivities. Antibiotics must be initiated.

7. If the patient is hemodynamically unstable, resuscitate aggressively and treat shock as outlined in Chapter 17.

8. Many centers advocate changing lines and line sites every 72 hours, which is a good guideline but occasionally is impractical in the patient in whom it is difficult to gain access.

Shortness of Breath After Insertion of a Central Line

Pneumothorax is a common complication of central line placement in IJ and subclavian sites. It should be suspected in a patient who has a central line in place that is recent. There are other, less common causes of SOB that must also be considered. See also Chapter 28 for a complete discussion on diagnosis and management of SOB.

■ PHONE CALL

Questions

1. **How long has the patient been short of breath?**
2. **How long has the line been in place?**
   Complications of central line placement may happen immediately after insertion or may be delayed by days.
3. **Did the patient undergo a surgical procedure, and if so, how long ago?**
4. **Are there any other symptoms?**
   Is the patient complaining of chest pain? Is the patient cyanotic or hypoxic?
5. **Are there any changes in vital signs?**
   Hypotension and increased respiratory rate are indicative of pneumothorax.

Orders

1. If the line is new, order posterior-to-anterior (PA) and lateral chest x-rays (CXRs) immediately.

This may be at the bedside if necessary. Order inspiratory and expiratory films, as pneumothorax is often best noted on the expiratory film.
2. Check oxygenation with a pulse oximeter, and treat hypoxia as necessary.
3. Treat hypotension with fluid resuscitation and pressors as necessary.
4. Have sterile gloves, dressing supplies, and 16-gauge needle at the bedside for diagnosis and treatment of tension pneumothorax.

Degree of Urgency

The patient must be evaluated immediately.

■ ELEVATOR THOUGHTS

What causes SOB after central line placement?
1. Local hematoma at a neck site causing pressure on the trachea
2. Pneumothorax (including tension pneumothorax)
3. Hemothorax
4. Tamponade
5. Air embolus
6. Pleural effusion

■ MAJOR THREAT TO LIFE

- Obstruction of the upper airway due to tracheal pressure
- Tamponade
- Tension pneumothorax
- Air embolus

■ BEDSIDE

Quick Look Test

Patients will tend to look sick. If tension pneumothorax, tamponade, or air embolus is present, the patient may look moribund.

Airway and Vital Signs

Tachypnea is generally apparent regardless of the cause. Tachycardia is present in tamponade and in tension pneumothorax and may be present simply because the patient is in distress. Hypotension is ominous and indicates tension pneumothorax or tamponade.

Selective Physical Examination

VS:	Check again now
HEENT:	Tracheal deviation and swelling at the insertion site in the neck (local hematoma)
CVS:	Pulsus paradoxus and elevated jugular venous distention (tamponade and tension pneumothorax)
	Muffled heart tones (tamponade or pericardial effusion)
Resp:	Unilateral decrease in breath sounds, and hyperresonance (pneumothorax)
	Dull to percussion (pleural effusion)
Line site:	Are connections tight? (air embolus)

■ MANAGEMENT

1. Each of these situations is life threatening; contact your resident immediately.
2. See Chapter 28 for evaluation and emergency treatment of tension pneumothorax and tamponade.
3. If there is upper airway obstruction, be prepared to intubate.
   Contact your resident and the intensive care unit (ICU) or the cardiac care unit team for airway protection and transfer of the patient.
4. Air embolism is treated by placement of the patient on the right side in Trendelenburg's position to sequester the air bubbles in the right ventricle.
   These will generally resorb, although some authors recommend aspiration of the air from the ventricle.

Placement of Intravascular Lines

■ STERILE TECHNIQUE

The major complication to intravascular access is that of infection locally at the insertion site, in the vessel itself, or as a widespread condition (line sepsis). The cleaner the insertion technique, the lower the risk of infectious complication. The following are some guidelines for establishing and maintaining a clean insertion.

1. **Make sure that the workspace is well lit and comfortable.**
    Sterility is often broken while having to reposition light-ing or a sterile field. Clear the area of objects that might catch sleeves or feet, and have room in which to move.
2. **Make sure all the required instruments and equipment are within easy reach.**
    This requires planning but will soon become second na-ture.
3. **Have an assistant standing by, if necessary; make sure it is someone familiar with sterile technique.**
4. **Inform the patient that a sterile field is going to be used, and instruct that areas of sterility are not to be touched.**
    It is also important to explain that the drapes are going to cover the eyes or airway temporarily. Always explain if there are uncomfortable or painful steps in the process, and warn before they occur. Sterility is often broken when a patient startles after a painful stimulus such as a needle poke.
5. **Prepare the insertion site.**
    Use alcohol or an iodine-based disinfectant soap and clean (or prep) the area well. Solution on gauze or prepack-aged swab sticks may be used. Start from the center of the desired field and work outward, cleaning a wider area than anticipated. Repeat with fresh gauze or swab for a total of three cleanings. If desired, more than one area may be initially prepared, and a second site may be kept sterile with a drape while the first site is being used.
6. **Scrub your hands with a disinfectant soap.**
    Remove jewelry first, and don a mask and cap before scrubbing, especially if the line will be needed for a long time, or if the patient is immunocompromised.
7. **Don sterile gloves and gown.**
    Get help to learn how to do this in a sterile fashion.
8. **Drape the area with sterile towels.**
    Make sure that the only thing visible through the "window" made with the towels is "prepared" skin. The towel may already be fenestrated, or a window can be made by using two or more towels. Drapes can be held in place with towel clamps.
9. **Try not to move from the sterile field (unless absolutely necessary).**
    Once in place and working, be mindful of where nonster-ile areas of the body are (elbows, hair, and waist).
10. **Work quickly and carefully.**
11. **Admit freely if there has been a break in sterility.**
    Often the constraints of time and pride invite overlooking a minor break in sterility. Time saved, however, will be more than matched by time required to care for a sicker

patient if a complication arises. Do not hesitate to "break scrub," rewash, redrape, and begin again if sterility has been broken. Do not put the patient at risk.

12. **The procedure is not finished until the line is secured.**

    Secure the line by taping, suturing, or tying down. Do this before removing the drapes. Make sure the line is secure even if a CXR is required to assess placement of the line before its use.

13. **Protect the line.**

    Place a dressing, including an antimicrobial ointment, over the site. Confirm all connections and joints before careful removal of the drapes.

14. **Prepare and drape the area again if repositioning of the line is necessary.**

■ SELDINGER TECHNIQUE

Some intravascular access is achieved by using a preplaced guide wire. This technique is also useful for replacing existing lines with clean catheters.

1. **Use sterile technique.**
2. **Prepare the skin as above.**
3. **Infiltrate the site with lidocaine.**
4. **Puncture the skin with the needle (usually, 18 gauge) on a 10-ml syringe.**

    Insert while aspirating until there is easy backflow of blood. Often the vein is encountered on the way out, so aspirate also while withdrawing the needle.

5. **While holding the needle in place, gently remove the syringe.**

    Be careful to hold a finger over the hub of the needle to stop the outflow of blood, and be careful to avoid the inflow of air.

6. **Insert the guide wire gently.**

    It should go into the vessel in the same direction as the catheter will go. It should pass as easily as a wire passing through very soft butter. If the wire does not pass easily, **DO NOT FORCE IT.** Remove the needle and the guide wire together, and reposition the needle before reinsertion of the wire. Examination of the guide wire before starting will show that if the wire abuts against a wall it will bend toward the curve of the "J" (Fig. 19–1). This may be exploited when a difficult placement is anticipated. Insert the wire in the orientation such that it will tend to bend toward the desired direction.

7. **If the needle must be removed because of inability to**

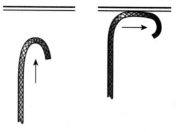

Figure 19–1 □ Typical bending pattern of J-wires.

pass the wire, DO NOT REMOVE THE WIRE FROM THE NEEDLE.

The bevel of the needle is sharp enough to shear off the end of the guide wire, which will remain in the vessel or in the tissues. Remove the needle and the guide wire simultaneously. Once out of the body, the guide wire may be removed by passing it completely through the needle from hub to tip.

8. **If the guide wire passes without resistance into the vessel, remove the needle over the wire.**

Always keep one hand on the wire to maintain its position in the vessel and to avoid the calamity of losing the wire completely in the vessel.

9. **Enlarge the insertion site, if necessary, by nicking the skin next to the wire** with a no. 11 blade scalpel.

This will be necessary if a dialysis catheter or an introducer sheath is going to be placed.

10. **Place a dilator over the wire to enlarge the passage through the tissues and into the vessel.**

Once the dilator is removed, the wound will bleed readily; be prepared to apply gentle pressure at the skin site with gauze. Be careful to maintain the wire position.

11. **Place the catheter or introducer over the wire into the vessel.**

- It is advisable to have flushed the lumens of the catheter with saline or a heparin-containing solution before placement.
- Maintain control of the wire.
- Remember to have removed the appropriate cap on multilumen catheters so that the wire passes through easily.
- Introducer sheaths should be introduced slowly, because they warm and become more compliant as they enter the body; they are also very large, and rapid movements can damage a wider area.
- Check each lumen by gently aspirating to confirm easy backflow of blood, and reinfuse with saline or heparin.

- If the catheter slides easily into the lumen of the vessel, remove the wire; hold a finger over the hub of the catheter until it is flushed and tightly capped.
- Confirm that each cap is in place and is tightly fastened.
12. **Secure the line and confirm the position by CXR, if necessary, before use.**

Forms of Intravascular Access

■ ARTERIAL LINES

Indications: Hemodynamic monitoring, arterial blood sampling, and frequent blood draw requirements. This is generally done in an ICU setting where the patient is under close observation.

Peripheral Arterial Line with Angiocatheter

The most straightforward approach involves use of a simple angiocatheter in the wrist. There are arterial line kits available that use the Seldinger (guide wire) technique that are also acceptable. The dorsalis pedis artery may also be used with this technique.

Placement

1. **Have all equipment ready.** You will need the following:
   - Skin preparation supplies (iodine, chlorhexidine, or alcohol)
   - Local anesthetic
   - Angiocatheter (20 or 22 gauge, 2 inches in length) or specific arterial line kit
   - Normal saline (NS) in a pressurized delivery system
   - Blood gas syringe if needed for arterial blood sampling
   - Additional 5-ml syringe with sterile NS
   - Suture for securing the catheter
   - Arm board with a small terry cloth roll to help secure line and prevent kinking
   - Equipment for continuous monitoring of arterial pressure
2. **Prepare the patient.**
   - Explain the procedure.
   - Explain the risks and the alternatives, and obtain informed consent if necessary.
   - Answer any questions.
3. **Select the site.**
   - Perform Allen's test to confirm the collateral circulation in the hand.
     Allen's test is performed by compression of both the

radial and the ulnar arteries until the palm blanches. Then release the ulnar artery, and confirm reperfusion of the palm. A delay of >5 seconds is considered abnormal, and another site should be chosen.

- Whenever possible, choose the patient's nondominant hand.

4. **Position the patient.**
   - The patient may be seated or supine.
     The selected wrist should be immobilized on an arm board with a roll under the wrist in slight dorsiflexion. Also get a chair to sit on, and confirm that all the equipment is available.

5. **Prepare the skin.**
   - Use sterile technique.
   - Prepare and drape the skin.
   - Infiltrate the entry site with 1 to 2% lidocaine.

6. **Insert the catheter.**
   - After confirming that adequate anesthesia has been achieved, locate the pulse with the index finger of your nondominant hand.
   - An optional step is to nick the skin over the entry site with a sterile scalpel, so as not to damage the catheter as it enters the skin.
   - While keeping the bevel down, insert the angiocatheter at a 30° to 45° angle to the artery, such that the tip of the catheter is more proximal to the heart than the hub.
   - When bright-red blood pumps freely into the catheter, continue to advance the catheter slowly until the flow just stops.
   - Back off slightly until the blood pumps again, and advance the catheter over the needle into the vessel.

7. **If blood does not flow immediately into the needle, do the following:**
   - Pull out, reconfirm the landmarks, reposition, and try again.
   - Occasionally, the needle must be flushed of clogging tissue before reinsertion; use a syringe of sterile NS.
   - If the catheter cannot be placed in three attempts, try another site.

8. **When the catheter is successfully placed, do the following:**
   - Secure the catheter to the skin with suture; some angiocatheters have wings for this purpose.
   - Obtain arterial blood samples as needed.
   - Attach to manometer for continuous monitoring.
   - Apply a sterile dressing.

9. **General considerations for use of arterial lines are as follows:**
   - Reassess the need for the arterial line daily.

- Confirm adequate blood flow to the hand and fingers daily.
- If fever occurs, remember to draw cultures from this site and other indwelling sites.
- If the site remains clean, the catheter should be changed over a wire every 3 to 5 days.

Femoral Arterial Line by Seldinger Technique

Arterial lines and especially femoral lines are for nonambulatory patients.

Placement

1. **Have all equipment ready.** You will need the following:
   - Skin preparation supplies (iodine, chlorhexidine, or alcohol)
   - Local anesthetic, i.e., lidocaine or a lidocaine and bupivacaine hydrochloride (lidocaine–Marcaine HCl) mixture
   - Supplies for Seldinger technique (or specific arterial line kit)
   - Needle (16 to 18 gauge)
   - 10-ml syringe
   - Guide wire
   - Scalpel
   - Dilator
   - Catheter
   - If the Seldinger technique is not used, a catheter-over-needle system may be used.
   - NS in a pressurized delivery system
   - Blood gas syringe if needed for arterial blood sampling
   - Suture for securing the catheter
   - Equipment for continuous monitoring of arterial pressure
2. **Prepare the patient.**
   - Explain the procedure.
   - Explain the risks and the alternatives, and obtain informed consent if necessary.
   - Answer any questions.
3. **Select the site.**
   - Palpate the groin pulse.
     It is found halfway between the anterior iliac spine and the symphysis pubis. Remember the following orientation of the artery to the vein: midline → vein → artery → nerve (Fig. 19–2).
   - Confirm distal pulses on the chosen side.
4. **Position the patient.**
   - Place the patient in supine position, elevate the bed to a comfortable height, and confirm that all the equipment is available.

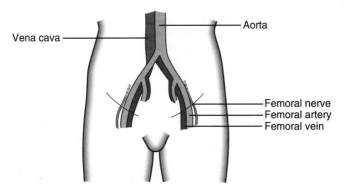

Figure 19–2 □ Anatomy of groin vasculature.

5. **Prepare the skin.**
   - Use sterile technique.
   - Prepare and drape the skin; shaving may be necessary.
   - Infiltrate the entry site with 1 to 2% lidocaine.
6. **Insert the catheter.**
   - Confirm that adequate anesthesia has been achieved.
   - Place the 10-ml syringe on the needle, and locate the pulse with the index finger of your nondominant hand.
   - With the bevel down, insert the needle at a 45° angle to the artery such that the tip of the catheter is more proximal to the heart than the hub.
     Aspirate during insertion (approximately 3–4 cm) **and** during withdrawal, as often the vessel is encountered on the way out.
   - When bright-red blood pumps freely into the syringe, remove the syringe and place a finger over the hub of the needle immediately.
   - Place the guide wire through the needle as per the Seldinger technique, and **make sure that the wire passes without resistance.**
   - Nick the skin at the entry site with a scalpel.
   - Place the dilator over the wire, and then remove.
     Watch for increased bleeding at the skin site. This is easily controlled with gentle pressure.
   - Place the catheter over the wire into the wound.
   - Remove the wire, confirm appropriate placement by brief observation of bright-red pulsatile blood emitting from the catheter hub, and cap the catheter.
7. **If blood does not flow immediately into the needle, do the following:**
   - Pull out, reconfirm landmarks, reposition, and try again.

- Occasionally, the needle must be flushed of clogging tissue before reinsertion; use a syringe of sterile NS.
- If the catheter cannot be placed in three attempts, try another site.

8. **When the catheter is successfully placed, do the following:**
   - Secure the catheter to the skin with suture.
   - Obtain arterial blood samples as needed.
   - Attach to manometer for continuous monitoring.
   - Apply a sterile dressing.

9. **General considerations for use of femoral arterial lines are as follows:**
   - Reassess the need for the arterial line daily.
   - Confirm adequate blood flow to the extremity daily.
   - Check the site daily for infection.
   - If fever occurs, remember to draw cultures from this site and other indwelling sites.
   - If the site remains clean, the catheter should be changed over a wire every 3 to 5 days.

Removal of Arterial Lines

1. Have scissors or blade, and gauze and tape ready.
2. Always wear gloves when there is a potential for exposure to blood or other bodily fluids.
3. Remove the sutures.
4. Remove the catheter.
5. Apply firm pressure at the entry site for 10 minutes (by the clock), or longer if the lumen was large or if the patient was anticoagulated.
6. After 10 minutes, confirm that bleeding has stopped.
7. Place a pressure dressing.
8. Check the site, and confirm adequate blood flow to the extremity.

Complications of Arterial Lines Procedures

1. Nonplacement of the line
2. Entry site infection
3. Vessel thrombosis (transient occlusion is common, occurring in about 10% of placements, and it is treated by removal of the line)
4. Suppurative thrombophlebitis
5. Distal ischemia
6. Hemorrhage

Problems of Arterial Lines

1. Complication of placement or removal
2. Bleeding from the placement site. (Be sure to check the

connections. Under arterial pressures, a poor coupling of lines can result in rapid exsanguination.)
3. Nonfunction
4. Infection at the site

■ CENTRAL VENOUS LINES

These include hemodynamic lines such as central venous pressure (CVP) lines and Swan-Ganz catheters, dialysis ports, and lines with multiple lumens for TPN or prolonged medication delivery. Venous blood sampling may also be possible through these sites.

Indications: Delivery of high concentrations of nutrition or medication; requirement for prolonged delivery of medication; requirement for hemodialysis; hemodynamic monitoring of CVP.

Subclavian Approach

This is a common approach to central venous access. It is the most comfortable for the awake patient, it is an easy and a relatively safe placement technique, and it is a very easy site to keep clean and protected. There is a higher risk of pneumothorax during placement of this line than IJ or femoral lines.

Anatomic Landmarks (Fig. 19–3)

1. The subclavian vein is found anterior to the first rib and the anterior scalene muscle.
2. The vein lies posterior to the clavicle and crosses under it medially and superiorly at the distal third of the clavicle and joins the internal jugular vein at the base of the neck.
3. If right-sided heart cannulation is desired, the left subclavian is more desirable than the right side, because this allows a more smooth arc of the catheter once in place.
4. The most common approach is from an infraclavicular site, although it is possible to approach from a supraclavicular site.
5. The insertion site is generally from a point 1 cm inferior to the distal third of the clavicle (Fig. 19–4).

Placement

1. **Use sterile Seldinger technique.**
   Kits have specific instructions.
2. **Have all equipment ready.** You will need the following:
   ■ Skin preparation supplies (iodine, chlorhexidine, or alcohol)

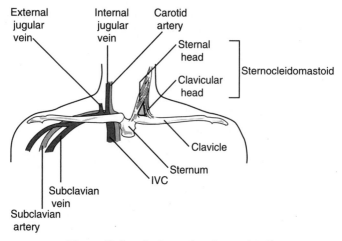

Figure 19–3 □ Anatomy of neck vasculature.

- Local anesthetic, i.e., lidocaine or a lidocaine and bupiva-caine hydrochloride (lidocaine–Marcaine HCl) mixture.
- Supplies for Seldinger technique (or specific central line kit)
- Needle (16 to 18 gauge)
- 10-ml syringe
- Guide wire
- Scalpel
- Dilator
- Catheter
- A catheter-over-needle system if the Seldinger technique is not used

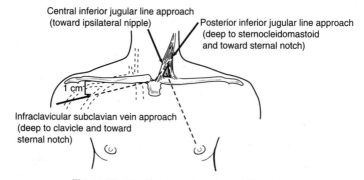

Figure 19–4 □ Needle entry site and directions.

- NS or a heparin-containing solution for flushing the catheter
- Suture for securing the catheter
- Equipment for continuous monitoring of venous pressure, if desired

3. **Prepare the patient.**
   - Explain the procedure.
   - Explain the risks and the alternatives, and obtain informed consent if necessary.
   - Answer any questions.

4. **Select the site.**

5. **Position the patient.**
   - Place the patient supine and at 15° Trendelenburg to increase the venous filling of the subclavian vein.
   - Place a small rolled towel between the shoulder blades.
   - Elevate the bed to a comfortable height.
   - Turn the patient's head away from the chosen site.
   - Confirm that all equipment is available.

6. **Prepare the skin.**
   - Use sterile technique.
   - Prepare and drape the skin.
   - Infiltrate the entry site as above with 1 to 2% lidocaine; then infiltrate toward the clavicle. Once the clavicle is reached, march stepwise down the bone, infiltrating the periosteum.
   - Get an estimate of the length of catheter required to reach the SVC by placing the catheter on the sterile field and approximating its anatomic position after placement.

7. **Insert the catheter.**
   - Confirm that adequate anesthesia has been achieved.
   - Place the 10-ml syringe on the needle.
   - With the bevel down, insert the needle at a 20° to 30° angle to the skin; direct the needle superiorly and medially toward the suprasternal notch (see Fig. 19–4).

     A finger may be placed here over the drapes to define a landmark. Insert the needle just below the clavicle such that it is necessary to progressively step down the bone with the needle tip to find the space just below the clavicle (Fig. 19–5). Advance along the dorsal surface of the bone and aspirate during insertion (approximately 5 cm).
   - If the vessel is not encountered during insertion, withdraw slowly while aspirating, as often the vessel is found on the way out.
   - When dark venous blood flows freely into the syringe, rotate the needle 90° such that the bevel now faces the patient's feet and remove the syringe from the needle.

     Immediately place your finger over the hub of the needle to avoid air embolus.

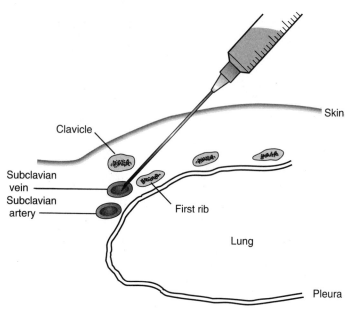

Figure 19–5 □ Infraclavicular approach to subclavian vein cannulation.

- Place the guide wire through the needle according to the Seldinger technique. **Make sure that the wire passes without resistance.**
- Nick the skin at the entry site with a scalpel.
- Remember to hold the wire at all times to avoid losing it in the vessel.
- Place the dilator over the wire, and then remove.
  Watch for increased bleeding at the skin site. This is easily controlled with gentle pressure.
- Place the catheter over the wire into the wound.
- Remove the wire, confirm appropriate placement by aspiration of blood through each lumen followed by flushing each lumen with saline or a heparin-containing solution, and cap the catheter.
8. **If blood does not flow immediately into the needle, do the following:**
   - Pull out, reconfirm landmarks, reposition, and try again.
   - Occasionally, the needle must be flushed of clogging tissue before reinsertion; use a syringe of sterile NS.
   - If the catheter cannot be placed in three attempts, try another site.

9. **If arterial blood is encountered, do the following:**
   - Remove the needle immediately, and discontinue the procedure.
   - Obtain an upright CXR immediately, and repeat in 12 to 24 hours.
   - Apply local pressure. Because of the anatomy of this site, significant bleeding can occur despite pressure applied to the skin.
   - Monitor the patient carefully for the next 24 hours to watch for signs of respiratory distress or severe blood loss.

10. **If air is encountered, do the following:**
    - Remove the needle immediately, and discontinue the procedure.
    - Obtain upright CXRs immediately, PA and lateral, inspiratory and expiratory, and repeat in 12 to 24 hours.
    - Monitor the patient carefully for the next 24 hours to watch for signs of pneumothorax.

11. **When the catheter is successfully placed, do the following:**
    - Secure the catheter to the skin with suture.
    - Obtain blood samples as needed.
    - Apply a sterile dressing.
    - Obtain an upright CXR to confirm placement before infusion of fluids. Correct placement is in the SVC, just above the right atrium.
    - Reposition as needed based on the CXR results.
    - Attach to manometer for continuous monitoring, if desired.

12. **General considerations for use of subclavian lines are as follows:**
    - Reassess the need for the intravenous line daily.
    - Check the site for infection daily.
    - If fever occurs, remember to draw cultures from this site and other indwelling sites.
    - If the site remains clean, the catheter should be changed over a wire every 3 to 5 days.

Inferior Jugular Vein Approach

This is a common approach. The line is not as comfortable for the patient as the subclavian once in place, but for many operators it is a simpler approach.

Anatomic Landmarks (see Fig. 19–3)

1. The IJ vein exits the skull and runs posteriorly and laterally to the carotid artery.
2. The vein runs medial to the sternocleidomastoid muscle at

the top of the neck, and then passes under the muscle to join the subclavian vein behind the medial clavicle.

3. At the base of the neck a triangle is defined by the two heads of the sternocleidomastoid muscle, medially by the sternal head, and laterally by the clavicular head. The base of the triangle is defined by the medial clavicle. The IJ vein enters this triangle at the apex and runs laterally to the sternal head of the muscle.

4. Insertion site for the middle or central approach is at the apex of the triangle, aiming toward the ipsilateral nipple (see Fig. 19–4).

5. Insertion site for the posterior approach is lateral to the sternocleidomastoid muscle starting 4 to 5 cm above the clavicle and aiming toward the suprasternal notch (see Fig. 19–4).

Placement

The general steps are similar to the subclavian approach. Refer to the placement of that line. Where steps differ, they are outlined here.

1. **Use sterile Seldinger technique.**
   Kits have specific instructions.
2. **Have all equipment ready.**
3. **Prepare the patient.**
4. **Select the site.**
5. **Position the patient.**
   - No scapula roll is necessary for this approach.
6. **Prepare the skin.**
   - Use sterile technique.
   - Prepare and drape the skin.
     The drape may cover the face of the patient; make sure the patient is comfortable and is able to breathe.
   - Infiltrate the entry site as above with 1 to 2% lidocaine.
   - Get an estimate of the length of catheter required to reach the SVC by placing the catheter on the sterile field and approximating its anatomic position after placement.
7. **Insert the catheter.**
   - Confirm that adequate anesthesia has been achieved.
   - Place the 10-ml syringe on the needle.
   - With your nondominant hand, palpate the carotid pulse.
     Put gentle pressure medially on the carotid to retract it away from the insertion site.
   - With the bevel down, insert the needle at a 20° to 30° angle to the skin (see Fig. 19–4).
     If the middle or central approach is used, direct the needle inferiorly and laterally toward the nipple on the ipsilateral side, and aspirate during insertion (approximately 4 cm).

- If the posterior approach is used, direct the needle inferiorly and anteriorly toward the suprasternal notch (approximately 5 cm; see Fig. 19–4).
- If the vessel is not encountered during insertion, withdraw slowly while aspirating, as often the vessel is found on the way out.
- When dark venous blood flows freely into the syringe, remove the syringe from the needle.

  Immediately place a finger over the hub of the needle to avoid air embolus.
- Place the guide wire through the needle, and complete the procedure according to the Seldinger technique.

8. **If blood does not flow immediately into the needle, do the following:**
   - Pull out, reconfirm landmarks, reposition, and try again.
   - Occasionally, the needle must be flushed of clogging tissue before reinsertion; use a syringe of sterile NS.
   - If the catheter cannot be placed in three attempts, try another site.

9. **If arterial blood is encountered, do the following:**
   - Remove the needle immediately, and discontinue the procedure.
   - Hold pressure at the site for 10 minutes (by the clock).
   - Obtain an upright CXR immediately, and repeat in 12 to 24 hours.
   - Resume the procedure once bleeding has been controlled locally.
   - Monitor the patient carefully for the next 24 hours to watch for signs of respiratory distress or severe blood loss.

10. **If air is encountered, do the following:**
    - Remove the needle immediately, and discontinue the procedure.
    - Obtain upright CXRs immediately, PA and lateral, inspiratory and expiratory, and repeat in 12 to 24 hours.
    - Monitor the patient carefully for the next 24 hours to watch for signs of pneumothorax.

11. **When the catheter is successfully placed, do the following:**
    - Secure the catheter to the skin with suture.
    - Obtain blood samples as needed.
    - Apply a sterile dressing.
    - Obtain an upright CXR to confirm placement before infusion of fluids. Correct placement is in the SVC, just above the right atrium.
    - Reposition as needed based on the CXR results.
    - Attach to manometer for continuous monitoring, if desired.

12. **General considerations for use of the inferior jugular vein approach are as follows:**
    - Reassess the need for the intravenous line daily.
    - Check the site for infection daily.
    - If fever occurs, remember to draw cultures from this site and other indwelling sites.
    - If the site remains clean, the catheter should be changed over a wire every 3 to 5 days.

Femoral Vein Approach

This is the easiest of lines to place. The tip of the line will reside in the inferior vena cava, and this is not a good placement for an ambulatory patient or for one in whom pulmonary wedge pressures might need to be monitored.

Anatomic Landmarks (see Fig. 19–2)

1. The vein is found halfway between the anterior iliac spine and the symphysis pubis.
2. Remember the following orientation of the artery to the vein: midline → vein → artery → nerve. (The vein lies between the pulse and the pubis.)

Placement

The general steps are similar to the subclavian approach. Refer to the placement of that line. Where steps differ, they are outlined here.

1. **Use sterile Seldinger technique.**
   Kits have specific instructions.
2. **Have all equipment ready.**
3. **Prepare the patient.**
4. **Select the site.**
5. **Position the patient.**
6. **Prepare the skin.**
   - Use sterile technique.
   - Prepare and drape the skin; shaving may be necessary.
   - Infiltrate the entry site as above with 1 to 2% lidocaine.
7. **Insert the catheter.**
   - Confirm that adequate anesthesia has been achieved.
   - Place the 10-ml syringe on the needle.
   - With your nondominant hand, palpate the femoral pulse.
   - With the bevel down, insert the needle at a 30° to 40° angle to the skin, medially to the pulse.
     Direct the needle superiorly. Aspirate during insertion (approximately 4 cm).
   - If the vessel is not encountered during insertion, withdraw slowly while aspirating, as often the vessel is found on the way out.

- When dark venous blood flows freely into the syringe, remove the syringe from the needle.
  Immediately place a finger over the hub of the needle to avoid air embolus.
- Place the guide wire through the needle, and complete the procedure according to the Seldinger technique.

8. **If blood does not flow immediately into the needle, do the following:**
   - Pull out, reconfirm landmarks, reposition, and try again.
   - Occasionally, the needle needs to be flushed of clogging tissue before reinsertion; use a syringe of sterile NS.
   - If the catheter cannot be placed in three attempts, try another site.

9. **If arterial blood is encountered, do the following:**
   - Remove the needle immediately, and discontinue the procedure.
   - Hold pressure at the site for 10 minutes (by the clock).
   - Once bleeding has been controlled locally, the procedure may be resumed.

10. **When the catheter is successfully placed, do the following:**
    - Secure the catheter to the skin with suture.
    - Obtain blood samples as needed.
    - Apply a sterile dressing.
    - Attach to manometer for continuous monitoring, if desired.

11. **General considerations for use of the femoral vein approach are as follows:**
    - Reassess the need for the intravenous line daily.
    - Check the site for infection daily.
    - If fever occurs, remember to draw cultures from this site and other indwelling sites.
    - If the site remains clean, the catheter should be changed over a wire every 3 to 5 days.

Removal of Central Venous Lines

1. Make sure the patient has no need for continued central venous access.
2. If a peripheral line is necessary, make sure it is in place and patent.
3. Have scissors or blade, and gauze and tape ready.
4. Always wear gloves when there is a potential for exposure to blood or other bodily fluids.
5. Position the patient supine. This decreases the risk of air embolus.
6. Remove the sutures.
7. Remove the catheter.

Prior to removal, have the patient inhale and hold his or her breath. This creates positive pressure in the chest cavity and decreases the risk of air embolism. Culture the tip if necessary. If the catheter is a longer term type and has a subcutaneous cuff, such as a Hickman or others, then it will be necessary to break the adhesions between the subcutaneous tissues and the cuff situated a short distance from the skin insertion site. If the distance is short, the adhesions may be broken with a hemostat through the orifice of the insertion site, after adequate local anesthesia and site cleansing. Occasionally, a separate skin incision is required over the palpable portion of the cuff, and adhesions must be bluntly dissected through that incision.

8. Apply firm pressure at the entry site and at the site of entry into the vessel for 10 minutes (by the clock), or longer if the lumen was large or if the patient was anticoagulated.
9. After 10 minutes, confirm that bleeding has stopped.
10. Check the site the next day for evidence of infection or continued bleeding.

Complications of Central Venous Line Procedures

1. Venous air embolism
2. Pneumothorax
3. Guide wire embolism
4. Arterial puncture
5. Nonplacement of the line
6. Misplacement of the line
7. Entry site infection
8. Vessel thrombosis
9. Thrombophlebitis
10. Hemorrhage

Problems of Central Venous Lines

1. Complication of placement or removal
2. Bleeding from the placement site
3. Nonfunction
4. Infection at the site

■ PERIPHERAL VENOUS LINES

This is the most common access and is used for routine fluid replacement and medication delivery.

Indications: Requirement of intravenous fluid replacement for maintenance or rehydration purposes; delivery of medication or nutrition.

Placement

1. **Use clean technique.**
   Wear gloves. Do not contaminate sterile portions of the catheter.
2. **Have all equipment ready.** You will need the following:
   - Skin preparation supplies (iodine, chlorhexidine, or alcohol)
   - Angiocatheter (18- to 22-gauge needles are commonly used)
   - NS or a heparin-containing solution for flushing the catheter
   - 10-ml syringe for flushing the catheter
   - Tape for securing the catheter
   - Local anesthetic (optional)
3. **Prepare the patient.**
   - Explain the procedure, including that all needle punctures may be painful.
   - Explain the risks and alternatives.
   - Answer any questions.
4. **Select the site.**
   - Most frequently, distal upper extremity sites are chosen. It is best to start more distally and then move proximally.
   - Palpable veins are often more easy to cannulate than visible ones.
   - If no veins are apparent, try to warm the extremity or place it in a dependent position to increase venous dilation.
   - In supine, nonambulatory patients, the lower extremity may be used.
   - Whenever possible, try to avoid sites that would be inconvenient to the patient. These might include the dorsum of the patient's dominant hand, antecubital veins, or painful sites such as the volar surface of the forearm.
5. **Position the patient.**
   - The patient should be comfortable, sitting or supine; occasionally armboards are required to immobilize sites such as the dorsum of the hand or the antecubital site. Also get a chair to sit on, and confirm that all the equipment is available.
6. **Prepare the skin.**
   - If the patient desires, or if a large needle is to be used, consider infiltration of the entry site with 1 to 2% lidocaine.

7. **Apply the tourniquet.**
   - Apply the tourniquet on the upper arm, because this gives better dilation of the distal superficial venous system.
   - Do not apply so tightly that the arterial flow into the extremity is impaired.
8. **Insert the catheter.**
   - After confirming that adequate anesthesia has been achieved (if used), palpate the vein with the index finger of the nondominant hand; apply gentle pressure to stretch the vein away from yourself.
   - An optional step is to nick the skin over the entry site with a sterile scalpel, so as not to damage the catheter as it enters the skin.
   - Keeping the bevel down, insert the angiocatheter at a 30° to 45° angle to the vein such that the tip of the catheter is more proximal to the heart than to the hub.
   - When dark venous blood flows freely into the catheter, continue to advance the catheter slowly until the flow just stops.
   - Back off slightly until the blood flows again, and advance the catheter over the needle into the vessel.
9. **If blood does not flow immediately into the needle, do the following:**
   - Pull back but not completely out of the skin, reconfirm the landmarks, reposition, and try again.
   - Occasionally, the needle must be flushed of clogging tissue before reinsertion; use a syringe of sterile NS.
   - If the catheter cannot be placed in three attempts, try another site.
     To avoid venous bleeding from the unsuccessful site, leave the catheter in the skin wound, and retry with a fresh angiocatheter. The unsuccessful angiocatheters may be removed later after the tourniquet is removed.
10. **When the catheter is successfully placed, do the following:**
    - Remember to remove the tourniquet.
    - Secure the catheter to the skin with tape.
    - Attach tubing for delivery of appropriate intravenous fluid.

Removal of Peripheral Lines

1. Make sure the patient no longer needs the site.
2. Always wear gloves when there is a potential for exposure to blood or other bodily fluids.
3. Remove securing tapes.
4. Remove the catheter.

5. Apply firm pressure at the entry site for 5 to 10 minutes, or longer if the lumen was large or if the patient was anticoagulated.
6. Confirm that bleeding has stopped.
7. Place a clean dressing.
8. Check the site the next day.

Complications of Peripheral Lines

1. Nonplacement of the line
2. Entry site infection
3. Vessel thrombosis
4. Suppurative thrombophlebitis
5. Hemorrhage (usually minor)
6. Infiltration of IV fluids

Problems of Peripheral Lines

1. Complication of placement or removal
2. Bleeding from the placement site
3. Nonfunction
4. Infection at the site

20

LEG PAIN

Leg pain is common with lower extremity surgery, trauma, vascular problems, inflammatory or degenerative conditions, infection, or referred pain. Some of these conditions can be managed by telephone, whereas others require that you examine the patient. A careful discussion with the RN will help to show which patients should be examined.

■ PHONE CALL

Questions

1. **What area of the leg is painful?**

   Pain in the region of a joint may be indicative of an inflammatory or an infectious process, but pain in the calf may suggest a vascular cause of the pain.

2. **What are the vital signs? Is there any shortness of breath (SOB)?**

   Deep venous thrombosis (DVT) and subsequent pulmonary embolus may first present with leg pain. SOB with a history of recent leg pain may suggest pulmonary embolus.

3. **Did the patient have surgery or a traumatic accident? If the patient had surgery, what type of operation was performed, and when was it performed?**

   Surgery on the lower extremities, the pelvis, and the abdominal wall predisposes a patient to development of DVTs. Investigate a traumatic cause of leg pain with a clinical examination and appropriate radiographs.

4. **Why was the patient admitted? Is there any history of recent trauma?**

   Pelvic and lower extremity trauma may be associated with leg pain and increased risk of DVTs. Posttraumatic leg pain in the presence of a loss of pulses may suggest an arterial injury.

5. **Is there a pulse in the leg? Is there swelling or discoloration of the skin?**

   An acute loss of pulses in a lower extremity represents an emergency. It often suggests acute embolism or thrombosis. Leg pain and pallor of the skin may suggest insufficiency of arterial inflow. This may accompany arterial injury, thrombosis, or compartmental syndrome. Bluish discoloration of the skin with or without leg pain suggests venous insufficiency.

6. **Has the patient lost any sensation in the leg acutely?**

   An acute loss of sensation suggests arterial insufficiency or compartmental syndrome.

7. **Is there a dressing or a cast in place on the leg?**

   Increasing pain in the presence of a cast or a dressing usually requires investigation. A dressing may be covering an infected wound; a cast may be too tight.

8. **Does the patient have known medical problems?**

   A patient who has known atherosclerosis, degenerative changes of the lower extremity, or history of DVT may be more likely to present with leg pain.

Inform RN

"Will arrive at the bedside in . . . minutes."

Sudden-onset, severe leg pain may be a sign of arterial or venous compromise and should be assessed immediately. Leg pain associated with fever, loss of pulses, new-onset swelling, or SOB may represent a limb-threatening or life-threatening process and requires immediate evaluation.

■ ELEVATOR THOUGHTS

What causes leg pain?
1. Vascular diseases
   - DVT
   - Acute arterial insufficiency (thrombus and embolus)
   - Arterial vasospasm
   - Chronic arterial insufficiency (arteriosclerosis obliterans)
   - Buerger's disease
   - Popliteal artery entrapment
   - Ischemia due to constrictive dressing or cast
   - Superficial thrombophlebitis
   - Venous stasis disease
2. Inflammatory and degenerative diseases
   - Degenerative arthritis (hips, knees, and ankles)
   - Lumbar disk disease (sciatica)
   - Acute gout and pseudogout
   - Rheumatoid arthritis
   - Systemic lupus erythematosus
   - Periostitis
3. Infectious processes
   - Cellulitis
   - Septic arthritis
   - Septic thrombophlebitis
   - Necrotizing fasciitis

- Osteomyelitis
4. Soft-tissue and bone processes
   - Compartmental syndrome
   - Neuropathy (diabetic)
   - Erythema nodosum
   - Neuroma or other soft-tissue mass
   - Skeletal tumors
   - Benign leg cramps
   - Postsurgical pain
   - Traumatic causes of pain

■ MAJOR THREAT TO LIFE

The following are either limb-threatening or life-threatening processes:
1. Arterial occlusion
2. Pulmonary embolus resulting from DVT
3. Infectious processes
   - Septic arthritis
   - Septic thrombophlebitis
   - Necrotizing infection
4. Compartmental syndrome

Acute arterial insufficiency: Acute arterial insufficiency often presents with an acute increase in pain, pallor, and loss of pulses in the affected extremity. In the lower extremity, it most frequently affects the foot. If circulation is not reestablished rapidly (within 6 hours), irreversible tissue damage and loss of limb may result.

Deep venous thrombosis: DVT is very common in postsurgical and bedridden patients, and it represents a great liability to the on-call physician. Although DVTs originate in the leg or pelvis, they may become blood borne and travel to the pulmonary artery. This may lead to a life-threatening pulmonary embolus.

Infectious processes: Infectious processes of the lower extremity may involve joints, blood vessels, and other soft tissues. Many of these processes are rapidly progressive due to the poor blood supply to the lower extremities in patients with vascular disease. Diabetic patients are particularly susceptible to infectious processes of the lower extremities. Diabetics generally have a component of small-vessel and large-vessel disease, with decreased blood flow to the legs. These patients often have neuropathies, making trauma and late detection of skin breakdown commonplace. The decreased immune function of diabetic patients makes infections especially troublesome and may lead to blood-borne infection and sepsis.

Compartmental syndrome: Compartmental syndrome may follow leg trauma or reperfusion of an ischemic extremity. Failure to recognize elevated lower extremity compartmental pressures may result in soft-tissue necrosis and ultimate limb loss.

■ BEDSIDE

Although the list of causes of leg pain is long, careful discussion of the on-call problem with the RN will help determine if examination and treatment of the patient is necessary. Loss of lower extremity pulses and foot pain (acute ischemia) is an emergency. New-onset lower extremity swelling must also be evaluated immediately and may represent DVT or compartmental syndrome. Fever and leg pain may indicate infection or DVT; this presentation requires your evaluation.

Quick Look Test

Most patients with leg pain will give a history that helps to provide a narrowed differential diagnosis. Patients with infectious processes often look sick, and patients with ischemia or DVT appear uncomfortable.

Airway and Vital Signs

By itself, leg pain should not lead to instability of the vital signs. However, when SOB, severe pain, or infection is associated with leg pain, changes in vital signs may be seen.

Heart Rate, Blood Pressure, and Respiratory Rate

Severe leg pain is stressful to patients, and it may lead to tachycardia, tachypnea, and hypertension. A DVT that migrates from the lower extremity to the pulmonary vessels may cause acute SOB and tachypnea.

Temperature

Leg pain associated with an infectious process often presents with fever. DVT may present with leg pain, fever, and swelling.

Selective History and Chart Review

Does the patient have a history of leg pain? Is the current pain similar to or worse than prior pain episodes?

Many patients with advanced atherosclerosis of the lower extremity vessels will have a history of intermittent claudication and foot pain. Patients with inflammatory or degenerative conditions will often give a history of chronic pain. It is important to establish a baseline to allow comparison with the patient's current leg pain. Pain very different or more severe than prior pain episodes requires you to perform a careful examination of the leg.

Is there a history of prior vascular surgery?

Patients who have undergone revascularization of the leg generally have significant peripheral vascular occlusive disease. These patients may have reocclusion of their bypass grafts or occlusion of arteries acutely in the other lower extremity.

Does the patient have a history of atrial fibrillation? Does the patient have prosthetic heart valves?

Atrial fibrillation is a leading cause of embolization and acute arterial occlusion in the lower extremities. Other causes of embolization include embolism from prosthetic heart valves or peripheral emboli (aortic and other vessels).

Is there a history of deep venous thrombosis or venous disease of the lower extremities?

Patients who have had prior DVTs are at an increased risk for having another one. Patients with a hypercoagulable state (e.g., cancer, pregnancy, and congenital conditions) are more likely to develop DVTs. Any history of venous insufficiency or venous stasis disease should be ascertained. Prolonged surgical procedures also predispose a patient to DVT formation.

Selective Physical Examination

The physical examination is directed toward finding a cause for the leg pain. Examination will be directed at looking for signs of inflammation, infection, arterial insufficiency, or venous disease.

VS: Obtain a set of vital signs; look for signs of fever (infection and DVT).

Resp: If the patient has SOB, listen for friction rub or evidence of pulmonary effusion (pulmonary embolus).

CVS: Look for pulse regularity; irregularity of the rhythm and rate suggests atrial fibrillation. Listen for evidence of a prosthetic heart valve (metallic click).

Extrem: Perform a complete vascular examination of the lower extremities, including an evaluation of femoral, popliteal, dorsalis pedis, and posterior tibial arteries. Recall that the posterior tibial vessels and the great saphenous vein are on the medial aspect of the ankle, with the posterior tibial vessels posterior to the medial malleolus and the saphenous vein about 1 cm anterior to the medial malleolus (Fig. 20–1). Evaluate for

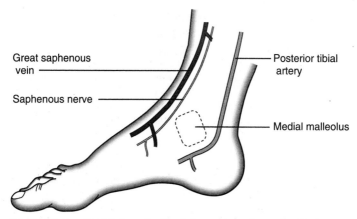

Figure 20–1 □ Medial view of ankle region and structures of major importance.

	tenderness, sensory function, and motor strength, and compare results with those of the opposite leg.
Skin:	Look for erythema, cyanotic changes, mottling, pallor, and edema.

■ MANAGEMENT

Management is directed at treating the cause of the leg pain, as follows.

Vascular Diseases

■ ACUTE ARTERIAL INSUFFICIENCY

Selective History

Is there a history of peripheral vascular disease or intermittent claudication?

Is there a history of cardiac or vascular disease (e.g., atrial fibrillation, prior embolus, prosthetic heart valve, left ventricular aneurysm, or aortic disease)?

Was pain, temperature change, or color change in the leg of sudden onset?

How does the symptomatic leg compare with the other leg?

Selective Physical Examination

Look for the "five Ps" for evidence of acute arterial occlusion, as follows:

Pain:	An early sign of ischemia
Pallor:	An early sign of ischemia
Pulselessness:	An early sign of gross arterial occlusion
Paresthesia:	Sensory loss in ischemic region
Paralysis:	Usually a late finding and indicative of tissue damage

In addition, look for the following:

VS:	Signs of shock, hypovolemia, or orthostasis
Skin:	Pallor, mottling, gangrenous changes, and chronic changes including hair loss, thin skin, and shiny skin
CVS:	Heart sounds: listen for regularity; pulse examination: radial, femoral, popliteal, dorsalis pedis, and posterior tibial; comparison of symmetry with other leg; use of Doppler probe if pulses not palpable
Neuro:	Evaluation of light touch sensation (first neurologic deficit seen in ischemia); evaluation of muscle strengths

The diagnosis of acute arterial insufficiency or occlusion is best made by history taking and careful physical examination. Always compare the symptomatic leg with the nonsymptomatic leg.

Patients who are sensate will often complain of leg pain in the presence of an acute arterial occlusion. Temperature changes and skin changes are also seen shortly after acute arterial occlusion. The leg will often show a distinct line of demarcation, below which the skin temperature is cooler and more mottled or pale than the region proximal to the suspected occlusion. Mark the line of demarcation, and evaluate the lower extremity pulses to see if pulse changes correspond to other changes.

Take care when treating patients undergoing cardiac catheterization or other invasive arterial procedures. These patients are at risk for embolization and may shower emboli to the lower extremity. Common locations for emboli include the foot and the toes. When circulation to the foot is compromised by an embolus, a cold foot or "trash foot" results. A cold foot represents an emergency that requires rapid action. Recent arterial catheterization may also lead to pseudoaneurysm formation at the insertion site and result in occlusion.

Management

Acute arterial occlusion is an emergency. In the event of acute occlusion, observe the following protocol:

1. Notify the chief resident or attending physician immediately.
2. If there are no contraindications, start heparinization immediately. The patient may be given **5000 to 10,000 U heparin intravenous (IV) bolus, followed by a continuous infusion of 1000 U/hr (18 mg/kg/hr).** Adjust the infusion rate to keep the partial thromboplastin time (PTT) at 70 to 80 seconds.
3. Arrange for an arteriogram immediately.
4. Review the case with the attending physician and a consulting vascular surgeon.

The patient will likely require emergent angiography and either surgical embolectomy or angioplasty. Fibrinolytic therapy is used only for surgically inaccessible peripheral arterial occlusions.

Do not confuse acute arterial insufficiency with chronic arterial insufficiency. Patients with long-standing arteriosclerosis and chronic intermittent claudication may present with pain at rest. If there is no concern with limb viability, the patient may be treated with analgesics and by having the leg placed in a more dependent position. Consultation with a vascular surgeon may be made on a nonemergent basis.

■ DEEP VENOUS THROMBOSIS

Selective History

Is there a history of prior DVT or coagulopathy?

Is there a history of trauma or surgery to the lower extremity or pelvis?

Is there a history of abdominal cancer?

Is there a history of prolonged immobilization?

Remember that the incidence of DVT is increased in the following patients:

1. Postoperative patients
2. Patients undergoing major orthopedic procedures
3. Patients >40 years of age
4. Obese or immobilized patients
5. Patients undergoing pelvic surgery or abdominal cancer surgery
6. Patients with pelvic or lower extremity fractures
7. Pregnant patients or those taking estrogen-based medications

Selective Physical Examination

VS: Rule out tachypnea and blood pressure changes suggestive of a pulmonary embolus.

Extrem: Evaluate lower leg and foot for new-onset edema; use a measuring tape if available to document a difference in size of the two extremities; look for erythema and warmth of the skin; palpate calf posteriorly and medially to feel for venous cords; gently compress the calf muscles against the tibia to evaluate for tenderness; also palpate the popliteal space, the adductor canal, and the groin to evaluate for tenderness; tenderness over a thrombosed vein is usually present if palpated.

Test for   With patient supine, straighten the leg and
Homans'   dorsiflex the foot; passive stretching of gas-
sign: trocnemius and soleus muscles occurs with this maneuver, which may elicit pain in the presence of a deep calf venous thrombosis.

DVT is a difficult diagnostic and therapeutic problem that can lead to pulmonary embolus. The most common veins affected are veins associated with the deep system of the lower extremity or veins within the pelvis (Fig. 20–2). It is generally difficult to

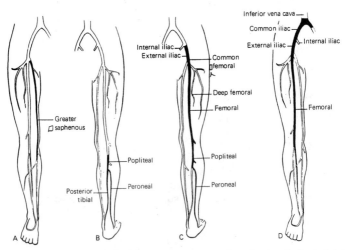

Figure 20–2 □ Common patterns of venous thrombosis. *A,* Superficial thrombophlebitis. *B,* The most common form of deep thrombophlebitis. *C* and *D,* Deep thrombophlebitis from the calf to the iliac veins. These patterns produce phlegmasia alba dolens, or if more complete, phlegmasia cerulea dolens. The usual locations of thrombosis in milk leg are shown in *C.* (From Haller JA Jr: Deep Thrombophlebitis: Pathophysiology and Treatment. Philadelphia, WB Saunders Co, 1967, p 12.)

palpate these structures directly. Diagnosis is made by clinical signs (e.g., noting new-onset edema in one extremity) and a high level of suspicion.

Diagnostic Testing

Ultrasound studies (duplex) are the most accurate noninvasive test for diagnosing proximal DVT. However, duplex is less accurate at diagnosing isolated calf venous thrombosis. Another reliable noninvasive technique for diagnosing proximal thrombosis is **impedance plethysmography. Contrast venography** is the most reliable technique for diagnosing DVT. However, this technique is invasive and has fallen out of favor as a first-line diagnostic procedure.

Management

Patients with a significant venous thrombosis of the lower extremity require bed rest, elevation of the affected extremity, and anticoagulation. Although isolated venous thromboses of the calf can eventually extend proximally in up to 20% of cases, some physicians treat small, isolated DVTs with bed rest, elevation, and observation alone.

Patients with proximal DVT should receive anticoagulation with IV heparin. Therapy can be initiated with a bolus of **5000 U heparin IV (60–80 U/bolus/kg of body weight) followed by a continuous infusion starting at 1000 U/hr (18 U/hr/kg of body weight).** Check PTT 6 hours after initiating therapy and every 6 to 8 hours thereafter until a steady state is reached. The goal of therapy is to achieve a PTT value 1.5 to 2.0 times the control value. This is usually a PTT of 50 to 80 seconds. Adjust the hourly rate of infusion accordingly. Most patients require 800 to 1600 U/hr.

By the second day of IV heparin therapy, consider starting patients on warfarin sodium (Coumadin) therapy. Patients may be given **warfarin sodium 10 mg/day** for the first several days. Recall that warfarin interferes with the vitamin K–dependent carboxylation of clotting factors. It generally takes several days to see the effects of warfarin. Remember that the prothrombin time (PT) reflects a warfarin dose given about 48 hours earlier. Follow anticoagulation by evaluating the PT on a daily basis. As the PT value begins to rise, consider decreasing the dose of warfarin. Many patients do well with about **5.0 mg/day.** Elderly patients and patients with liver disease often require smaller daily doses. The international normalized ratio (INR) has been calculated to standardize warfarin anticoagulation. An INR of 2.0 to 3.0 is generally therapeutic. Once a patient is adequately anticoagulated on warfarin, IV heparin therapy may be stopped.

There are risks in using heparin or warfarin. Bleeding is a serious complication. Avoid these anticoagulants in acute trauma patients, neurosurgical patients, or patients with active peptic ulcer disease. In addition, avoid the use of warfarin in pregnant patients. Warfarin crosses the placenta and causes birth defects. Also beware of the numerous drugs that may interact with warfarin and alter PT. A list of some of the common drugs that alter PT are listed in Table 20–1.

Perioperative Prophylaxis for DVTs

- Thigh-high TED hose and sequential compression devices should be used on the patient intraoperatively if the operation is expected to last more than 2 hours.
- **Subcutaneous heparin 5000 mg twice a day** may also be used. Discuss the heparin dose with a resident or attending physician prior to administering it.

Inflammatory and Degenerative Diseases

■ ACUTE GOUT AND PSEUDOGOUT

Acute Gout

Acute gout is an extremely painful condition in which monosodium urate crystals are released into the joint space from the synovium. Definitive diagnosis is made by demonstrating negatively birefringent monosodium urate crystals by using polarizing microscopy. Gout most commonly affects the foot and ankle. Patients may be managed with the nonsteroidal anti-inflamma-

Table 20–1 □ COMMON DRUGS THAT INTERACT WITH WARFARIN AND ALTER PROTHROMBIN TIME

Increases Prothrombin Time	Decreases Prothrombin Time
Metronidazole	Cholestyramine
Trimethoprim and sulfamethoxazole	Barbiturates
Disulfiram	Rifampin
Amiodarone	Carbamazepine
Omeprazole	Griseofulvin
Cimetidine	Penicillins
Some cephalosporins	
Heparin	
Thyroxine	
Clofibrate	

tory drug (NSAID) **indomethacin 100 mg orally (PO) followed by 50 mg PO every 6 hours. Ketorolac tromethamine (Toradol) 30 mg intramuscularly (IM), followed by 15–30 mg IM every 6 hours** may be used for pain control in more severe cases. An alternative is **colchicine 0.5 to 0.6 mg PO every 1 to 2 hours, which may be repeated until gastrointestinal side effects occur or when a maximum dose of 6 mg has been given in a 24-hour period.**

Pseudogout

Pseudogout is caused by the release of calcium pyrophosphate crystals from the joint surface into the joint space. Joint aspiration shows weakly positive birefringent rods in the joint fluid. Patients may also be managed with an NSAID such as indomethacin. Intra-articular steroids may be used in patients in which NSAIDs are contraindicated. As an alternative, **prednisone 40 to 60 mg PO every day** may be given for several days until a response is obtained and then rapidly tapered.

Soft-Tissue and Bone Processes

■ COMPARTMENTAL SYNDROME

Compartmental syndrome is a group of signs and symptoms resulting from increased pressures in the compartments of the lower extremity. The diagnosis is based on clinical examination and history. Patients usually present with pain, diminished sensation, and weakness or diminished muscle function. Clinical examination also shows tenseness and tenderness in compartment(s) of the lower extremity. Passively stretching the foot (dorsiflexion and plantarflexion) will often cause severe pain.

Close observation and repeated examinations spaced no more than 30 minutes apart is important for demonstrating progression. Symptoms that worsen progressively suggest increasing compartmental pressures and the need for compartmental release. The most common causes of compartmental syndrome are trauma and reperfusion injury. Table 20–2 lists injuries known to cause compartmental syndrome of the lower extremity.

Selective Physical Examination

Clinical examination is the key to diagnosis. Rate the status and the function of the following:

1. Muscle function should be graded from 0 to 5 and followed serially.

Table 20–2 □ COMMON CAUSES FOR COMPARTMENTAL
SYNDROME OF THE LEG

Vascular	Other
Bleeding into a compartment	Infection
Reperfusion edema	Tight casts
Venous obstruction	Lying on limb
Intra-arterial drug injection	
Traumatic	
Fracture	
Tissue crush	
Contusion	
Burns	
Snakebite and spider bite	

2. Sensation should be evaluated as normal, slightly diminished, significantly diminished, or absent.
   Sensation should be tested by both pinprick and two-point discrimination.
3. Tenseness is palpated and recorded as normal, slightly increased, significantly increased, or rock-hard.

Clinical findings alone are generally used to diagnose compartmental syndrome. However, in patients in whom the diagnosis cannot be made or ruled out by clinical examination (e.g., unconscious patient), evaluate the compartmental pressures. If you are rotating on a surgery service, ask the senior resident for help with measuring compartmental pressures. In some hospitals, orthopedic surgery performs these measurements, and a consultation can be obtained immediately.

Two common techniques for measuring compartmental pressures include the infusion technique and the wick catheter technique. Both techniques involve inserting either a needle or a catheter into the leg compartment and measuring pressures with the aid of a transducer. A knowledge of the anatomy of the leg is also essential to interpreting the results of these tests. The lower leg is divided into three compartments by projections of fascia, tibia, fibula, and interosseous membrane. These compartments contain muscles, nerves, arteries, and deep veins. Figure 20–3 shows the cross-sectional anatomy and compartments of the lower leg.

Management

Fasciotomy is recommended when compartmental pressures approach 30 mm Hg, or when the pressure is within 20 mm Hg of the diastolic blood pressure. In most cases, however, the decision to perform decompressing fasciotomy will be based on the progression of symptoms and the clinical picture. If a patient

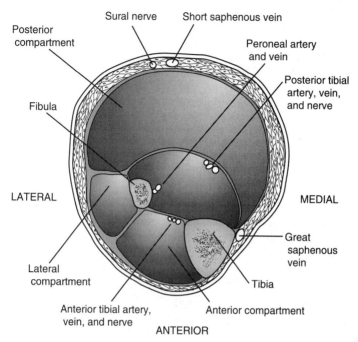

Figure 20–3 □ Cross-sectional anatomy and compartments of the lower leg.

requires surgical treatment, general surgery, orthopedic surgery, or plastic surgery services can perform fasciotomies of the lower extremity. It is critical to not postpone fasciotomy if indicated. Delayed surgical treatment may result in muscle necrosis and permanent nerve damage.

Infectious Processes

■ CELLULITIS

Common cellulitis in otherwise healthy patients usually involves *Staphylococcus aureus* or *Streptococcus* species. The first-generation cephalosporins, such as **cefazolin 1 g IV every 8 hours,** are effective against staphylococcus. Adding **penicillin G potassium 2 to 3 million units IV every 4 hours** to a first-generation cephalosporin adds good *Streptococcus* coverage. **Nafcillin 1 to 2 g IV every 6 hours** covers both *Staphylococcus* and

Streptococcus. Diabetic patients or patients with compromised lower extremity circulation have a higher incidence of gram-negative and anaerobic infections. For these patients, consider a broader spectrum antibiotic, such as **ticarcillin disodium (Timentin) 3.1 g IV every 6 hours** or **ampicillin sodium and sulbactam (Unasyn) 2.1 g IV every 6 hours.** Elevate the cellulitic extremity and treat with appropriate analgesics.

■ SEPTIC ARTHRITIS

Selective History

Septic arthritis may lead to systemic sepsis and permanent joint dysfunction. Patients usually present with a tender, erythematous, swollen joint. The affected joint is usually painful to both passive and active flexion. The patient will often have a fever. In a patient with a polyarticular rheumatologic disorder, a joint that is acutely inflamed significantly out of proportion to the other joints may be infected.

Septic arthritis is usually divided into nongonococcal or gonococcal disease. Nongonococcal septic arthritis is most often caused by *Staphylococcus aureus* and *Streptococcus* species and is most common in immunocompromised patients or in those with joint trauma. Gonococcal disease accounts for more than one-half of all septic arthritis in otherwise healthy, sexually active adults.

Look for predisposing factors.

Has there been recent joint pain, discomfort with movement of the extremities, or recent skin rash?

The cardinal signs of a gonococcal arthritis are migratory or additive polyarthralgias, tenosynovitis (inflammation of the tendons), and dermatitis.

Is there a history of penetrating trauma in the region of a joint?

Trauma to a joint may introduce organisms and lead to tissue injury. Open joint trauma greatly increases the incidence of *Staphylococcus* and *Streptococcus* infections.

Does the patient have a joint prosthesis?

Septic arthritis in the presence of a prosthetic joint is disastrous, and usually, removal of the prosthesis is required. Consult an orthopedic surgeon in these cases.

Management

1. Using sterile technique, aspirate the joint.

   If unsure of how to aspirate the joint, call the chief resident, or a consulting rheumatologist or an orthopedic surgeon. Collect fluid for an immediate Gram stain, culture

(aerobic and anaerobic, gonococcal, and tuberculous), white blood cell (WBC) count and differential, and glucose levels. In septic arthritis, the joint fluid is usually cloudy or turbid. The WBC count is usually >10, 000 cells/mm^3.
2. Send for blood cultures and serum glucose; the synovial glucose will be <50% of the serum glucose in a true septic joint.
3. Start IV antibiotics immediately.
   Remember that a negative Gram stain does not mean the patient does not have bacterial infection. Gram stain is frequently negative in culture-positive gonococcal arthritis.

Gram-Positive for Organisms

Gram-positive cocci:	Consider **nafcillin 1 to 2 g IV every 4 hours** or **vancomycin 1 g every 12 hours**
Gram-negative bacilli:	Initial coverage, consider **ceftriaxone 2 g IV every 24 hours**. If suspect *Pseudomonas*, consider **piperacillin 2 to 3 g IV every 4 to 6 hours plus gentamicin 1 mg/kg IV every 8 hours.**

Gram-Negative for Organisms

Otherwise healthy adult:	Consider antistaphylococcal agent. If patient is at risk for gonococcal infection, add **ceftriaxone 1 g IV every 24 hours** or **penicillin G potassium 2 to 3 million units IV every 4 hours.**
Immunocompromised adult:	Consider *Staphylococcus* and Gram-negative coverage.

4. Elevate and splint the joint.
5. Consider surgical drainage in the following situations:
   - Septic hip joint
   - Loculated joint abscess
   - Prosthetic joint infection
   - Osteomyelitis or joint cartilage infection concomitant with septic arthritis

■ NECROTIZING FASCIITIS

Selective History

This devastating, life-threatening infection involves extensive necrosis of the superficial fascia, with wide undermining of the skin and sepsis. Most of these cases are caused by mixed infections of beta-hemolytic streptococci and staphylococci; however, either of these groups of pathogens alone can cause necrotizing fasciitis. Gram-negative organisms are responsible for about 10% of cases.

Most cases of necrotizing fasciitis occur as secondary infections of abrasions, cuts, insect bites, and bruises. Susceptible patients include those with diabetes and peripheral vascular disease.

Look for predisposing factors.

Is there a history of a skin trauma?

Does the patient have diabetes, peripheral vascular disease, or an immunologically compromised state?

Selective Physical Examination

VS: Fever, tachycardia, and hypotension
Skin: Edema (mild to massive); cellulitis is usually present; color is often pale red without distinct borders (early); color becomes purple, and may turn black later in the rapid course; bullae and blisters frequently present; serosanguineous exudate or seropurulent exudate; rapidly advancing involvement of tissue

Management

The mortality rate in necrotizing fasciitis exceeds 30%. Treatment must be definitive and rapid.

1. Start IV antibiotic therapy.
   Consider triple antibiotic coverage (ampicillin, gentamicin, and metronidazole) until cultures demonstrate a specific flora to which to direct therapy.
2. Contact your chief resident or attending physician immediately.
3. Obtain a general surgery consultation by a senior-level resident immediately.
   Patients with necrotizing fasciitis require aggressive surgical debridement in the operating room. All undermined, necrotic fascia must be debrided and wounds must be opened. Frequent redebridements are generally required. Definitive culture and Gram stain can be taken in the operating room. Frequently, organisms will grow in culture despite the initiation of IV antibiotics several hours earlier.

21

MENTAL STATUS CHANGES

The cognitive functioning of a patient is the most complex of all physiologic processes, and it is therefore affected by derangements in many organ systems. Appropriate assessment of mental status changes requires a knowledge of a prior mental status examination. This information may be available from the chart or from the bedside caregiver. It is useful to organize your thinking according to that baseline and how the patient appears. The etiologies of confusion fall into two major categories: delirium and dementia.

Delirium is an acute change and is characterized by clouded sensorium, agitation, confusion, and misinterpretations of the environment (hallucinations, illusions, and delusions). Delirium is potentially reversible and may be recurrent. For example, a common cause of a confusion in a postoperative patient is hypoperfusion. Remember that mental status is one of the three readily identifiable end-organ functions that are acutely affected by shock (the others being skin perfusion and urine output). Correction of the hypoperfusion will, in many cases, also reverse the confusion. Untreated, delirium increases morbidity and mortality.

Dementia is an irreversible state of loss of memory, loss of cognitive function, and recognition. This is a baseline finding and should be well documented in the chart. A patient who has elements of dementia may still become delirious. It is necessary to compare the current state with how the patient was described at the time of his or her best recent cognitive functioning.

Most concerning are mental status changes in patients after recent neurosurgical procedures or in patients at risk for sepsis.

■ PHONE CALL

Questions

1. **What symptoms is the patient exhibiting?**
   Clarify whether the patient is a risk to him- or herself or to others.
2. **Is this level of consciousness a change?**
   What was the baseline level of consciousness? Has the patient exhibited this sort of behavior before?
3. **Are there other medical problems?**
   This may include metabolic derangements such as diabe-

tes, hypocalcemia, hypomagnesemia, or thyroid malfunction; primary central nervous system (CNS) disease such as seizure disorder, stroke, or organic brain syndrome; or infectious disease such as meningitis or sepsis.

4. **What medications is the patient currently taking?**
   Many will cause a change in mental status.
5. **Has the patient undergone a surgical procedure, and if so, how long ago?**
   If this was a neurosurgical procedure, consider ordering a noncontrast computed tomographic (CT) head scan immediately. If the patient is taking narcotic medication, depressed cognitive functioning may result.
6. **Did the patient fall?**
   See Chapter 10.
7. **Are there any other symptoms?**
8. **Are there any changes in vital signs?**

Orders

1. Make sure the patient and the bedside caregivers are safe. Often delirious patients exhibit combative behavior.
2. Order a bedside finger stick glucose level check immediately. Send for complete blood count and electrolyte level immediately.
3. Check oxygen saturation of arterial blood (SaO_2) with pulse oximetry.
   Supply O_2 if necessary. Be careful when delivering O_2 to patients with chronic obstructive pulmonary disease (COPD).
4. Hold all medications that could further alter the patient's sensorium.
5. If the patient is currently taking narcotic medication, have **naloxone hydrochloride (Narcan) 2 mg for intravenous (IV) administration at the bedside.**

Degree of Urgency

The patient must be evaluated immediately. A recurrent benign problem that is well documented in the chart, or that is expected, may wait if there is more urgent work to do. If there is uncertainty in your mind, see the patient immediately.

■ ELEVATOR THOUGHTS

What causes a change in mental status?
- Central nervous system

Infection (meningitis, abscess, infected appliance, human immunodeficiency virus [HIV], and encephalitis)

Cerebral vascular accident and transient ischemic attack

Head trauma

Tumor

Primary dementia (Alzheimer's, multi-infarct dementia, and Parkinson's disease)

Encephalopathies (Wernicke's and alcoholic)

Seizures (petit mal and postictal state)

CNS vasculitis

- Medications
    Narcotics
    Sedatives
    Hypnotics
    Anesthetic agents
    Antidepressants
    Anticonvulsants
    Nonsteroidal anti-inflammatory drugs (NSAIDs)
    Steroids
    Other medications, e.g., histamine H_2 receptor antagonists, other antihistamines, lidocaine, and digoxin
- Medication withdrawal
    Alcohol
    Anxiolytics
- Metabolic derangements
    Hypoglycemia and hyperglycemia
    Hyponatremia and hypernatremia
    Hypercalcemia
    Acid–base disorders
    Endocrinopathies (hypothyroidism, hyperthyroidism, and adrenal malfunction)
- Organ failure
    Renal
    Liver (encephalopathy)
    Respiratory system (hypoxia and hypercapnia)
    Circulatory system (hypoperfusion)
    Multiorgan failure
- Other global infection or serious illness
    Sepsis
    Polytrauma

■ MAJOR THREAT TO LIFE

- Alcohol withdrawal
- CNS mass lesion (herniation, tumor, and epidural or subdural fluid collections)
- Hypoxia
- Medication overdose

- CNS infection
- Sepsis

■ BEDSIDE

Quick Look Test

The degree of change in a patient's mental status is an indication of the severity of the underlying condition. A patient may be described as

Awake and alert
Lethargic
Stuporous
Comatose

Patients who need emergent treatment include those for whom lethargy, stupor, or coma is an acute change.

A Glasgow Coma scale is often used (Table 21–1).

Airway and Vital Signs

Confirm adequate air movement and oxygenation. Check a pulse oximeter reading and supply supplemental O_2 as required. Remember that supplemental O_2 may cause respiratory failure in patients with COPD. Early sepsis may present with tachycardia and hypotension. The febrile patient may be delirious just by virtue of the fever. Hypoxic patients may hyperventilate; patients who are narcotized will hypoventilate.

Table 21–1 □ GLASGOW COMA SCALE

Function	Response	Score
Eye opening (E)	Spontaneously	4
	To voice	3
	To pain	2
	None	1
	Eyes swollen closed	C
Best motor response (M)	Obeys commands	6
	Localizes pain	5
	Withdraws from pain	4
	Decorticate to pain	3
	Decerebrate to pain	2
	None	1
Best verbal response (V)	Oriented, appropriate	5
	Confused	4
	Inappropriate words	3
	Incomprehensible sounds	2
	None	1
	Intubated/trach	T

Initial Management

1. Support ventilation and oxygenation if necessary.
2. Support circulation and blood pressure if necessary.
3. Check blood glucose result, and correct if necessary.
4. Perform and document a complete neurologic examination (see below).

Selective History and Chart Review

- Look for causes of mental status changes (see Elevator Thoughts).
- Review the patient's current medications.
    Look also at the list of medications normally taken at home. Was an important medication forgotten in the hospital orders?
- Compare the most recent neurologic examination to previous ones in the chart.

Selective Physical Examination

VS:	Repeat now.
HEENT:	Is there papilledema (see Fig. 15–1) or nuchal rigidity (meningitis)? What are pupil size and reactivity? (Pinpoint pupils suggest narcosis. Dilated pupils suggest sympathomimetic medications. Unequal pupils suggest intracranial mass lesion.) Is there evidence of head injury secondary to a fall (bruises, abrasions, skull bony abnormalities, or blood behind the tympanic membrane)?
Skin:	Is it cool and clammy (poor perfusion)? Is there icterus? Are there spider angiomata (organ failure)?
MS:	A complete mental status examination is required for the assessment of a confused or lethargic patient. Document this well. This may not always be possible for patients who are stuporous or comatose.
1. Consciousness:	Is the patient alert, lethargic, stuporous, or comatose?
2. General appearance:	What is the behavior, and what is the physical condition?
3. Mood:	Is the patient depressed, restless, agitated, or labile?
4. Form of thought:	How does information flow? Are there loose associations, flights of ideas, or perseverations?

5. Content of thought:	What is the information that flows? Is it composed of delusions or concrete ideations?
6. Perceptions:	Is the environment being misinterpreted? Are there illusions, or hallucinations (auditory or visual)?
7. Orientation:	Does the patient know who and where he or she is and what the time and the date are?
8. Registration:	Is the patient able to take in and repeat new information?
9. Recall:	Is the patient able to repeat the new information in short- and long-term fashions?
10. Long-term memory:	Is the patient able to recognize famous dates or famous people?
11. Language:	How is language used? Is it understood (spoken and written)?
12. Judgment:	What is the response to hypothetical situations?
Neuro:	A complete physical and neurologic examination is also important to evaluate for lateralizing signs that might suggest a CNS lesion or disease. Compare this with other neurologic examinations documented in the chart.
Tubes:	Does the patient have a CNS drain such as a ventricular shunt? Is it functioning? Has the disoriented patient removed other important lines or drains?
Wound:	Is the dressing intact?
Additional tests:	Perform additional tests as indicated.

■ MANAGEMENT

Further management is dictated by the suspected diagnosis. The treatments of sepsis, hypoxemia, metabolic derangement, and seizures are covered elsewhere in this book.

Medications

If a specific medication can be identified as the cause of the confusion, stop the drug and replace it with another appropriate medication as necessary. Often in elderly patients, a simple dose adjustment is necessary. Many medications require individualization of dosages.

If there has been a change in renal or liver function, look at the medications that are excreted or detoxified by these organs and make adjustments as necessary. It is important to review all the medications that a patient is taking—not just those that affect mental status, but also those that are nephrotoxic or hepatotoxic and other medications that are affected by a change in organ function. In these cases, a consultation with a nephrologist or a hepatologist is often helpful.

If a patient requires a medication that was omitted from the admission record or the postoperative orders, readminister it.

Some medications have antidotes that may be administered. Before treatment with further medication, be certain that the drug to be reversed is responsible for the change in mental status.

Narcotic Medication

- Administer **naloxone hydrochloride (Narcan) 0.2 to 2.0 mg IV, intramuscularly (IM), subcutaneously (SC), or by endotracheal tube (ET) every 5 minutes until there is a response (to a total of 10 mg); the effective dose may be repeated every 20 to 60 minutes.**

Benzodiazepine Medication

- Administer **flumazenil (Romazicon) 0.2 mg IV over 30 seconds.** If there is an initial response in 30 seconds after the first dose, **an additional 0.3 mg may be given over 30 seconds.** If there is still no response, further doses of **0.5 mg may be administered every 1 minute to a total dose of 3 to 5 mg**. The effective dose may **be repeated every 20 minutes at a rate of 0.2 mg/min (to a total of 3 mg/hr).** Administration of flumazenil is associated with a risk of seizure, and it should be given carefully.

Specific Drug Overdose

Consult a pharmacology text, and contact the poison control department in your county to determine specific therapy. Treatment may include activated charcoal, ipecac, dialysis, and psychiatric consultation in addition to support of the patient's respiration and circulation.

Herniation or Mass Lesion

Patients who have lateralizing signs on neurologic examination (unequal pupils and unilateral loss of sensation or motor function) require a noncontrast head CT scan immediately. This is especially true of patients after recent neurosurgical procedures or of those who have had serious head trauma. If necessary, make sure that the patient's airway and circulatory system are supported. If the CT scan is abnormal or changed from baseline, contact the resident. Neurosurgical consultation may be required to drain fluid collections or to place a bolt for pressure manometry. These patients will require surgical therapy and transfer to the intensive care unit or the cardiac care unit.

Alcohol Withdrawal

This is a potentially fatal complication of a hospitalized patient. It is important to establish a history of drinking, because withdrawal symptoms occur 24 to 48 hours after the last drink. Medical or psychiatric consultation is often required to help in the treatment of these patients.

Signs and Symptoms

- Change in mental status (insomnia, hallucinations, restlessness, and anxiety)
- Autonomic hyperactivity (sweating and tachycardia)
- Nausea and vomiting
- Hand tremors: coarse, fast frequency, and made worse with activity
- Delirium tremens (DTs)
- Seizures
- Korsakoff's psychosis or Wernicke's encephalopathy

Management

1. **Benzodiazepines**
   - **Chlordiazepoxide hydrochloride (Librium) at 25 to 100 mg IM or IV every 6 hours. Do not exceed 300 mg in a 24-hour period.**
     Or
   - **Diazepam (Valium) at 5 to 10 mg orally (PO) every 6 hours.**
     Maintain the administration of these medications for 24 hours, and then begin to reduce, as possible, by 20% per day over 5 to 7 days. Additional doses may be used to control agitation as necessary.
2. **Fluid and electrolyte support**
3. **Thiamine 100 mg IM or IV; repeat dose every day** until a regular diet is resumed
4. **Folate 1 mg PO every day for 4 days**
5. **Multivitamin 1 PO every day**
6. **Magnesium sulfate and antiepileptics** (may be useful to help control postwithdrawal seizures)
7. **Haloperidol lactate (Haldol) 2 to 5 mg PO/IM twice per day** (useful to control symptoms of withdrawal psychosis [DTs])
8. **Enlist medical or psychiatric consultation as needed to help care for the patient.**

Complications

- Seizures
- Aspiration

Primary Psychiatric Disease

Psychosis, schizophrenia, depression, mania, or other organic brain dysfunction is an additional diagnosis that will affect the treatment and the healing potential of the patient. These diagnoses require evaluation and treatment by a specialist. Do not hesitate to enlist the help of psychiatric colleagues.

■ SPECIAL SURGICAL CONSIDERATIONS

Preoperative Considerations

1. An acute change in mental status may affect a scheduled elective procedure.
   Check with the chief resident or the attending physician about canceling the procedure if necessary.
2. A history of cyclic changes in mental status, such as "sundowning" in elderly patients, is common and will be exacerbated postoperatively.
   Anticipate this, and make sure the patient is safe and the staff is made aware.
3. Many preoperative sedatives will affect mental status.

Postoperative Considerations

1. Many postoperative medications, such as anesthetic agents, narcotics, and sedatives, affect mental status.
   Expect some drowsiness and disorientation in any patient for a day after a general anesthetic, and expect a longer recuperation and more severe symptoms in elderly patients.
2. Postoperative neurosurgical patients should have well-documented neurologic examinations in the chart, which should be used as standards of comparison.
   A significant change in mental status requires a noncontrast head CT scan immediately to rule out mass lesion.
3. Postoperative neurosurgical patients also may have appliances in place to drain fluid collections or to monitor intracranial pressures.
   These can be a source of CNS infection or they may malfunction, causing increased intracranial pressure. In addition, a normally functioning drain does not preclude the presence of problematic fluid collections elsewhere in the skull.

Remember

1. High fever can be a source of delirium.
2. Sleep deprivation is a source of disorientation.

22

NAUSEA AND VOMITING

Nausea and vomiting are common on-call problems. There are many causes of nausea and vomiting. It is believed that the medulla contains two distinct centers that mediate vomiting, a chemoreceptor zone and a vomiting center. Toxic substances, drugs, and input from the cerebral cortex, the gastrointestinal (GI) tract, and other organs stimulate these centers to induce nausea and vomiting. Surgical patients are frequently exposed to medications that can stimulate the chemoreceptor zone. In addition, patients undergoing abdominal surgery frequently have a functional ileus and changes in GI function that predispose them to nausea. To be effective on call, you must know the common causes of and the treatments for nausea and vomiting.

■ PHONE CALL

Questions

1. **How severe is the nausea, and did the patient vomit?**

   Clarify the severity of the nausea and whether the patient has vomited. A patient who has mild nausea may benefit from orally (PO), rectally (PR), or intramuscularly (IM) administered antinausea medication. These methods of medication delivery are effective, yet they require time for the medication to be absorbed. A patient who has severe nausea and active vomiting may benefit more quickly from medication delivered intravenously (IV).

2. **Was anything associated with the nausea and the vomiting?**

   Did the patient recently eat a meal? Did the patient recently receive a medication or general anesthesia? Has the patient recently received chemotherapy?

3. **Has this patient had surgery? If so, what was the operation, and when was it performed?**

   It is critical to know what type of surgery and when the surgery was performed. Some types of surgery are associated with changes in GI function. For example, abdominal surgery frequently causes a postoperative ileus. Nausea and vomiting are common after major abdominal surgery unless decompression with a nasogastric (NG) tube is performed. Knowing exactly when surgery was performed is also important when dealing appropriately with nausea or vomiting problems. Patients are frequently nauseated in the first 12 hours postoperatively. This is often due to postanesthetic recovery. Many currently used anesthetic agents require several hours for anesthetic metabolism. Patients are frequently nauseated during this early postoperative period. Although anesthesiologists frequently give patients an antiemetic agent at the end of an operation, the antiemetic agent dosing may need to be repeated.

4. Has the patient had abdominal surgery?

Always suspect that a patient who has had abdominal surgery may have a functional ileus. As discussed in Chapter 6, a functional ileus may last 4 to 5 days or longer. Patients having upper abdominal surgery are generally maintained with nothing by mouth (kept NPO) and are decompressed with an NG tube until they pass flatus. Patients having lower colonic surgery are usually kept NPO, but they generally do not need NG tube decompression.

5. Has the patient recently had an NG tube?

After abdominal surgery or certain GI problems (e.g., bowel obstruction), NG tubes are placed. NG tubes are removed when it is believed that acceptable GI function has returned (patient is passing flatus). Frequently, NG tubes are removed prematurely, and patients become nauseated. If the patient vomits repeatedly, replacement of the NG tube may be warranted.

6. Is there hematemesis or coffee-ground emesis?

Hematemesis may indicate active bleeding; suspect GI bleeding. Hematemesis of bright-red or dark blood indicates that the source is proximal to the ligament of Treitz. This bleeding is frequently from the esophagus or the stomach, and it often indicates GI bleeding (see Chapter 13). Coffee-ground emesis indicates that old blood has been metabolized in the stomach by gastric acid. Blood is a strong emetic agent.

7. Are there any changes in vital signs?

A patient who has been vomiting repeatedly may become dehydrated and suffer from acid–base imbalance. The patient may also have a severe electrolyte disturbance or suffer from diabetic ketoacidosis.

8. Does the patient have an IV? Does the patient have any drug allergies? What are the patient's weight and age?

Check to see if the patient has IV access. If the patient has been vomiting repeatedly and is dehydrated, he or she will need IV fluids. In addition, many effective antiemetic medications may be delivered by an IV route. Also, clarify if the patient has any drug allergies. Some patients may have adverse reactions to antiemetic medications. Finally, have the nurse give the patient's weight and age. These will help to determine the dosing of an appropriate antiemetic agent. Beware of using inappropriate doses of antiemetic agents in children or in elderly patients.

Inform RN

"Will arrive at the bedside in . . . minutes."

Many of the calls for nausea and vomiting will be routine and do not require examination of the patient. However, if a patient has unstable vital signs, hematemesis, or significant distress, inform the RN that you will be coming to evaluate the patient.

■ ELEVATOR THOUGHTS

What causes nausea and vomiting?
- Gastroenteritis
  - Viral illness
  - Food poisoning (e.g., *Staphylococcus* and *Salmonella*)
- Drugs
  - Narcotics (e.g., morphine and meperidine hydrochloride)
  - Common therapeutic drugs (e.g., digoxin and theophylline)
  - Chemotherapeutic agents
  - Recovery from anesthesia (anesthetics)
- Abdominal causes
  - Functional ileus
  - Bowel obstruction
  - Inflammation or irritation of GI tract structures
  - Hepatobiliary and pancreatic disorders
- Electrolyte, endocrine, and metabolic disturbances
  - Acidosis
  - Hypernatremia
  - Hyponatremia
  - Hypercalcemia
  - Diabetic acidosis
  - Pregnancy
  - Uremia
- Associations with shock
  - Hypotension
  - Sepsis
  - Acute myocardial infarction
- Central nervous system (CNS) disorders
  - CNS infection, e.g., meningitis or encephalitis
  - Subarachnoid hemorrhage and stroke
  - Increased intracranial pressure secondary to trauma
  - Intracranial mass
- Conditions related to the inner ear
  - Infection

Motion sickness
Meniere's syndrome
- Psychiatric conditions
  Anxiety disorder
  Anorexia nervosa
  Bulimia
  Psychosis

■ MAJOR THREAT TO LIFE

- Aspiration pneumonia
- Intractable vomiting leading to GI bleeding (e.g., Mallory-Weiss tear)
- Unrecognized electrolyte or metabolic emergency (e.g., diabetic ketoacidosis)
- Postemetic rupture of the esophagus

A weakened patient or a patient with altered mental status is at high risk for aspiration. **Aspiration pneumonia** is a common cause of morbidity and death in debilitated patients. Severe and prolonged nausea and vomiting should be treated aggressively. Life-threatening complications of forceful vomiting include severe **GI bleeding** and **esophageal rupture.** In addition, it is important to identify and to treat **dehydration** and **electrolyte abnormalities** in vomiting patients. Frequently, nausea and vomiting signal serious electrolyte and metabolic disturbances.

■ BEDSIDE

It is necessary to examine and to evaluate patients with nausea and vomiting who also show signs of significant dehydration, hematemesis, or alterations in normal vital signs.

Quick Look Test

Does the patient look well (mildly nauseated), sick (very distressed), or critical (about to die)?
Patients with all types of medical problems will present with nausea and vomiting. A patient who is vomiting in response to a life-threatening problem (e.g., severe ketoacidosis, CNS bleeding, and hypotension) will often have an altered mental status and will look sick. If the patient is mildly nauseated with a normal mental status, the patient is probably stable.

Airway and Vital Signs

The airway is of concern in weakened patients or in patients with altered mental status. If these patients vomit, they are likely to aspirate. Aspiration may cause airway obstruction, tachypnea, hypoxemia, chemical pneumonitis, or pneumonia. You should make sure that the airway is clear after a compromised patient has vomited. With a gloved hand, sweep any vomitus from the mouth and the throat. Use bedside suction and a large suction tip to clear the airway. Once the airway is clear, the patient should be positioned in a lateral decubitus position. Any additional emesis will tend to drain from the mouth and not be aspirated. A patient in respiratory failure may need to be intubated.

Patients who have had severe and repeated bouts of vomiting may demonstrate changes in vital signs. They may show signs of dehydration and acidosis. On examination, look for tachycardia, tachypnea, and hypotension.

Selective History

Are there changes in neurologic status?

A patient who starts vomiting and who demonstrates a change in neurologic status may have a life-threatening problem. Consider stroke, meningitis, and increased intracranial pressure. Also, examine the abdomen quickly to look for abdominal distention and tenderness.

Selective Physical Examination

HEENT: Nuchal rigidity may indicate meningitis or subarachnoid hemorrhage. Papilledema indicates increased intracranial pressure (see Fig. 15–1).

Neuro: Assess mental status. Look for pupil symmetry and equal muscle strength on both sides of the body. A change in mental status, the finding of pupil asymmetry, or focal weakness may represent a neurosurgical emergency. Call a neurosurgeon for these problems.

GI: Assess if the abdomen is distended or tender. Abdominal distention may indicate a functional ileus. Abdominal tenderness may indicate peritoneal irritation, bowel obstruction, or peritonitis.

■ MANAGEMENT

The Unstable Patient with Severe Vomiting

1. Management should begin by stabilization of the vital signs. An unstable, vomiting patient who shows signs of hypo-

volemia or acidosis should be resuscitated with IV fluids (lactated Ringer's or normal saline). However, be careful not to fluid resuscitate patients who show evidence of increased intracranial pressure.

2. Make sure the airway is secure.

Do what is possible to minimize the chance that the patient will aspirate. Consider intubating a patient who has both respiratory distress and intractable, severe vomiting. Use a cuffed endotracheal tube, which will protect the airway from vomitus.

3. Look for electrolyte or metabolic causes of vomiting.

Once resuscitation with IV fluids has begun, draw an electrolyte panel, a complete blood count, and a glucose level. Be sure to draw the blood from a site distal to or away from the IV. Correct any electrolyte or glucose abnormalities.

4. Look for mechanical causes of the vomiting.

Has the patient had recent abdominal surgery? Should the patient have an NG tube? If a patient is vomiting repeatedly and has evidence of obstruction or ileus, place an NG tube to decompress the stomach and to remove residual gastric contents. **Do not place an NG tube if the patient has had recent esophageal or stomach surgery (to avoid the risk of perforation through the suture line).** In these patients, NG tubes must be placed with fluoroscopic guidance.

The Stable Patient with Nausea and Vomiting

1. Many patients with a self-limited illness such as viral gastroenteritis will need no therapy. These patients benefit from a clear liquid diet.

2. Look for mechanical causes of vomiting.

If the patient appears to have a functional ileus or a bowel obstruction, an NG tube will decompress the upper GI tract and the patient will feel better. If possible, discuss the need to place an NG tube with the patient before attempting to place it.

3. Look for any adverse drug reactions.

Frequently, morphine, meperidine hydrochloride, and other drugs induce nausea. Simply discontinuing the offending drug will often stop or slow the nausea and vomiting. If the patient requires a narcotic for adequate analgesia, combining an antiemetic agent with the narcotic may be effective; for example, meperidine is frequently combined with promethazine hydrochloride (Phenergan) for IM administration.

4. Look for electrolyte or metabolic disturbances that can explain the nausea and vomiting.

Table 22–1 □ COMMON ANTIEMETIC AGENTS

Drug Name	Drug Type	Dose
Promethazine hydrochloride (Phenergan)	Phenothiazine	25–50 mg PO, PR every 4–6 hr 25 mg IM every 4–6 hr 12.5 mg IV every 4–6 hr Peds: 0.5–1.0 mg/kg/dose PO, PR, or IM
Prochlorperazine maleate (Compazine)	Phenothiazine	5–10 mg PO, PR 3 or 4 times per day 5 mg IV over 2–3 min Peds: 0.13 mg/kg/dose
Trimethobenzamide hydrochloride (Tigan)	Related central agent	250 mg PO 3 times per day 200 mg PR, IM every 6–8 hr Peds: 100 mg/dose if patient is >30 lb
Metoclopramide monohydrochloride monohydrate (Reglan)	Dopamine antagonist	10 mg PO, IM, IV 1 hr before meals and at bedtime
Cisapride (Propulsid)	Prokinetic agent	10–20 mg PO before meals and at bedtime
Ondansetron hydrochloride (Zofran)	Serotonin 5-HT$_3$ blocker	8 mg PO, IV 3 times per day IV form may be given in a single 32-mg dose every day if desired

PO = orally; PR = rectally; IM = intramuscularly; IV = intravenously; Peds = pediatric.

Draw an electrolyte panel and a glucose level. Correct any significant abnormalities.

5. Consider providing an antiemetic drug. These agents may be given IV, IM, PO, or PR. They fall into four distinct classes. See Table 22–1 for a list of common antiemetic agents.

23

PAIN MANAGEMENT

Surgical patients have pain. As an on-call physician, you will receive many calls requesting pain medication for patients. Many of these calls are for reordering of medications. However, some of the calls will be for new-onset or poorly controlled pain. It is important to know how to control pain. Having an understanding of the various analgesic agents and delivery systems will allow you to order appropriate pain medication for patients.

■ PHONE CALL

Questions

1. **Where is the patient's pain, and how severe is the pain?**
   It is important to know what hurts the patient. Frequently, a patient will have pain in a location unrelated to the main medical problem or surgical site; for example, patients may develop back pain from prolonged bed rest. In addition, you should ask about the severity of a patient's pain. Severe pain is treated differently than mild pain.

2. **Has the patient had surgery? If so, what operation did the patient have, and when was it performed?**
   A patient who has had recent surgery or a traumatic injury will have pain. It is important that you know what type of operation the patient had and when it was done. This will help you decide what treatment to offer.

3. **Does the patient have any drug allergies?**
   You should know about any allergies or adverse drug reactions in a patient's history. You do not want to order a pain medication that will cause complications or allergic reactions. Also avoid ordering analgesic medications that have given a patient significant side effects or unpleasant experiences.

4. **What pain medication, if any, is the patient taking now?**
   It is important to know whether a patient is currently taking pain medication and whether the patient has pain while taking the medication. This will help you decide what changes to make in dosing or in analgesic selection.

5. **What is the patient's weight and age?**
   Elderly patients and pediatric patients are especially sensitive to narcotics. It is important to know the age and the weight of a patient when prescribing pain medication. For

pediatric patients of <75 lb (35 kg), dose medications by kilograms of body weight. For elderly debilitated patients, consider reducing the normal adult dose. Use your best judgment; you can always supplement with additional pain medication if necessary.

6. **Does the patient have a history of chronic pain?**

    Patients with chronic pain present significant challenges to the on-call physician. These patients are frequently demanding and will ask specifically for a particular medication (usually a narcotic). Try to assess what pain medications have been used recently in their care. Remember that non-narcotic preparations should be used to treat chronic pain whenever possible. Try to limit use of the narcotic pain medications to treat acute pain or acute pain episodes within the baseline chronic pain.

7. **Does the patient have a history of renal or liver disease or any history of peptic ulcer disease?**

    Avoid the use of acetaminophen in patients with liver disease. Acetaminophen can cause serious liver damage in these patients. Aspirin may cause gastrointestinal (GI) bleeding in patients with peptic ulcer disease. Although nonsteroidal anti-inflammatory drugs (NSAIDs) are generally safe and effective analgesics, they may cause adverse GI and renal effects; dyspepsia, gastritis, and peptic ulceration may occur with the use of NSAIDs. Although infrequent, reversible impairment of renal filtration, nephritis, papillary necrosis, and acute renal failure can occur with use of NSAIDs; avoid use of NSAIDs in patients having impaired renal function.

Orders

1. If pain is severe and not controlled by oral (PO) or intramuscular (IM) analgesics, ask the RN to place an intravenous (IV) line.
2. After ordering an appropriate pain medication, ask the RN to phone back in an hour if the pain has not been relieved by the medication.
3. If ordering high-dose or IV narcotic agents, ask the RN to monitor the patient's respiratory rate (RR), blood pressure (BP), and heart rate (HR).

Inform RN

"Will arrive at the bedside in . . . minutes."

If a patient has new-onset pain, previously undiagnosed pain, or pain significantly greater than you might expect otherwise, you need to examine the patient. For example, a stable ward patient complaining of sudden-onset, severe abdominal pain radiating to the back may have an expanding abdominal aortic aneurysm. Only by examining the patient will you find a pulsatile mass characteristic of an abdominal aortic aneurysm. Thus, make a habit of examining patients who have pain uncharacteristic of a particular medical problem or operation.

■ ELEVATOR THOUGHTS

What causes pain?
- Postoperative conditions
    Incisional wound
    Expanding hematoma
- Infections
    Cellulitis
    Abscess
    Osteomyelitis
- Inflammatory conditions
    Arthritis
    Neuritis and neuropathies
    Erythema nodosum
    Reflex sympathetic dystrophy
- Traumatic injuries
    Fractures
    Contusions
    Open wounds
    Posttraumatic inflammation
    Compartmental syndrome
- Skeletal system
    Lumbar disk disease (sciatica)
    Metastatic tumors to bone
    Primary skeletal tumors
    Expansile bone lesions
- Vascular disease
    Angina or myocardial infarction
    Arterial occlusion
    Venous thrombosis or thrombophlebitis
    Thromboangiitis (Buerger's disease)
- Psychological factors
    Chronic pain disorder
    Narcotic dependence

■ MAJOR THREAT TO LIFE

- Pain that is classic for a life-threatening medical problem (e.g., myocardial infarction, aortic aneurysm, and stroke)

- Untreated, severe, stressful pain leading to arrythmia or myocardial infarction

■ BEDSIDE

The purpose of evaluating a patient at the bedside is to rule out the major threats to life. Pain is a classic presentation for a variety of severe medical problems. Start your evaluation of the patient at the bedside by obtaining a pertinent history and performing a quick chart review.

Quick Look Test

Does the patient look well (mild pain), sick (moderate pain and distressed), or critical (severe pain and about to die)?

If a patient's pain is far greater than you would expect based on the operation or medical problem, rule out a major threat to life before treating with an analgesic. Severe pain associated with pale appearance, altered mental status, and overall distress may signal a severe problem such as dissecting or expanding aneurysm, contained ruptured vessel, expanding hematoma, stroke, myocardial infarction, or other emergency.

Airway and Vital Signs

Poorly treated pain may make a patient tachycardic and hypertensive. This occurs because pain may lead to sympathetic nervous system activation. In addition, abdominal pain (epigastric or subcostal) or musculoskeletal chest wall pain may contribute to shallow breathing and splinting. However, pain should not compromise the vital signs. Hypotension, bradycardia, or hypoxia generally indicate an underlying, significant medical problem or process. When evaluating the airway and vital signs, ask the following:

What is the HR, and is it regular or irregular?

Sinus tachycardia is common in patients with poorly treated pain. However, tachycardia associated with hypotension or irregular rhythm may signal a severe medical problem. For example, leg pain or chest pain associated with tachycardia and shortness of breath could be the presentation of pulmonary embolus.

What is the patient's temperature?

Pain alone does not cause fever. When pain is associated with fever, there are several types of processes to think about. For example, in postoperative surgical patients, incisional pain frequently leads to immobilization. Atelectasis is common in these patients and is a likely cause of fever. Other common causes of fever and pain include infectious or inflammatory processes.

Selective History and Chart Review

Where is the pain?

It is important to have the patient pinpoint the location of the pain. This will give you insight as to the likely cause.

When did the pain start, and has the patient experienced similar pain before?

Quickly review the chart noting the patient's medical history, date of surgery (if any), and postoperative course. Review the analgesics that the patient has been taking.

Selective Physical Examination

The goal of this examination is to rule out a serious medical problem that could be responsible for the pain. The examination should include a careful evaluation of both the site of the pain and the major organ systems.

VS:	HR, BP, RR, and temperature
HEENT:	Site of pain or surgical site
CVS:	Pulse volume
	Skin temperature and color
	Capillary refill (should be <2 seconds)
Resp:	Equal breath sounds
	Rales or rhonchi
Abd:	Softness
	Tenderness
	Rebound
Neuro:	Mental status
	Movement of all extremities
	Symmetric muscle strengths
Surgical site:	Examine for evidence of erythema, swelling, infection, dehiscence

■ MANAGEMENT

Once you have ruled out a major threat to life and have diagnosed the cause of the pain, you may treat the patient with an appropriate analgesic. The most common analgesics used in hospitals fall into the following three categories:

- Nonnarcotic agents

  These are best for mild to moderate pain, and they include acetaminophen and NSAIDs.

- Combination agents
  These agents are best for moderate pain, and they include oral agents that contain both a nonnarcotic (acetaminophen or aspirin) and a narcotic.
- Narcotic agents
  These drugs are for moderate to severe pain, and they include morphine, meperidine hydrochloride, and fentanyl.

Nonnarcotic Agents

These drugs are very useful for managing mild to moderate pain. Most are available for PO use. Acetaminophen is useful for mild pain and headache. It has analgesic and antipyretic properties but no anti-inflammatory properties. The NSAIDs are very useful for both analgesia and anti-inflammatory purposes. They are commonly used for musculoskeletal and arthritic pain. Most of these agents are in PO form, and one of these agents (ketorolac) is available in both IM and PO forms. Table 23–1 provides a list of some of the more popular nonnarcotic agents.

Combination Agents

These drugs combine oral narcotics with nonnarcotic analgesics. The combination of these two types of agents gives a synergistic effect. These are effective and potent drugs for moderate pain. The nonnarcotic component is either acetaminophen or aspirin. Choose the agent based on both the nonnarcotic and the narcotic ingredients. Remember to avoid ordering aspirin-containing combination agents in preoperative patients (aspirin interferes with platelet aggregation). In addition, do not use aspirin-containing drugs in the immediate postoperative period because of the increased risk of postoperative bleeding. Table 23–2 provides common combination agents. Note that some of these agents are available in different strengths. The strengths vary based on the narcotic component. Combination agents, especially the hydromorphone- and the oxymorphone-containing agents, have the potential for abuse.

Narcotic Agents

The narcotics are best reserved for moderate to severe pain. Some of these drugs are available in PO form and others are limited to parenteral use. Table 23–3 provides a list of commonly used narcotics.

The narcotic agents are generally class II or III substances, and they require triplicate prescription forms for outpatient use. All of the narcotics generally have side effects, which include sedation, respiratory depression, and nausea. In overdose, severe respira-

Table 23–1 □ COMMON NONNARCOTIC ANALGESICS

Drug	Dose and Route (Adult)	Comments
Acetaminophen (Tylenol)	650 mg PO or PR every 4 hr Pediatric dose: 10 mg/kg/dose	Avoid in patients with liver disease
Aspirin (Bayer varieties and Ecotrin)	650 mg PO every 4–6 hr	Avoid in patients with peptic ulcer disease Antiplatelet aggregation action
Ibuprofen (Motrin and Advil)	300–800 mg PO 4 times per day	NSAID Avoid in patients with liver or renal disease Avoid in patients with peptic ulcer disease Some antiplatelet aggregation action
Indomethacin (Indocin)	25–50 mg PO 3 times per day	NSAID
Sulindac (Clinoril)	150–200 mg PO twice per day	NSAID
Diflunisal (Dolobid)	1000 mg PO initially, then 500 mg PO twice per day	NSAID
Naproxen (Naprosyn)	200–500 mg PO 2 or 3 times per day	NSAID
Ketorolac	30 mg IM loading, followed by 15–30 mg IM every 6 hr or 10 mg PO every 6 hr	Potent parenteral NSAID Approved for short-term use (5 days)

PO = orally; PR = rectally; NSAID = nonsteroidal anti-inflammatory drug; IM = intramuscularly.

Table 23–2 □ **COMMON COMBINATION ANALGESICS**

Drug	Dose and Route (Adult)	Comments
Tylenol with Codeine	No. 2: 300 mg aceta + 15 mg codeine	2 strengths
	No. 3: 300 mg aceta + 30 mg codeine	
	1–2 tablets PO every 4 hr	
Darvocet-N	50: 325 aceta + 50 mg propoxyphene napsylate	2 strengths
	100: 325 aceta + 100 mg propoxyphene napsylate	
	1–2 tablets PO every 4 hr	
Darvon Compound-65	325 mg ASA + 65 mg propoxyphene napsylate	
	1–2 tablets PO every 4 hr	
Fiorinal	325 mg ASA + butalbital 50 mg + 40 g caffeine	
	1–2 tablets PO every 4 hr	
Vicodin or Vicodin ES	500 mg aceta + 5 mg hydrocodone bitartrate	2 strengths
	ES: 500 g aceta + 7.5 hydrocodone bitartrate	
	1–2 tablets PO every 4–6 hr	
Lortab	500 aceta + 2.5 or 5.0 or 7.5 mg hydrocodone bitartrate	3 strengths
	1–2 tablets PO every 4–6 hr	
Tylox	500 mg aceta + 5 mg oxycodone HCl	
	1 capsule PO every 6 hr	
Percocet	325 mg aceta + 5 oxycodone HCl	
	1 tablet PO every 6 hr	
Percodan	325 mg ASA + 5 mg oxycodone HCl	
	1 tablet PO every 6 hr	

aceta = acetaminophen; PO = orally; ASA = acetylsalicylic acid.

tory depression, altered mental status, and hypotension can result. Care must be used when administering parenteral narcotics. Frequent nursing checks of the patient's level of sedation and vital signs should be performed.

Narcotic drugs are usually given parenterally (IM or IV) to hospitalized patients. Table 23–4 compares IM and IV routes for administration of a narcotic drug.

One of the best ways to administer a narcotic IV is to use a patient-controlled analgesia (PCA) pump. A PCA pump is a device that allows a patient to self-administer a narcotic based on need. The patient presses a button that is attached to the pump,

Table 23-3 □ COMMON NARCOTICS FOR TREATING PAIN

Drug	Dose and Route (Adult)	Comments
Fentanyl citrate (Sublimaze)	2–3 µg/kg IV, to 50 µg	Short-duration IV, but very effective; 1–2-hr duration
	Transdermal patches: one 2.5-mg patch every 3 days	
Hydromorphone hydrochloride (Dilaudid)	1–2 mg PO, IM, PR every 4–6 hr	4–5-hr duration
Meperidine hydrochloride (Demerol HCl)	25-mg increments IV	More idiosyncratic rxns when given IV; 2–4-hr duration
	1.0–1.5 mg/kg, to 150 mg maximum IM, PO	Good for chronic pain and narcotic withdrawal; 4–6-hr duration
Methadone hydrochloride (Dolophine HCl)	1.5–10 mg PO, IM every 3–6 hr	
Morphine sulfate	0.1–0.2 mg/kg, to 2–4-mg IV increments	The "gold standard"; 2–4-hr duration
Sustained release morphine sulfate (MS Contin)	10–30 mg PO every 8–12 hr	Good for chronic pain 8–12-hr duration
Nalbuphine hydrochloride (Nubain)	5–10 mg IV, IM every 3–6 hr	3–6-hr duration
Pentazocine	30 mg IV, IM every 3–4 hr	2–3-hr duration
Propoxyphene hydrochloride	65 mg PO every 4 hr	Mild pain; 4–6-hr duration

IV = intravenously; PO = orally; IM = intramuscularly; PR = rectally.

Table 23–4 □ **COMPARISON OF INTRAMUSCULAR AND INTRAVENOUS ROUTES OF NARCOTIC ADMINISTRATION**

IM administration	Onset of action of narcotic is 15 to 20 minutes after injection
	Lower peak effect than IV administration
	Longer duration of action compared with IV route due to slower absorption
	Slower onset of narcotic side effects (e.g., respiratory depression)
IV administration	Immediate onset of action
	Greater peak effect than IM administration
	Shorter duration of action compared with IV route
	More rapid onset of potential side effects

IM = intramuscular; IV = intravenous.

and when the button is pressed, a measured dose of narcotic is delivered to the patient. The pump allows regulation of the narcotic to be used, frequency (maximum doses per hour), dose (milligrams per dose), maximum narcotic delivered per hour (milligram maximum per hour), and basal rate (base rate of narcotic in milligrams per hour).

If properly used, the PCA pump is a safe narcotic delivery system. If the dosing or frequency settings are deliberately set a little too high, the patient will become sedate and less likely to continue self-administering dosing. However, only the patient should be allowed to give him- or herself narcotic doses; a patient can be overdosed on narcotics with a PCA if family members or friends press the dose button and give an already sedate patient additional drug. Frequent nursing checks of the patient's level of sedation and vital signs should be performed. In addition, you must make sure that a narcotic antagonist (naloxone hydrochloride [Narcan]) is available on the ward. Table 23–5 gives typical settings for a PCA pump using three different narcotics.

Table 23–5 □ **TYPICAL PCA SETTINGS**

Narcotic	Dose	Lockout Interval	Basal Rate (Low Dose)
Morphine	1–3 mg	every 10–15 min	None to 2 mg/hr
Meperidine hydrochloride (Demerol HCl)	5–15 mg	every 10–15 min	None to 15 mg/hr
Fentanyl	15–25 μg	every 10–15 min	None to 25 μg/hr

PCA = patient-controlled analgesia.

Dose

Select a dose that gives the patient measurable relief of pain without excessive sedation. If the patient does not obtain pain relief from your initial PCA set dose, try increasing the dose of narcotic without changing the lockout interval. If the patient's pain is relieved without excessive sedation or change in vital signs, the pain is being managed appropriately. Record the amount used during the shift.

Lockout Interval

If the patient achieves pain relief with activation of a dose, but the pain returns before the end of the lockout period, shorten the lockout period. Many patients will need a PCA lockout in the 10-minute range. Some patients may do best with a lockout interval of <10 minutes. You can always start the lockout interval in the 10- to 15-minute range and shorten the interval if needed.

Basal Rate

This feature of a PCA allows you to run a narcotic drip to supplement the patient-controlled dosing. A basal rate offers the advantage of allowing the patient a level of continuous analgesia. However, a basal rate also introduces some risks. If the basal rate of narcotic is excessive, a patient may develop respiratory depression and excessive sedation. If you are going to run a basal rate, it is suggested that it be at a relatively low and safe dose. Higher doses can be used safely only in continuously monitored units or the intensive care unit.

Narcotic Antagonists

If you are going to use parenteral narcotics, narcotic antagonists must be available. These agents are usually competitive inhibitors that act on the opiate receptors. If a patient receiving parenteral narcotics becomes oversedated, hypotensive, or hypoxic or has significant respiratory depression, you should consider reversing the narcotic agent with an antagonist. Use **naloxone hydrochloride (Narcan) 0.4 to 2.0 mg IV, IM, subcutaneously, or by endotracheal tube.** IV naloxone is most likely to give the most rapid reversal.

Other Pain Management Options

There are other strategies for managing pain while on call. Many hospitals have a pain service run by anesthesiologists, and consulting with them can be very useful. They can help manage pain with a variety of therapies including epidural catheters, IV lidocaine, and long-acting nerve blocks.

Patients having thoracic or abdominal surgery can frequently benefit from epidural anesthesia. An epidural catheter is usually placed at the time of surgery by an anesthesiologist. An epidural can also be placed postoperatively. Either a narcotic infusion or a local anesthetic infusion can be run through the epidural catheter to provide profound analgesia. The epidural catheter is usually placed and managed by the anesthesiology service. There are risks associated with epidural catheters, including infection, bleeding, and hypotension. Discuss the case with your chief resident or attending physician before consulting anesthesiology for placement of an epidural catheter.

24

PREOPERATIVE PREPARATION

Ideally, a patient is prepared preoperatively for a procedure by the primary care team. Occasionally, an on-call physician will be asked to complete a workup or to check a laboratory result. Preoperative preparation encompasses those precautions that are aimed at decreasing the inherent risks of a procedure. A patient must be readied both physically and psychologically.

■ NUTRITION

Extensive surgical procedures are followed by an obligate catabolic period, the length of which is influenced by the extent of the operation, the natural history of the disease state, and the general health of the patient. Urgent and emergent conditions do not allow for the shoring up of metabolic stores. But in elective cases, enteral supplementation, especially with protein-rich foods, or even total parenteral nutrition may be beneficial. The diets of patients with documented malnutrition (albumin of <3.0 g/dl or a 15% weight loss) should be supplemented. There is value in supplementation in elderly patients or in patients with other degenerative diseases such as cardiac cachexia or pulmonary insufficiency. Benefit is measurable in 5 to 7 days.

■ HYDRATION

Surgery is associated with intravascular volume depletion. This may include fluid losses such as bleeding and insensible losses due to exposure of surgical fields to the air, and hemodynamic changes due to anesthetic agents. Patients should be well hydrated preoperatively to account for potential losses. In addition, patients may present with fluid deficits. Intra-abdominal infections and generalized sepsis are associated with sequestration of fluids or "third spacing." Intravascular volume may be further depleted by vomiting, diarrhea, or anorexia before presentation. Correction of preexisting fluid deficits should be added to hydration before a surgical procedure. Fluid replacement therapy is covered more fully in Chapters 12 and 17. Follow moderate fluid replacement therapy closely with adequate hemodynamic, urine output, and electrolyte monitoring. Care should be used when hydrating a patient with suspected congestive heart disease.

■ PROPHYLACTIC ANTIBIOTICS

Prophylactic antibiotic treatment has documented efficacy in many but not all surgical procedures. Table 24–1 lists those instances in which the inherent costs and risks of antibiotic therapy are outweighed by the potential costs and risks of infectious complications. Antibiotics should be delivered at least 30 minutes before the skin incision to ensure adequate tissue levels of the agent. Additional doses should be given at appropriate intervals postoperatively for 24 hours. Attending surgeons often have their own preferences as to when antibiotics should be used and which agent is appropriate; for example, many physicians prefer the use of second-generation cephalosporins before bowel surgery. Always ask. Shaving, if necessary, should be done immediately before the incision.

■ MECHANICAL BOWEL PREPARATION

Alimentary tract cases, as described above, are contaminated with enteric bacteria. To decrease the risk of infection and compli-

Table 24–1 □ OPERATIONS FOR WHICH PROPHYLACTIC ANTIBIOTICS ARE FOUND TO BE BENEFICIAL

Procedure	Antibiotic
Oropharyngeal	Penicillin
Esophageal (includes hiatal hernia)	1st-generation cephalosporin
Gastroduodenal	1st-generation cephalosporin
Biliary tract (high risk) Age >70 yr Cholecystitis Required choledochostomy	Mechanical bowel preparation and 2nd-generation cephalosporin
Bowel resection (small or large)	Mechanical bowel preparation and 2nd-generation cephalosporin
Laparotomy for penetrating abdominal trauma	1st-generation cephalosporin
Colorectal	Mechanical bowel preparation and 1st-generation cephalosporin
Appendicitis with suspected perforation	2nd-generation cephalosporin
Hysterectomy	1st-generation cephalosporin
Abdominal or lower extremity revascularization	1st-generation cephalosporin
Foreign body implantation Cardiac valve Prosthetic joint	1st-generation cephalosporin

cation of abscess formation, mechanical bowel preparation is beneficial. This is performed the day before surgery. The patient is instructed to remain on a clear liquid diet. Four liters of electrolyte solution (e.g., GoLYTELY or Colyte) is administered by mouth and should be completely taken within the space of 1 hour. A nasogastric tube may be required for administration. If the efflux does not clear, supplemental saline enemas may be useful. Enemas may be the sole agent required for rectal surgery. In addition, oral antibiotics are administered, as follows:

Neomycin 1 g and erythromycin base 1 g by mouth at 1 P.M., 3 P.M., and 11 P.M. on the day before surgery. Always administer the oral antibiotics well in advance of or after the electrolyte solution, as any pills in the gastrointestinal tract will get washed out. The goal of mechanical bowel preparation is not to completely sterilize the bowel contents, but to decrease the bacterial count. The patient should be maintained with nothing by mouth for 6 to 8 hours before surgery to ensure adequate stomach emptying and to decrease aspiration risk. Be sure to maintain adequate intravenous hydration during this time. Routine medications may be given the morning of surgery with a small sip of water.

■ PREOPERATIVE LABORATORY STUDIES

Blood is generally drawn preoperatively to evaluate potential risks of the procedure to the patient, for example, for measurement of hemoglobin and hematocrit when anemia is suspected. Another purpose is to establish a baseline for comparison, if the same study will be used to follow the patient postoperatively, for such things as tumor markers, or Ca^{2+} before parathyroid resection. Clotting studies (prothrombin time, partial thromboplastin time, Ivy bleeding time, and platelet count) are important for patients with liver failure, renal failure, or bleeding diathesis, and also for those patients treated with anticoagulants (including aspirin) or those who may require blood product replacement. Other studies (e.g., chest x-ray and electrocardiogram) may be considered as the patient's clinical condition indicates.

■ BLOOD PRODUCT REPLACEMENT

The blood required postoperatively is determined by the patient's cardiovascular reserve, the amount of blood lost during the procedure, and the ongoing postoperative losses due to leaks or hypocoagulability states. The need to have blood or products available is dependent on the type of surgery planned and the preferences of the surgeon. The blood bank requires a clot tube to be drawn well in advance of need so that the patient's serum can be matched with the product. There are several options for ensuring the availability of blood (Table 24–2). Check with the hospital blood bank for more information regarding specific times of preparation and the time interval for which each option is valid.

Patients may also have blood available from other sources. Autologous blood is that which has been donated by the patient in the weeks before in preparation for elective surgery. Directed donor blood has been donated by a friend or a relative of the patient and is crossmatched to the patient. It is important to confirm the readiness of these types of blood with the blood bank. Also, individual blood banks may have protocols for specific surgical procedures. If you know of a greater blood need before a procedure, let the blood bank know well in advance.

■ OTHER CONSIDERATIONS

Patients with concurrent illnesses may have special requirements for pre- and postoperative care. Cardiovascular evaluation is important in patients who are elderly or who have a history of heart disease. This is especially important after myocardial infarction (MI). A general surgical procedure within 6 weeks of an MI carries a 50% risk of a second MI. The risk of death approaches 25%. Elective procedures should be postponed for at least 6 months after MI, if possible, to decrease the risk of subsequent cardiac events. If this is not possible because of urgency, appropriate care should be used, including afterload reduction, cardiovascular and hemodynamic monitoring, and arrhythmia precautions.

Specific diseases require selective preparation. For example, a patient to be operated on for removal of pheochromocytoma must

Table 24–2 □ **OPTIONS FOR ENSURING THE AVAILABILITY OF PREOPERATIVE BLOOD**

Type only	This gives only the ABO blood type and the Rh status of the patient.
Type and hold (no. of units)	This types the patient's blood and reserves the blood for use in the future. The blood may be released for use in another patient if it is not used.
Type and crossmatch (no. of units)	This types the patient's blood and prepares the units of blood for subsequent administration. The blood cannot be released for use in any other patient.

first be adequately hydrated, treated with nitroprusside, and then treated with alpha and beta blockade to protect against catecholamine storm. In a similar manner, patients with thyroid storm require beta blockade and antithyroid measures.

Patients treated with recent or chronic steroid replacement therapy will require stress doses of hydrocortisone to bolster the physiologic postoperative adrenal response (Table 24–3). Do not hesitate to enlist specialists to help handle a complex series of problems, as your primary care team allows.

■ PSYCHOLOGICAL PREPARATION

Along with physiologic changes, the patient will also undergo psychological changes after a surgical procedure. Anticipation of these changes and proper preparation of the patient will make the postoperative period smoother for both patient and physician. Patients may already be depressed and frightened at the new onset of illness or the prospect of surgery. Listen to patients carefully; they often communicate their fears. Answer questions fully and honestly. Make enough time to talk. Be optimistic but not unrealistic. Explain to each patient and to significant others the full procedure, the risks, the alternatives, and the goals. Include descriptions of the scar and any disfiguring aspects of the procedure (including drains or tubes). Be sure to describe what the postoperative recovery period will be like and what will be expected of the patient. Include descriptions of what to expect with regard to pain and its management, incentive spirometry, bowel function, ambulation, and diet.

Expect the patient to be depressed for 2 or 3 days after the procedure. Encourage support from family and significant others during this time. Anticipate a psychological regression, which is common with anyone who enters the hospital. Hospitals, by their nature, remove part of a patient's individuality and reduce even strong-willed people to the common denominators of nursing

---

Table 24–3 □ PERIOPERATIVE STEROID REPLACEMENT REGIMEN

Preoperative	100 mg hydrocortisone IV at midnight and 2 hr before surgery
Postoperative	100 mg hydrocortisone IV immediately postoperative, again in 8 hr, and again in 12 hr
POD 1	100 mg hydrocortisone IV every 12 hr
POD 2	50 mg hydrocortisone IV or PO every 12 hr
POD 3	Continue to taper rapidly over 4–5 days unless replacement steroids are necessary

IV = intravenously; POD = postoperative day; PO = by mouth.

schedules and bodily functions. Encourage questions; remind the patient to write questions down, because they may be difficult to remember later when the care team is making rounds. Most important is maintaining openness and approachability. Each patient will have different needs.

The night before surgery, patients often require a sedative for sleep. More important may be a reassuring visit from the attending surgeon to answer any last-minute questions.

■ PREOPERATIVE NOTE

All the above information should be summarized in a brief preoperative note. The following is an example:

Preop Note
Procedure anticipated:
Attending surgeon:
List of routine medications/therapies:
List of significant preoperative exam findings:
List of preoperative lab and study results:
Bowel preparation (if needed):
Diet orders:
Blood products available:
"On call to OR" instructions:
   Void:
   Preoperative medications:
Consent signed and witnessed:
PAR (a brief statement that the procedure has been discussed with the patient, e.g.: "Procedure, alternatives, and risks described in detail to the patient, questions were answered to his/her satisfaction. He/She elects to proceed. Consent signed."):

25

PRONOUNCING DEATH

One of the most unpleasant requirements of on-call responsibilities is pronouncing death. This important task represents a significant medicolegal responsibility. You may not have had much experience evaluating recently deceased persons, and there is some controversy as to what exactly constitutes the legal definition of death. This chapter provides a guide of the steps to follow when declaring a patient deceased.

Different states in the United States may have differing criteria for declaring death. However, most states and neighboring countries, including Canada and Mexico, have adopted the concepts of both physiologic death and brain death. Physiologic death refers to absence of any spontaneous cardiac activity, no blood pressure, and no evidence of respiration. Pronouncing brain death is more complicated and is usually managed by neurology or neurosurgery services. There is more variability regionally as to what constitutes brain death. Remember that declaring death is a serious medicolegal responsibility. Be careful and studious in your evaluation of the person presumed deceased.

When you are paged by the RN to pronounce a patient dead, it is advisable that you come equipped with a stethoscope and a penlight. The most important thing to ascertain is that the patient has no spontaneous circulation or respiratory function. It is also important to perform a brief assessment of the neurologic system. Table 25–1 indicates the key criteria for declaring death. Using these criteria to declare death requires that the person presumed deceased has a body temperature of at least 34°C to 35°C. If the body is very cold, you may have to warm it before legally pronouncing death. Recall that hypothermia slows metabolic rate, heart rate, and respiratory rate. Hypothermic critically ill patients have been mistaken for dead. Also make sure that there is no history of use of paralytic drugs or sedatives within a reasonable time period. If paralytic drugs were used within the last 6 to 8 hours before the presumed death, a paralytic reversing agent such as neostigmine methylsulfate (Prostigmin) should be administered.

■ STEPS FOR PRONOUNCING DEATH: THE NONVENTILATED PATIENT

1. Overview the chart briefly.
   Make sure that in examining the presumed deceased you

Table 25–1 □ KEY CRITERIA FOR PRONOUNCING DEATH

No cardiac activity (asystole)
No blood pressure
No respiratory activity

will incur no infectious risk (e.g. human immunodeficiency virus or hepatitis).

2. Check the identity of the patient by looking at the identification bracelet worn on the wrist.

   Make sure you know who you are pronouncing dead.

3. Make sure that the patient does not respond to verbal or tactile stimuli.

   You may want to perform a sternal rub to satisfy yourself that the presumed deceased does not respond to painful stimuli.

4. Check for radial and carotid pulses.

   The deceased patient will have no pulses anywhere.

5. Check the blood pressure.

   The deceased patient will have no blood pressure.

6. Listen for heart sounds; listen carefully over the entire precordium.

   You will hear no heart sounds in a deceased patient. You may also want to listen over the carotid artery in the neck. If the patient is in the intensive care unit and is attached to monitoring leads, you may wish to evaluate the rhythm strip, although this is not necessary.

7. Listen for spontaneous respirations over both lung fields.

   A deceased patient will have no air movement whatsoever.

8. Examine the pupils.

   The pupils of a deceased patient will be fixed, and they will also often be dilated, but not always. The pupils will not respond to light.

■ STEPS FOR PRONOUNCING DEATH: THE VENTILATED PATIENT

If a mechanically ventilated patient has lost cardiac activity and has no blood pressure, you must alter the procedure by which you declare death. First, contact the attending physician for consent to turn off the ventilator. Once there is agreement to terminate mechanical ventilation, proceed to disconnect the ventilator. First, however, make sure that all the electrocardiographic (ECG) leads are properly connected and that the monitoring equipment is functioning. You do not want to disconnect from the ventilator a patient who actually does have cardiac activity. In addition, make sure that the patient has not been given any paralytic drugs within 6 to 8 hours of the examination.

1. After you have verified that the ECG monitoring equipment is functioning and all the connections are intact, proceed to disconnect the ventilator from the patient; leave the endotracheal tube in place.
2. Follow the procedure outlined in steps 1 to 8 in the preceding section for declaring death.
3. Observe the patient for a full 3 minutes for evidence of spontaneous respiration.
4. Record in the medical record that mechanical ventilation was terminated after consultation with the attending physician and after all evidence of circulatory function had ceased. Document the rest of your examination. Give a time and a date when you declared death.

■ AFTER YOUR EXAMINATION

Always remember to document your examination in the chart. Carefully list what your examination found. The time of death is the time you complete your examination. Record the time of death and the date. Sign the note. You may also be required to fill out and sign the death certificate. Some hospitals will also ask that you call the medical examiner's office to notify them of the death.

It is appropriate to contact your supervising resident or the attending physician as soon as you pronounce the patient dead. Ask your superiors if they want you to contact the next of kin. It is appropriate to notify the family as soon as practically possible. Also ascertain from the attending physician whether an autopsy is necessary or appropriate. The attending physician may want to consult the family about this option.

If you are going to notify the family of the deceased and you did not know the patient, take some time to review the medical history and the recent events. Talk to the nursing staff about the family members who have visited the patient. Become aware of any difficult family situations that may be important.

First, contact the family member closest to the patient. Sometimes the RN will know which family member is the spokesperson for the family. You may also see a notation in the chart as to who is the next of kin. Once you have made telephone contact with the family member, identify yourself and the hospital where you work. In an apologetic and conciliatory tone, inform the family member that their loved one has passed away. Frequently, the family member will want to know the time of death and the circumstances. If appropriate, you may wish to offer the reassur-

Table 25–2 □ CRITERIA FOR PRONOUNCING BRAIN DEATH

No cerebral or brain stem function
   Fixed pupils
   No response (including reflexes) to noxious stimuli
   Apneic during oxygenation (for 10 min)
   No oculovestibular responses (50-ml ice-water calorics)
   Spinal reflexes may be intact
   Circulatory function may be intact
Coma of known cause and duration
   Known structural damage or disease
   Known irreversible metabolic disease
   No hypothermia, sedation, paralytic drugs, or drug intoxication
   Minimum 6-hr observation of no brain function; if drugs or alcohol were
      involved, a minimum of 24 hr of observation of no brain function and
      a negative toxicology screen is required
Optional criteria
   No cerebral circulation on angiogram
   Electroencephalogram isoelectric for 30 min at maximal gain
   Auditory evoked responses show no brain stem function

ance that death was painless and peaceful. Do not be shocked if a family member is not surprised or too upset. Many families have watched a loved one deal with chronic illness, pain, and suffering for many years. They are often relieved when they hear that the loved one has passed away. Other families may show obvious grief and despair at the notification of the death of their loved one. Try to be supportive, and understand that distinct cultures deal with death in different ways.

■ BRAIN DEATH AND ORGAN DONATION

As the on-call physician, it is not your responsibility to pronounce brain death. This is a more complicated task than declaring physiologic death. Consult neurology or neurosurgery for help with this task. The declaration of brain death is important for obtaining legal clearance for organ donation. If you believe that a brain-dead patient may be a good candidate for organ donation and the family is supportive, contact the organ transplant program at your hospital or in your city. There is usually a transplant coordinator on call 24 hours a day to help make arrangements. You should maintain the brain-dead patient on supportive hydration and ventilation until the transplant service takes over the management of the organ donor.

The concept of brain death has been accepted throughout the United States, Canada, Mexico, and much of the world. The diagnostic criteria followed by most hospitals are shown in Table 25–2.

26

POSTOPERATIVE BLEEDING

Bleeding in the postoperative period is a concern for the on-call physician. You must decide whether the bleeding has a surgical cause (major vessel bleeding) or a medical cause (abnormal coagulation status). Some patients will require a return to the operating room for control of bleeding. Other patients may require bedside care or transfusion of blood products. Guidelines for evaluation of bleeding patients and for management of postoperative bleeding problems are discussed in this chapter.

■ PHONE CALL

1. **What are the patient's vital signs?**

   Rapid postoperative bleeding is usually associated with hypotension and tachycardia.

2. **How severe is the bleeding?**

   Ask the RN to describe the bleeding site. Is the dressing or the wound slowly oozing blood, or is there a large amount of blood on the dressing or in the patient's bed? Also ask the RN if the surgical site appears markedly swollen or bruised (hematoma).

3. **What operation did the patient have, and when was the operation performed?**

   Knowing the surgical site is critical when managing bleeding patients. For example, a bleeding patient who has undergone abdominal, chest, or pelvic surgery can easily bleed into the potential spaces of these anatomic areas.

4. **Does the patient have known bleeding problems, and is the patient taking anticoagulant medication?**

   Ask the RN if the patient has a history of bleeding diathesis (e.g., alcoholic liver disease). Also find out if the patient is taking, or has recently taken, aspirin, warfarin sodium, or other medication that interferes with normal blood clotting.

5. **Does the patient have recent blood count and coagulation studies? Is there blood available for this patient in the blood bank?**

   If a postoperative patient is already anemic from a surgical procedure, significant postoperative bleeding is likely to lead to decompensation. Recent coagulation studies are important to help you rule out coagulopathy as a cause of bleeding. Make sure that blood is available for any patient with significant postoperative bleeding.

Orders

1. Order intravenous (IV) line access.

    For patients with significant bleeding, ask the RN to establish an IV if a functional IV is not present. For patients with significant bleeding, one or two large-bore (14- to 16-gauge) antecubital IVs are necessary. Large antecubital IVs are generally better than central lines for fluid resuscitation.

2. Give IV fluids.

    Order a 500-ml fluid bolus (normal saline [NS] or lactated Ringer's [LR]) if a patient has hemodynamic compromise associated with active bleeding.

3. Order hematocrit immediately.

    Ask the RN to draw a hematocrit immediately if possible. The RN should be sure to draw blood from a site distal to the IV or from the opposite upper extremity. If a patient has bleeding associated with hemodynamic compromise, blood should be drawn only after IV access and fluid resuscitation have been initiated.

4. Order platelet count and coagulation studies (prothrombin time [PT] and partial thromboplastin time [PTT]) immediately.

Inform RN

"Will be at the bedside in . . . minutes."

Postoperative bleeding requires immediate bedside evaluation. The amount of bleeding may be underestimated by the RN.

■ ELEVATOR THOUGHTS

What are the causes of postoperative bleeding?

Surgical Causes

- Technical surgical errors
    1. Ties coming off vessels
    2. Inadequate coagulation of vessels
    3. Unrecognized vessel injury (traumatic or iatrogenic)
    4. Transected vessels not bleeding at the time of surgery (vasospasm)
- Bleeding from surgical sites
    1. Bleeding associated with coughing or hypertension
    2. Bleeding from vessel anastamoses (vascular surgery)

Medical Causes

- Platelets
    1. Thrombocytopenia

   2. Platelet dysfunction
         von Willebrand's disease
         Uremia
         Nonsteroidal anti-inflammatory drugs (NSAIDs) and
            other drugs
- Soluble blood clotting factors
   1. Coagulopathy of liver disease
   2. Other coagulation factor deficiencies
         Hemophilia A and B (factors VIII and IX, respectively)
   3. Vitamin K deficiency
   4. Disseminated intravascular coagulation (DIC)
   5. Dilutional coagulopathy
   6. Coagulopathy associated with drugs
         Heparin
         Warfarin sodium (Coumadin)

■ MAJOR THREAT TO LIFE

- Major surgical bleeding (large vessel)
- Bleeding in the neck leading to airway compromise
- Intracranial bleeding leading to increased intracranial pressure or herniation
- Severe coagulopathy or DIC

■ BEDSIDE

Quick Look Test

Does the patient look well (comfortable), sick (uncomfortable or distressed), or critical (about to die)?
   Patients who have significant postoperative bleeding usually look distressed or critical. Rapid intravascular blood loss leads to activation of the sympathetic nervous system with resulting tachycardia and peripheral vasoconstriction. These patients may appear pale and may be hypotensive. If a patient appears to have rapid, surgical-type bleeding, attend to the patient personally. Have the RN call for backup help from a senior or chief resident.

Airway and Vital Signs

   Check that the patient has a patent, nonobstructed airway. Patients with significant bleeding in the upper aerodigestive tract are at high risk for aspiration of blood, and they may need to be intubated.

What is the respiratory rate?

Tachypnea may suggest airway compromise or impending shock.

What is the heart rate (HR)?

Tachycardia in the presence of significant bleeding suggests intravascular volume depletion and impending hypotension.

What is the blood pressure (BP)?

Sympathetic activation in the presence of postoperative bleeding causes tachycardia and peripheral vasoconstriction in an attempt to maintain a normotensive blood pressure. Rapid or extensive blood loss overcomes the sympathetic drive and leads to hypotension.

What is the temperature?

Measuring the temperature is important, as abnormally low body temperature (hypothermia) interferes with normal blood coagulation.

Selective History and Chart Review

An actively bleeding patient requires immediate bedside evaluation. Have the RN bring the patient's chart to the bedside, and review the type of surgical procedure performed, the date of surgery, the known blood coagulation status and recent hematocrit, and any anticoagulant medication that the patient has been taking.

Selective Physical Examination

The goals of the selective examination are to assess the patient's hemodynamic stability and evaluate the site of bleeding.

VS:	Repeat now.
HEENT:	Look for sites of bleeding with the aid of good lighting and suction.
Resp/CVS:	Evaluate the drainage from chest tubes or mediastinal tubes. Ask the RN if the tubes are putting out a more bloody fluid. Is there frank blood draining from these tubes?
Wound:	Using sterile technique, remove any dressing from the wound site. Evaluate for frank bleeding, swelling or increase in girth, hematoma, or discoloration of the skin.

■ MANAGEMENT

Surgical Bleeding

Life-Threatening Postoperative Hemorrhage

Severe postoperative bleeding associated with hemodynamic compromise is a problem that must be dealt with quickly and emphatically. Follow a logical treatment plan, and obtain help from other physicians on duty immediately.

The first priority is to stabilize the patient hemodynamically. Intravascular fluid resuscitation is extremely important. For patients with hypotension, tachycardia, or other signs of impending circulatory shock, run a 500-ml bolus of NS or LR wide open. Have the RN take the vital signs every 2 minutes. Give more fluid or adjust the fluid rate based on the normalization of the patient's BP and HR. Some patients may require a bolus of several liters of IV fluid.

Assess the airway and breathing. If bleeding is associated with severe hypotension and shock, consider intubation.

Control external hemorrhaging with direct pressure if possible. Internal hemorrhaging is best treated in the operating room.

Trendelenburg's positioning may help maintain central perfusion in the presence of hemorrhaging and hypotension.

Consider immediate transfusion of packed red blood cells (PRBCs) in the presence of massive hemorrhage. Have a member of the team run to the blood bank to obtain crossmatched (if available) or uncrossmatched (if no crossmatched blood is available) O type, Rh negative blood. Begin transfusion immediately. While waiting for blood products, maintain BP with crystalloid or colloid infusion.

Have a team member set up suction and adequate lighting. Using sterile technique, try to visualize the source of bleeding. Sometimes, significant bleeding is superficial enough that it can be controlled directly and easily with a stitch or a Kelly clamp. If the bleeding is from an extremity, use a BP cuff or tourniquet to help slow the bleeding.

If the bleeding source appears to be internal, do not attempt to control bleeding at the bedside. Frequently, a large internal hematoma may tamponade bleeding. Disrupting this tamponade may exacerbate hemorrhaging. Treating the patient with fluid and PRBCs is the best support you can give at the bedside. Major internal bleeding requires control in the operating room. Consider emergent return and surgical reexploration for major internal bleeding.

There are some cases in which widely opening a surgical wound at the bedside may be appropriate. If a patient develops airway compromise associated with bleeding after head and neck surgery, a hematoma may be compressing the trachea. This wound should be opened immediately to evacuate the hematoma. Direct pressure on the bleeding can be applied until surgical control can be achieved. If a patient is near arrest or has arrested at the bedside, it is also appropriate to widely open a surgical wound. A good example would be a cardiac surgery patient who has developed cardiac tamponade.

Always keep in mind that bleeding into large potential spaces (pleural, abdominal, pelvic, and thigh) can lead to exsanguination. Control of bleeding into these spaces requires immediate surgical exploration.

Minor Postoperative Bleeding

These calls are very common. Many postoperative patients will have minor oozing from surgical sites. These patients are hemodynamically stable and generally show blood spotting on outer dressings.

Consult the attending surgeon or chief resident before rendering any treatment. If the attending surgeon feels it is appropriate, and using proper lighting and sterile technique, remove the outer dressing, exposing the surgical incision line or wound. Evaluate the wound for evidence of direct bleeding. Frequently, skin bleeding will be easily visualized. A simple stitch or a figure eight stitch will usually stop bleeding.

If the wound is open and bleeding appears to be coming from very small vessels in a diffuse area, apply a pressure dressing to the area. If the wound is closed and bleeding is coming from the incision line, apply manual pressure for 10 minutes and apply a sterile pressure dressing to the area. Sterile gauze sponges, ABD pads, Elastoplast adhesive tape, and Ace wraps are very helpful in creating these dressings.

If a hematoma is present, apply a pressure dressing and contact the chief resident. Hematoma evacuation may require a nonemergent trip to the operating room.

Medical Bleeding

Medical bleeding is caused by coagulopathy. Bleeding tends to be diffuse from all cut surfaces. Normally, vasoconstriction and platelet action tend to stop bleeding by creating a platelet plug in cut vessels. In the presence of thrombocytopenia or platelet dysfunction, normal numbers of platelet plugs are not formed. In the absence of adequate soluble blood clotting factors, an organized clot cannot be formed. This also leads to continued, prolonged postoperative bleeding. To best manage medical bleeding, identify whether the bleeding problem is related to platelets, soluble blood clotting factors, or both.

Platelets

Thrombocytopenia. Platelet counts of $<30,000/\mu l$ may cause prolonged bleeding in postoperative patients. Postoperative bleeding associated with a platelet count of $<30,000/\mu l$ should be treated with a platelet transfusion. Thrombocytopenia may be caused by dilution, decreased marrow production, or increased peripheral destruction of platelets.

It is a good idea to give at least a six-pack of platelets if bleeding is significant. For dilutional thrombocytopenia, a general rule is that 8 units of platelets should be given for each 10 to 12 units of blood transfused. Although many of the platelets transfused are sequestered rapidly by the spleen, they usually act long enough to create a platelet plug.

Platelet Dysfunction. Many drugs including NSAIDs interfere with platelet aggregation. Other conditions including renal failure (uremia) and von Willebrand's disease inhibit platelet function. Platelet function may be tested with a bleeding time. A normal bleeding time (Ivy bleeding time test) is <7 minutes.

Patients with significant postoperative bleeding who have a history of platelet dysfunction, a prolonged bleeding time, or known ingestion of drugs that interfere with platelet activity may require a platelet transfusion. Patients with known von Willebrand's disease may be treated with cryoprecipitate, factor VIII, or desmopressin acetate (DDAVP). If possible, contact the chief resident or attending physician before giving platelet transfusions. Anticoagulation is sometimes desirable in vascular or microsurgical postoperative management.

Soluble Blood Clotting Factors

When blood clotting factor production or concentration is low, prolonged postoperative bleeding results. There are many causes of low clotting factor activity. However, in an acutely bleeding patient, most of these are treated by fresh frozen plasma (FFP) transfusion. Usually a minimum of 2 to 3 units of FFP is required to observe clinical improvement of the coagulopathy. Indications for the transfusion of FFP include the following:

1. Bleeding patients on warfarin (Coumadin) therapy
   Warfarin depletes the vitamin K–dependent blood clotting factors. FFP reverses the effects of warfarin rapidly. Administration of vitamin K generally corrects the effects of warfarin slowly.
2. As an adjunct to massive blood transfusions
   A bleeding patient whose entire blood volume has been replaced over a short time generally will need FFP to have acceptable (<50% greater than normal) PT and PTT values. Frequently, these patients will also require platelet transfusions.
3. Bleeding patients with liver disease
4. Patients with dilutional coagulopathy
   Hemodilution may lead to prolonged PT and PTT values. Bleeding patients with dilutional coagulopathy may require FFP and platelets. Patients with a history of congestive heart failure or who are already fluid overloaded can be given IV furosemide (Lasix) in conjunction with the FFP.

Postoperative Bleeding Associated with Heparin Therapy.
Some postoperative patients will be maintained on IV heparin
therapy. This is common practice in vascular surgery and micro-
surgery. If a patient develops postoperative bleeding on heparin
therapy, consider slowing the rate of heparin infusion or discontinuing heparin. Because the half-life of heparin is only 90 minutes, minor bleeding may resolve with this conservative approach. Patients with significant bleeding should be treated by
discontinuing the heparin therapy. If necessary, heparin effect can
be reversed with **protamine sulfate (1 mg/90 U heparin) given
IV slowly.** You can estimate the circulating amount of heparin by
calculating one-half of the previous hour's dose. For example, a
patient on a heparin infusion of 1000 U/hr should be given 5 mg
of protamine. No more than 50 mg of protamine should be given
in a single dose. Furthermore, protamine should be given over 10
to 15 minutes. Side effects of protamine include bradycardia,
hypotension, and flushing.

**Postoperative Bleeding in Patients with Known Clotting Fac-
tor Deficiencies.** Patients with a known clotting factor deficiency
are best managed with specific factor replacement. Most of these
factors are available as recombinant, purified proteins. If specific
clotting factors are not available, FFP or cryoprecipitate (containing factor VIII) may be useful. A consulting hematologist may
help with the management of these patients.

Disseminated Intravascular Coagulation. DIC is a poorly understood process in which diffuse bleeding is accompanied by a
rapid consumption of blood clotting factors. DIC is seen after
trauma, some types of surgery (lung, brain, or prostate), obstetric
complications, and septicemia. DIC commonly presents with diffuse bleeding from surgical sites, IVs, and sites of recent needle
puncture. The PTT is significantly prolonged, fibrinogen values
are very low (<75 mg/dl), thrombin time is prolonged, and
fibrin degradation products are elevated. Treatment includes FFP,
cryoprecipitate, and platelet transfusions. Correction of the underlying cause is also mandatory.

27

SEIZURES

Seizure activity is a synchronous discharge of electrical activity in the brain. The locus in the brain dictates what clinical symptoms are noted. Generalized tonic–clonic seizure activity is the major symptom for which you will be called. Seizure activity is frightening and disturbing to witness. Patients actively having seizures can harm themselves, and the underlying abnormalities are often serious.

■ PHONE CALL

Questions

1. **Is the patient still having seizures?**
   This requires immediate attention. Patients who are actively having seizures are at risk for aspiration, for metabolic derangements, and for hypoxia.
2. **What is the type of seizure?**
   Is it a full-body tonic–clonic, a focal, or a petit mal seizure? Is the patient conscious or unconscious?
3. **Has the patient had a seizure before?**
   New-onset seizure activity is a medical emergency. An expected seizure such as in a patient with a known seizure disorder may need no specific evaluation other than ensuring the patient's safety and attention to specific injuries if present.
4. **Was there a change in the patient's mental status either before or after the seizure?**
   Be mindful that most tonic–clonic seizures are followed by an unconscious postictal period.
5. **Is the patient injured in some way?**
6. **Has the patient undergone a surgical procedure, and if so, how long ago?**
   Seizures are common after neurosurgical procedures, and they represent a significant change in mental status. It also may indicate malfunction in any shunting device present.
7. **Are there any other symptoms?**
8. **Are there any changes in vital signs?**

Orders

If the Patient Is Actively Having a Seizure

1. Order oxygen (O_2) and oximetry monitoring.
2. Confirm that intravenous (IV) access is available.

An IV will be very difficult to place during an active seizure. If IV access is not established and the seizure is prolonged, some medications (including diazepam) may be given intramuscularly (IM), rectally, or via endotracheal tube.

3. Observe seizure precautions (Table 27–1).

     Make the environment safe for the patient.

4. Have suction available at the bedside to handle secretions.

5. Observe aspiration precautions.

     Place the patient in a lateral decubitus position. Remove dentures and other oral objects if easily done. Have an oral airway at the bedside.

6. Have an IV insertion tray available at the bedside if an IV is not already started.

     Have 1 L normal saline (NS) available, and have the IV tubing preflushed.

7. Have the means to perform a finger stick glucose test at the bedside.

8. Have the following medications available at the bedside:

   - **Thiamine 100-mg vial for IM injection**
   - **50% dextrose in water 50 ml for IV injection**
   - **Diazepam (Valium) 20 mg vial for IV injection or**
   - **Lorazepam (Ativan) 4 mg vial for IV injection**

If the Patient Is Postictal

1. Check oximetry and deliver O_2 as necessary.
2. Check finger stick glucose test.
3. Observe seizure precautions; the patient may have another seizure.
4. Observe aspiration precautions.

Degree of Urgency

Patients who have unexpected seizure activity require immediate attention, whether they are actively having a seizure or they are in a postictal state.

Table 27–1 ◻ SEIZURE PRECAUTIONS

1. Put bed in lowest position.
2. Put oral airway at the head of the bed.
3. Pad side rails of the bed, and put rails up while the patient is in bed.
4. Make suction and oxygen available at the bedside.
5. Allow out-of-bed privileges (including bathroom visits, showers, and baths) with supervision only.
6. Take axillary temperatures only.
7. Provide supervision when patient uses potentially dangerous objects such as razors or scissors.

■ ELEVATOR THOUGHTS

What are the causes of seizure?

- Central nervous system
  1. Tumor

     The type of seizure noted depends somewhat on the location of the mass.
  2. Stroke

     Old scarring from a previous stroke or infarct may be a seizure focus. Ongoing stroke with active injury may cause seizure.
  3. Head injury

     As with previous stroke, other causes of neural tissue scarring can be a seizure focus.
  4. Recent cranial surgery

     Seizures are common after neurosurgical procedures; these may be because of injury to the brain or because of complicating bleeding or infection. Often neurosurgeons are quite specific regarding the treatment of patients with seizures. Do not give any medications until specifically told to do so by the resident or the attending physician. If the seizure activity is a new symptom, an immediate head computed tomographic (CT) scan without contrast is often required.
  5. Infection

     Infection may be from meningitis, abscess, or other causes of encephalitis.
  6. Primary epilepsy

     Primary epilepsy includes grand mal or petit mal seizures. Patients with a history of seizure disorders tend to have seizures.
- Metabolic (the "hypos")
  1. Hypoglycemia
  2. Hyponatremia
  3. Hypocalcemia
  4. Hypomagnesemia
  5. Hypoxia
  6. Acid–base derangements
- Medications
  1. Inappropriately low levels of antiepileptic medication
  2. Meperidine (Demerol) overdose

     This is common in elderly patients, especially in the postoperative period.
  3. Benzodiazepine intoxication or withdrawal
  4. Barbiturate withdrawal
  5. Alcohol withdrawal
  6. High-dose penicillins
  7. Lidocaine intoxication

8. Aminophylline intoxication
9. Neuroleptic intoxication
10. Isoniazid
11. Lithium carbonate or other antidepressants
12. Insulin
    Note that overmedication of diabetes mellitus with resultant hypoglycemia can be more dangerous than undermedication.
- Other
  1. Organ failure (e.g., hepatic and renal)
  2. Cerebral vasculitis
  3. Other encephalopathy or degeneration (e.g., hypertension and human immunodeficiency virus)
  4. Cerebral edema
  5. Nonseizure or pseudoseizure

■ MAJOR THREAT TO LIFE

- Hypoxia
- Aspiration
- Ongoing central nervous system (CNS) injury, i.e., extension of a stroke or a worsening cerebral edema

---

If the Patient Is Actively Having a Seizure

■ BEDSIDE

Quick Look Test

Don't Panic. A seizure is disturbing to witness, but the initial therapy follows common sense. Most seizures are self-limited and will resolve in 2 to 5 minutes. Bear in mind that many of those around you will also be fighting the urge to panic.

Airway and Vital Signs

Most at risk is the patient's ability to breathe. Evaluate the airway. Clear foreign bodies and secretions from the mouth, and confirm good aeration of the lungs. Insert an oral airway, if possible, to facilitate respiration and allow suctioning. Do not attempt to insert the airway if it is difficult to do so or if force is required.

Evaluate oxygenation by pulse oximetry. Deliver O_2 by nasal cannula or mask as necessary. Because of the high metabolic rate during seizure activity, do not rely on arterial blood gas (ABG) data. Many of the abnormalities noted on ABGs will resolve without additional treatment in the postictal state.

Confirm a femoral pulse. Do not attempt to restrain the patient (this includes application of blood pressure cuffs).

Initial Management

1. Have someone notify the resident.
   New-onset seizures are medical emergencies.
2. Place the patient into the lateral decubitus position.
3. Keep the airway clear, and maintain oxygenation.
4. Observe the seizure activity.
   Note if the whole body is involved or just a portion of it. Is the patient conscious? Has the patient lost bowel or bladder control? This should be well documented later.
5. Wait.
   No other therapy is initially required for seizures that last up to 3 minutes and then spontaneously resolve.

If the seizure lasts longer than 3 minutes:
1. Reevaluate airway and oxygenation status.
2. Confirm IV access.
   If no IV access is available, this is the time to start it. It may take several holders to immobilize a limb long enough to establish an IV. Speed of access is important, so defer to the most experienced hands.
3. Draw up to 20 ml of blood for hematology and chemistries.
   See Selective Physical Examination below.
4. Give **thiamine 100 mg by slow IV push over 3 to 5 minutes.**
5. Give **50% dextrose in water by slow IV push.**
   If hypoglycemia is the cause of the seizure, the activity may suddenly cease. Stop the infusion and switch to a 5% dextrose in water infusion. (Thiamine is administered before the glucose to avoid exacerbation of Wernicke's encephalopathy.)

If the seizure activity continues:
6. Administer **diazepam (Valium) at a rate of 2 mg/min IV until the seizure activity stops, to a total dose of 30 mg.** Whenever diazepam is administered, have resuscitation equipment nearby, because it is a respiratory depressant.
   Lorazepam (Ativan) in doses of **2 to 4 mg IV push over 3 to 5 minutes** may be used instead of diazepam. Lorazepam also has the advantage of being rapidly absorbed rectally and may be administered by this route, via red rubber catheter followed by an NS flush, if no IV access is available.

If the seizure activity continues despite 10 mg diazepam (one-half the total dose):
7. Begin to administer **phenytoin (Dilantin).**
   An additional IV will be required, because diazepam and

phenytoin are not compatible in the same IV line, nor is phenytoin compatible with dextrose-containing solutions. **Phenytoin** loading dose is **18 mg/kg by slow IV push, no faster than 25 to 50 mg/min.** Administration of phenytoin is associated with hypotension and cardiac dysrhythmias. If the patient is not on a cardiac monitor, keep a finger on the femoral pulse during the infusion. If dysrhythmias are noted or femoral pulse weakens, slow the infusion rate. If the seizure stops during the administration of phenytoin, stop the diazepam infusion but continue the phenytoin load until complete. A newer phenytoin derivative, fosphenytoin, is now available and may be administered more rapidly. See Management below for further care.

If the patient continues to have the seizure for >30 minutes:
8. This is a medical emergency.
     Status epilepticus is best treated by an intensivist or neurologist. Renotify the resident and arrange transfer to the intensive care unit for comprehensive care.

If the Patient Has Stopped Having the Seizure

■ BEDSIDE

Quick Look Test

Immediately after grand mal seizures, patients are generally in a postictal state (unconscious). Some focal seizures are also associated with loss of consciousness (i.e., complex seizures).

Airway and Vital Signs

Check vital signs and pulse oximetry, and treat with O_2 as necessary. It is not unusual for a patient to become acidotic during a seizure, so temporary compensatory tachypnea is common.

Initial Management

1. Observe seizure and aspiration precautions.
     The initial seizure may have stopped, but another seizure is possible. Make sure that the patient is in the lateral decubitus position and that the airway is clear. Suction the oral cavity as necessary. Confirm that an oral airway is at the bedside.
2. Make sure the patient has adequate IV access.
3. Draw blood for appropriate chemistries (see Selective Physical Examination below).

4. Check a finger stick glucose test.

Treat significant hypoglycemia (<60 mg/dl) with **50 ml 50% dextrose in water by slow IV infusion** or by constant administration of **5% dextrose in water.**

Selective History and Chart Review

- Is there a condition that would predispose to seizure activity? See Elevator Thoughts.
- What was the quality of the seizure?

    Did it start as focal and then secondarily generalize? Focal or partial complex seizures are more likely of primary CNS cause than other causes.
- Review the patient's medications.
- Review recent laboratory data with emphasis on electrolyte, Ca^{2+}, Mg^{2+}, and glucose levels.
- Review recent antiepileptic medication levels if any.

Selective Physical Examination

VS:	Repeat now.
MS:	Assess level of consciousness, i.e., response to pain and voice.
HEENT:	Examine for mouth lacerations, chipped teeth, and facial fractures.
	Remove dentures and other foreign objects from mouth.
Resp:	Check for adequate aeration and evidence of aspiration.
Skin:	Check for bruising or trauma.
Extrem:	Examine for fractures.
Neuro:	When the patient is awake, do a complete neurologic examination.
	Are there any focal neurologic findings?
Wound:	Are sutures intact? Is there any new bleeding or discharge?
Tubes:	Confirm that any necessary tubes are still in place and are well secured.

Additional tests:
1. Serum glucose
2. Electrolytes
3. Calcium
4. Magnesium
5. Blood urea nitrogen and creatinine
6. Albumin
7. Levels of appropriate antiepileptic medications
8. Complete blood count and differential

■ MANAGEMENT

1. Endeavor to find the cause.
   Seizures are a sign and not a diagnosis.
2. Treat any reversible causes such as hyponatremia or medication overdose.
3. Treat any identifiable injuries.
4. Maintain seizure and aspiration precautions and IV access for at least 24 to 48 hours past the last seizure.
5. Most seizures are self-limited and are single events. They often do not require long-term antiepileptic medication therapy.
6. Give antiepileptic medications.
   If further seizure activity is suspected, or if the patient has a known seizure disorder, make sure ongoing antiepileptic medication is within therapeutic range. If the patient is not currently taking antiepileptic medication, load with phenytoin as described above (if not already done). Once loaded with phenytoin, continue the dosing at 300 mg orally or IV per day, and adjust according to serum levels.
7. Order head CT scan without contrast immediately.
   If a structural lesion is suspected or if the seizure follows a neurosurgical procedure, a head CT scan without contrast is indicated.
8. If meningitis is suspected, a lumbar puncture should be performed and appropriate antibiotic started as indicated. Make sure to rule out cerebral herniation with a head CT scan or adequate fundi visualization before the lumbar puncture.
9. Follow up in the morning with appropriate laboratory and medication level checks.
10. Perform neurologic checks every hour. Then decrease the interval as the patient stabilizes. Instruct the bedside caregiver to notify you if any change occurs.

■ SPECIAL SURGICAL CONSIDERATIONS

Preoperative Considerations

New seizure activity is a medical emergency and preempts any elective procedure planned. Any metabolic derangements should be corrected before surgery.

Postoperative Considerations

Postoperative neurosurgical patients should be evaluated with an immediate head CT scan for any unexpected seizure activity or significant change in mental status. Always clear antiepileptic medication with the resident or attending physician before use. These medications alter the sensorium and may mask symptoms that indicate a serious change in mental status.

28

SHORTNESS OF BREATH

It is common to be asked to assess problems with a patient's breathing. Shortness of breath (SOB) has many causes. Most at risk to develop respiratory distress are patients who have had thoracic or upper abdominal procedures, elderly patients, obese patients, and poorly nourished patients.

■ PHONE CALL

Questions

1. **How long has the patient had SOB?**
2. **Was the onset slow or rapid?**
    A rapid onset suggests pneumothorax or pulmonary embolus.
3. **Is the patient cyanotic?**
4. **Is the patient already on oxygen (O_2)?**
5. **Does the patient have a history of chronic obstructive pulmonary disease (COPD)?**
    If the patient retains carbon dioxide (CO_2), the amount of oxygen that may be delivered is affected.
6. **Has the patient undergone a surgical procedure, and if so, how long ago?**
    Be especially mindful after placement of central lines.
7. **Are there any other symptoms such as chest pain, cough, or fever?**
8. **Are there any changes in vital signs?**

Orders

1. Measure arterial hemoglobin saturation (SaO_2) by pulse oximetry if not already done.
    As an alternative, have an arterial blood gas (ABG) kit at the bedside. This will give a rapid indication of the arterial partial pressure of oxygen (PaO_2).
2. Deliver oxygen as necessary.
    If the patient does not retain CO_2, O_2 may be safely delivered at a rate that keeps the O_2 saturation at $\geq 90\%$. See Table 28–1 for various regimens of O_2 delivery.
3. If the patient has a history of reactive airway disease (RAD) (COPD or asthma), order bronchodilator treatment if it has been >2 hours since the last treatment (Table 28–2).

Table 28–1 □ OXYGEN DELIVERY TECHNIQUES

System	Recommended Flow	Maximum FiO_2	Humidification	Control of FiO_2
Room air	N/A	0.28	Poor	N/A
Nasal cannula	1–6 L/min	0.44	Poor	Poor
Open face mask	8–10 L/min	0.44	Good	Good
Venturi mask	10 L/min	0.45	Poor	Great
Tight face mask	8–10 L/min	0.60	Poor	Good
Nonrebreather mask	10 L/min	1.0	Poor	Good
Endotracheal tube	N/A	1.0	Great	Great

FiO_2 = fraction of oxygen in inspired air.

Table 28–2 □ BRONCHODILATOR THERAPIES TO CONTROL REACTIVE AIRWAY DISEASE

Generic	Trade	Dosage	Interval
Beta-2 Agonists			
Albuterol	Proventil and Ventolin	2.5–5 mg in 3 ml NS	every 4–6 hr
		2 puffs of MDI	every 4–6 hr
		2–4 mg PO	every 6–8 hr
Fenoterol	Berotec	0.5–1.0 mg in 3 ml NS	every 4–6 hr
Isoetharine	Bronkosol	0.3 mg in 2.7 ml NS	every 4–6 hr
		2 puffs of MDI	every 4–6 hr
Metaproterenol	Alupent and Metaprel	0.3 mg in 2.7 ml NS	every 4–6 hr
		2 puffs of MDI	every 4–6 hr
		10 mg PO	every 6 hr
Terbutaline	Brethaire, Brethine, and Bricanyl	0.25–0.5 mg in 2.6 ml NS	every 6–8 hr
		2 puffs of MDI	every 6–8 hr
		2.5–5 mg PO	every 6–8 hr
Anticholinergics			
Ipratropium bromide	Atrovent	0.5 mg in 3 ml NS	every 6–8 hr
		2 puffs of MDI	every 6 hr
Atropine		0.5–1.0 mg in 3 ml Ns	every 8 hr

328

Injectable

Terbutaline	0.25–0.5 mg IM	every 6–8 hr
Epinephrine (1:1000)	0.25–0.5 mg IM	every 8–12 hr
Aminophylline		
Loading	5 mg/kg IV over 20–30 min	
Maintenance	0.6–0.9 mg/kg/hr IV (maintain levels at 10–20 µg/ml)	
PO form	6 mg/kg every 12 hr of the long-acting preparation	

Medication	IV Dose	PO Dose	Dose Equivalency*
Steroids			
Hydrocortisone	250 mg bolus	—	1
Methylprednisolone	3–5 mg/kg divided every 6 hr	—	5
Prednisone	1.0–1.5 mg/kg	1.0–1.5 mg/kg	4
Dexamethasone	0.1–0.2 mg/kg	5–10 mg	25–30

*Glucocorticoid potency compared with hydrocortisone milligram per milligram.
NS = normal saline; MDI = metered dose inhaler; PO = orally; IM = intramusculary; IV = intravenously.

Degree of Urgency

The patient must be evaluated immediately.

■ ELEVATOR THOUGHTS

What are the causes of shortness of breath?
- Cardiovascular causes
  1. CHF
  2. Pulmonary embolism
  3. Cardiac tamponade
- Pulmonary causes
  1. Atelectasis (usually 24 to 48 hours after a surgical procedure)
  2. RAD (e.g., COPD, asthma, or gastroesophageal [GE] reflux)
  3. Upper airway obstruction
  4. Pneumothorax
  5. Pleural effusion
  6. Pneumonia
  7. Aspiration of gastric contents
- Miscellaneous causes
  1. Anxiety
  2. Marked abdominal distention

■ MAJOR THREAT TO LIFE

- Hypoxia
- Myocardial infarction, as a cause of SOB or as a sequela of other causes of SOB

■ BEDSIDE

Quick Look Test

Hypoxia is evident by agitation and cyanosis. Patients with significant hypoxia will appear anxious and ill. CO_2 retention is evident by lethargy or obtundation.

Airway and Vital Signs

Confirm the patency of the upper airway. Remove any oral obstruction such as dentures or foreign bodies. Tachypnea (respiration rate [RR] >20 breaths/min) will be present if hypoxia, anxiety, pain, or acidosis is present. Slow RRs (<12 breaths/min) indicate a depression of the central nervous system (CNS) with medications (such as opiates) or primary cerebral lesion. If there is a cardiac cause, tachycardia or arrhythmia may also be present. Fever denotes an infectious cause but may also be present with atelectasis or pulmonary embolism. A drop in blood pressure (BP) may indicate pulmonary embolism, tension pneumothorax, congestive heart failure (CHF), or sepsis.

■ IF THE PATIENT IS HYPOXIC

Initial Management

1. Deliver adequate O_2.

   The delivery technique will vary by the situation. The factors that determine the delivery technique are as follows:
   - Amount of oxygen needed
   - Need for precise control of fraction of oxygen in inspired air (FiO_2)
   - Need for humidification
   - Patient comfort

   See Table 28–1. Remember that if the patient has a history of COPD and retains CO_2, the amount of O_2 delivered must be limited. Patients with baseline high partial pressure of carbon dioxide (PCO_2) levels do not have a hypercapnic drive for respiration and must rely on their hypoxic drive. FiO_2 levels at >0.28 may decrease their drive to breathe.

2. Evaluate the O_2 delivery by following pulse oximetry and periodic ABGs.

   Use the minimum amount of O_2 necessary to achieve the desired oxygenation. Pulse oximetry gives a good estimate of the arterial hemoglobin saturation (SaO_2), which is generally linked to the PaO_2 (Fig. 28–1). Remember, however, that the pulse oximeter will not evaluate PCO_2, bicarbonate ion (HCO_3^-), or pH of the serum.

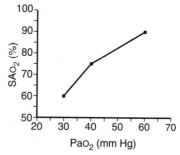

Figure 28–1 □ Approximate relationship between PaO_2 and SaO_2.

3. Be ready to resuscitate.

If the patient is severely hypoxic or in obvious distress, have a resuscitation cart nearby. Make sure the patient has a patent intravenous (IV) line.

Selective History and Chart Review

- Cardiovascular causes
  1. Congestive heart failure

     Are there symptoms of orthopnea or paroxysmal nocturnal dyspnea? Is there evidence of fluid overload from overzealous resuscitation or the mobilization of third-space fluids? CHF is a symptom, not a disease. **A cause must be sought.** Possible causes are listed in Table 28–3. Left-sided heart failure presents as pulmonary edema and SOB. Right-sided heart failure presents as peripheral edema and organomegaly. Most often, components of both are present.

  2. Pulmonary embolism

     Is the patient postoperative? Most perioperative deep vein thromboses of significance form intraoperatively on the operating table and are best prevented by preoperative application of support (thromboembolic disease [TED]) stockings and sequential compression boots. Were support stockings and sequential compression boots in place during surgery? Are they in place now? Is there a history of prior thromboembolic phenomena? Is the patient hypercoagulable (is there malignancy, inflammatory bowel disease, nephrotic syndrome, use of oral contraceptive pills, or deficiency of antithrombin III, protein C, or protein S)? Are there other risk factors for pulmonary embolism (prolonged bed rest, immobile limb, obesity, CHF, pregnancy, or vein trauma)? Do not expect to find the classic triad of chest pain, hemoptysis, and SOB. Rarely are they all present simultaneously.

  3. Tamponade

Table 28–3 □ CAUSES OF CONGESTIVE HEART FAILURE

Myocardial infarction	Sodium retention or salt overload
Hypertension	Dysrhythmia
Valvular heart disease	Beta blockade or other cardiac depressant
Congenital heart disease	Renal disease
Pericardial disease	Anemia
Cardiomyopathy	Fever and infection
Pulmonary embolism	Pregnancy
Fluid overload	Noncompliance with medications or diet

Was there a recent central line placement? Is there a history of penetrating chest trauma?

- Pulmonary causes
  1. Atelectasis

     This is a very common cause of postoperative SOB, hypoxia, and fever. Is the patient postoperative or taking pain medication? Another common cause is hyperoxygenation.

  2. Reactive airway disease

     Is there a history of COPD, asthma, or GE reflux? COPD may be present as chronic bronchitis (production of mucus on most days for 3 months of a year in 2 consecutive years) or as emphysema, or it may have components of both. Cigarette smoking is strongly linked with COPD. Is there a history of exposure to a specific asthma trigger (respiratory infection, irritant, allergen, or medication such as aspirin or beta blocker)? Is the patient taking steroids? Has the patient ever required mechanical ventilation in the past?

  3. Upper airway obstruction

     Is there a history of aspiration or sleep apnea? Causes include laryngeal edema, epiglottitis, vocal cord paralysis, and foreign body.

  4. Pneumothorax

     Was there a recent central line placement or thoracic surgery? Has a chest tube been removed recently? Is there a history of penetrating chest trauma or spontaneous pneumothorax?

  5. Pleural effusion

     Is there a history of pulmonary infection or abscess? Other risk factors are listed in Table 28–4.

  6. Pneumonia

     Risk factors include advanged age, immunosuppression, prolonged hospitalization, mechanical ventilation, aspiration of foodstuffs or vomitus, and preexisting cardiac, pulmonary, or CNS disease.

  7. Aspiration of gastric contents

Table 28–4 □ CAUSES OF PLEURAL EFFUSIONS

Congestive heart failure	Asbestos exposure
Organ failure (liver and kidney)	Chylothorax
Nephrotic syndrome	Pancreatitis
Malignancy	Superior vena cava syndrome
Pulmonary infection	Peritoneal dialysis
Abdominal abscess	Dressler's syndrome
Collagen vascular disease	Meigs's syndrome

This may lead to pneumonia or RAD symptoms. Is there decreased level of consciousness, hiatal hernia, vomiting, nasogastric (NG) tube in place, or history of chronic reflux?

- Miscellaneous causes
  1. Anxiety
     Is there a history of panic disorder?
  2. Marked abdominal distention
     Is there a history of liver failure, other forms of ascites, or bowel obstruction? Has there been any recent gastrointestinal (GI) surgery?

Selective Physical Examination

VS:	Repeat now; tachycardia (CHF and pulmonary embolus)
	Tachypnea (CHF)
	Fever/chills (atelectasis and pneumonia)
MS:	Agitation (hypoxia) and lethargy (hypercapnia)
HEENT:	Upper airway obstruction (foreign body)
	Elevated jugular venous distention (JVD) (tamponade, CHF, RAD, and pneumothorax)
	Deviated trachea (pneumothorax)
CVS:	Arrhythmia (CHF and pulmonary embolus)
	S_3 (this is the most specific finding for CHF)
	Loud P_2 (RAD)
	Cardiac murmur (CHF)
Resp:	Rales (CHF)
	Decreased aeration (pleural effusion or pneumothorax)
	Pleuritic chest pain (pneumonia)
	Pleural friction rub (pulmonary embolus)
	Pulmonary consolidation (pulmonary embolus or pneumonia)
	Pleural effusion (CHF, pulmonary embolus, and pneumonia)
	Use of accessory respiratory muscles (RAD)
	Wheezing (CHF, RAD, pneumonia, and pulmonary embolism)
	Prolonged expiratory phase (RAD)
Abd:	Distention and ascites (CHF and bowel obstruction)
	Hepatomegaly (CHF)

Skin:	Cyanosis (hypoxia and RAD)
Extrem:	Ankle or presacral edema (CHF)
	Tender or red calf (thromboembolism)
Tubes:	Chest tube in place or recent chest tube removal
	NG tube in place
	Recent central venous line placement
Special examinations:	Measurement of pulsus paradoxus may give an indication of the severity of airflow obstruction in RAD. To measure pulsus paradoxus, take a routine BP. Inflate the cuff to 30 mm Hg above the systolic pressure and slowly release. Note the BP at which Korotkoff's sounds are first noted. These sounds are initially heard only with exhalation. Then note the pressures at which the Korotkoff's sounds are audible during both inhalation and exhalation. The pulse will seem to double. If the difference between these two pressures is >10 mm Hg (pulsus paradoxus), there is a significant obstruction to airflow. This is also seen in significant cardiac output obstruction such as pulmonary embolus or tamponade.
Additional tests:	
1. CXR:	This may be done at the bedside immediately if necessary; see Table 28–5 for significant findings
2. ABG:	Gives rapid assessment of serum PaO_2, PCO_2, pH, and a calculation of HCO_3^-
3. CBC:	Evaluate hemoglobin and hematocrit
4. ECG:	Pulmonary embolism may give findings of tachycardia, dysrhythmia, or evidence of right ventricular strain: S_1, Q_3, right axis deviation, and right bundle branch block

■ MANAGEMENT

Congestive Heart Failure

1. Deliver oxygen as required.
2. Establish IV access.
    Run 5% dextrose in water to keep the vein open.
3. Sit the patient up to allow maximum aeration of the lungs.
4. Give **morphine sulfate (MSO₄) 2 to 4 mg IV every 5 to 10**

**Table 28–5 □ RADIOGRAPHIC FINDINGS IN COMMON
ETIOLOGIES OF SHORTNESS OF BREATH**

Congestive Heart Failure

Cardiomegaly
Perihilar congestion
Bilateral interstitial or alveolar infiltrates
Cephalization of flow (redistribution of lung markings)
Kerley's B lines
Pleural effusion

Pulmonary Embolism

Atelectasis
Unilateral wedge infiltrate
Unilateral pleural effusion
Raised hemidiaphragm
(May be normal)

Atelectasis

Volume loss
Basilar streaking or infiltrates
(May be normal)

Pneumothorax

(Exhalation film most useful)
Mediastinal shift (with tension pneumothorax)
Unilateral hyperaeration
Loss of lung tissue in hemithorax

Pneumonia

Infiltrates (unilateral, bilateral, patch, and lobar)
Pleural effusion
(May be unremarkable until the patient is fully hydrated)

Reactive Airway Disease

Hyperinflation of the lungs
Flattened diaphragms
Increased anterior–posterior diameter
Occasional infiltrates (with associated pneumonias, atelectasis,
pneumothorax, or pneumomediastinum)

---

minutes to 10 to 12 mg, which will pool the blood in the splanchnic circulation and decrease pulmonary edema.

Hold MSO$_4$ treatment if symptoms of decreased respiratory drive or hypotension are apparent. Reverse the effects of MSO$_4$ as necessary with **naloxone hydrochloride 0.2 to 2.0 mg IV, intramuscularly (IM), or subcutaneously (SC) to a total of 10 mg.** Note that the half-life of naloxone is shorter than that of most narcotics and that repeat doses may be necessary.

5. Give nitroglycerin (NTG), as follows:

Ointment	2.5 to 5.0 cm topically every 4 hours or
Tablets	0.3 to 0.6 μg sublingually (SL) every 5 minutes or
Spray	1 puff SL every 15 minutes

Hold NTG for systolic blood pressure (SBP) of <90 mm Hg. Adequate function of NTG is generally confirmed by a headache, which usually responds to **acetaminophen (Tylenol and others) 650 to 1000 mg orally (PO) or rectally (PR) every 4 hours as necessary.**

6. Give diuretic therapy, as follows:
   - **Furosemide (Lasix) 20 to 80 mg IV over 2 to 5 minutes.**
     The dose may be doubled and administered **every hour as needed to a total dose of 400 mg** if no response is noted. Be cautious in giving large doses of furosemide. Doses of **>100 mg** should be **given slowly (<4 mg/min)** to avoid ototoxicity. Also use caution when used in conjunction with aminoglycoside antibiotics.
   - **Hydrochlorothiazide 25 to 50 mg PO (a thiazide diuretic)** or **metolazone (Zaroxolyn) 5 to 10 mg PO** may be added **once or twice a day** to furosemide therapy (a loop diuretic) for more effective diuresis.
   - If furosemide therapy is ineffective, consider use of **ethacrynic acid (Edecrin) 50 mg IV every hour for 2 doses** or **bumetanide (Bumex) 1 to 10 mg IV over 1 to 2 minutes.**
   - Monitor diuretic therapy with intake/outake measurements (I/Os), frequent weight checks, and serum electrolyte evaluations. Replace K^+ as necessary.
7. Restrict sodium in the diet and in the IV fluids.

Pulmonary Embolism

1. Deliver oxygen as required.
2. Confirm the diagnosis.
   A ventilation–perfusion ($\dot{V}/\dot{Q}$) scan should be performed as soon as possible. A **high-probability** $\dot{V}/\dot{Q}$ scan confirms pulmonary embolism and indicates the need for anticoagulation. A **normal** $\dot{V}/\dot{Q}$ scan eliminates the possibility of pulmonary embolism. An **intermediate** or **low-probability** $\dot{V}/\dot{Q}$ scan is not as helpful, and anticoagulation must be started or continued based on the clinical condition of the patient. Pulmonary angiography is useful in settings of equivocal $\dot{V}/\dot{Q}$ scans or to implement local thrombolytic therapy.
3. Give anticoagulation.
   This must be started immediately (i.e., before the $\dot{V}/\dot{Q}$ scan) if the clinical suspicion is high enough. It may always be stopped later if the scan is normal. Proceed as follows:
   - Ensure that the patient has no potential bleeding problem

(other bleeding diathesis, tumor, peptic ulcer, fresh surgical wounds, or stroke).

If present, confirm the pulmonary embolus first with a $\dot{V}/\dot{Q}$ scan. Options other than anticoagulation may be available, such as interruption of the inferior vena cava with a filter or by direct ligation or surgical removal of the existing clot.

If there are no contraindications:

- Draw blood for complete blood count (CBC), prothrombin time (PT), partial thromboplastin time (PTT), and platelets.
- Bolus with **heparin 100 U/kg IV.**

  Follow with a maintenance administration of **heparin** at **1000 to 1600 U/hr IV.** Heparin orders should be written in very specific language (e.g., 25,000 U per 500 ml of 5% dextrose in water to run at 20 ml/hr so as to deliver 1000 U per hour). Make sure to double-check dosages and rates.
- Maintain the PTT in a therapeutic range (generally 1.8–2.8 times normal, but the attending physician may have a specific PTT in mind; ask if you are unsure).
- Follow each change in the rate of heparin in 4 to 6 hours with a PTT.

  When stable, PT, PTT, and international normalized ratios (INRs) may be checked daily. Platelet counts should be ordered at 2- to 3-day intervals to assess for heparin-induced thrombocytopenia. This generally occurs after 7 days of heparin therapy and is associated with the appearance of immunoglobulin G (IgG) in the serum. Treatment includes discontinuation of heparin and conversion to another form of anticoagulation (PO warfarin or IV dextran).
- If tolerated, heparin should be continued for at least 5 days.
- On the first or second day, begin **warfarin (Coumadin) therapy 10 mg PO.** Titrate the dose to achieve a therapeutic increase in the PT (generally 1.3–1.5 times normal, with an INR in the 2–3 range; again, check with the attending physician for a specific number). Decrease the daily warfarin dose as a therapeutic PT is reached.
- Attainment of a therapeutic PT/INR range will take about 5 days. When therapeutic range has been maintained for 48 to 72 hours, the heparin may be discontinued.
- Review the patient's medication list for any possible interactions with warfarin or heparin.
- Avoid IM injections or nonsteroidal anti-inflammatory drug (NSAID)-containing medications, sulfinpyrazone, dipyridamole, or thrombolytic agents while taking anticoagulants.
- Anticoagulation with warfarin should be maintained for

at least 6 to 12 weeks with PT/INR checks every 1 to 2 weeks when stable.

- Remember some rules of thumb when using anticoagulation:

    Heparin primarily prolongs the PTT but also prolongs the PT; a therapeutic PTT range due to heparin will also cause a 1- to 3-second increase in the PT.

    Warfarin primarily prolongs the PT but also prolongs the PTT; this effect is due to the effect on factors IX and X and prothrombin and is seen after a week of therapy.

    Always remember to order both PT and PTT when the patient is taking both warfarin and heparin.

4. Find the source.

    Most pulmonary emboli originate in the lower extremities. Deep vein clots may be present in the absence of thrombophlebitis. Clinical suspicion is heightened by the presence of Homan's sign (pain behind the knee with dorsiflexion of the foot) or a swollen, tender leg. Studies to evaluate the deep venous system include noninvasive techniques such as Doppler ultrasonography and impedance plethysmography. Doppler ultrasonography is good for completely occluded veins but is limited in its evaluation of partially occluded veins or in settings of venous collateralization or edema. Impedance plethysmography is especially good at evaluation of the iliofemoral and popliteal systems but is limited in its ability to localize disease. Invasive techniques include IV contrast or radioisotope venography.

5. Give thrombolysis.

    In selected patients, thrombolysis with streptokinase or urokinase may be indicated. **Thrombolysis should not be done on a postoperative patient, because there is a significant risk of bleeding or anastomotic leak.** If appropriate, this technique should be done by those specifically trained in the technique, such as interventional radiologists.

Tamponade

1. Deliver oxygen as required.
2. Confirm the diagnosis.

    This potentially fatal complication usually follows penetrating trauma to the chest, thoracic surgery, or, rarely, central line placement. It may also be slowly progressive in settings of pericarditis. Findings in tamponade include progressive cardiac outflow obstruction with Beck's triad of distended neck veins, muffled heart sounds, and decreased BP. Kussmaul's sign of a paradoxical increase in JVD with inspiration may also be present. Pulsus paradoxus should be present at 10 to 15 mm Hg. Chest x-ray (CXR) may not be helpful, as the average tamponade is only about 200 ml in volume and does not significantly increase the size of the heart silhouette. Occasionally a "water bottle" sign is present, which suggests pericardial effusion. Electrocardiography (ECG) is also nonspecific. Emergency echo is the most specific for diagnosis of tamponade.

3. Volume load.

Increasing the preload is important to maintain adequate cardiac output. Give a 1-L bolus of NS.

4. Give emergent pericardiocentesis.

If clinical suspicion is high, diagnosis and treatment may be affected by pericardiocentesis. This is a **code** situation and should be done at the bedside only if the patient has hemodynamic collapse. Notify your resident immediately. Defer to the most experienced person. Contact the intensive care unit (ICU) or cardiac care unit (CCU) for assistance in the procedure.

- The patient should be on continuous ECG monitoring and is best placed in a 30° semi-Fowler position if possible.

  Attach a V lead to the pericardiocentesis needle for more sensitivity. An insulated wire with alligator clips at each end works well.
- Prepare the skin over the xiphoid area with iodine, chlorhexidine, or alcohol.
- Puncture the skin with a blade 2 cm below the costal margin, adjacent to the xiphoid.
- Insert an 18-gauge 10-cm spinal needle, and direct the needle upward and backward at a 45° angle for 4 to 5 cm. Mentally aim toward the right or the left scapular tip; the right is preferable as the risk of right ventricular penetration is lessened.
- Aspirate frequently as the needle is advanced. Continue to advance the needle until fluid is encountered, until cardiac pulsations are noticeable, or until ST elevation is noted on the ECG monitor. You may have a sensation of entering a cavity.
- Most blood in a hemopericardium is clotted, so usually only 5 to 10 ml is removable. If 20 ml or more is easily withdrawn, the needle is most likely in the right ventricle.
- A small aspiration of fluid often makes a big difference in cardiac function. If blood is encountered and is clotted, or if no hemodynamic change is apparent after aspiration, the patient may need a thoracotomy or local pericardial window excision.
- A sample of fluid should be sent to the laboratory for Gram stain, culture (bacterial, fungal, and mycobacterial), hematologic cell count, cytology, protein, and glucose.

Other studies as indicated may include rheumatoid factor, antinuclear antibodies, or complement levels.

Atelectasis

1. Deliver oxygen as required.
   Maintain the lowest FiO_2 necessary.
2. Alter the patient's pain medication as necessary to achieve a better balance between adequate relief and somnolence.
   The patient must be able to breathe deeply, ambulate, and cough effectively.
3. Order assisted ambulation.
   Make sure the patient is adequately mobilized. Order ambulation with assistance if necessary.
4. Stimulate and encourage coughing.
   This requires adequate pain relief and instruction to the patient on how to support the wound to avoid undue discomfort.
5. Vigorous chest physiotherapy (CPT) may be useful in patients with copious secretions or COPD.
6. Bronchodilators may be useful for those patients with a component of RAD (see Table 28–2).
7. Order supplemental nutrition as necessary.
8. Consider bronchoscopy.
   On occasion, severe atelectasis responds to bronchoscopy, especially where there is segmental or large regions of collapse.

Reactive Airway Disease (Asthma and COPD)

1. Supply oxygen as necessary.
   Use the minimum FiO_2 required to maintain an SaO_2 at $\geq 90\%$.
2. Order bronchodilators as outlined in Table 28–2.
   With adequate cardiac monitoring and precautions, the **beta-2 agonists may be given as frequently as every 1 to 2 hours as needed.** Also, some benefit may be derived from alternating between different types of beta-2 agonists in a combined therapy approach. Note that steroids should be started early, as their effects may not be noticed for many hours after initiation of therapy. Steroid therapy in excess of 15 days should be slowly tapered over several days.
3. Mobilize secretions with CPT.
4. Maintain adequate hydration.
5. Look for medications that impair smooth muscle responsiveness to beta-2 agonists, such as beta blockers or cholinergics.
6. Look for and treat triggers to asthma, as follows:

- Respiratory infection (this is the most common)
- Irritation (including cigarette smoke)
- Allergy
- Drugs (aspirin and beta blockers)
- GE reflux

7. Order ventilator support as indicated for respiratory failure (see below).

Pneumothorax

1. Confirm the diagnosis.

   Findings may include decreased breath sounds and hyper-resonance of the hemithorax, deviation of the trachea, hypoxia, and chest pain. In cases of tension pneumothorax, progressive cardiac outflow obstruction is apparent.

2. Give O_2 at 100%.

   Many small pneumothoraces will resolve spontaneously by increasing the FiO_2. This acts by replacing the air in the pleural space with oxygen, which is absorbed through the tissues much more rapidly than nitrogen.

3. Treat tension pneumothorax with immediate insertion of an 18-gauge needle into the second intercostal space anteriorly at the midclavicular line on the affected side.

   This will confirm the diagnosis and allow some relief of symptoms until adequate chest tube drainage can be implemented.

4. Place a tube thoracostomy.

   If the air leak is small, a small to moderately sized chest tube (12–24 Fr) may be placed in an anterior position from a high intercostal space in the midaxillary line. Occasionally, it is preferable to place the tube in the second intercostal space in the midclavicular line anteriorly to facilitate patient comfort.

   - Placement and management of chest tubes is outlined in Chapter 30.
   - Confirm tube placement by immediate bedside upright posterior-to-anterior and lateral CXR.
   - Reposition as necessary.
   - Daily CXRs are recommended to follow the course of therapy and to confirm continued adequate placement of the tube.
   - The tube insertion site will remain uncomfortable until the tube is removed; make sure the patient has adequate pain relief.
   - Pulmonary toilet is important in a patient with chest tubes.
     Make an incentive spirometer available, and instruct the patient as to its use and importance.

5. Know when to go to the operating room (OR).

Pneumothoraces that do not respond to tube thoracostomy may require surgical repair.

Pleural Effusion

1. Deliver oxygen as required.
2. Confirm the diagnosis by CXR and thoracentesis.
3. Determine the cause.

   See Table 28–4. The treatment will include reversal of the underlying condition.
4. Order thoracentesis.

   If the patient is in respiratory distress, a thoracentesis will significantly improve the patient's ability to oxygenate by increasing lung inflation. Do not remove (tap) >1500 ml of fluid in a single procedure to avoid reinflation pulmonary edema. A sample of the pleural fluid should be sent to the laboratory for the following studies as indicated:

   - Gram stain, cultures (aerobic and anaerobic bacterial, fungal, and mycoplasma)
   - Ziehl-Neelsen (ZN) stain and TB culture
   - Cell count and differential
   - Lactate dehydrogenase (LDH)
   - Protein
   - Glucose
   - Cytology for malignant cells
   - Other studies as appropriate (amylase, triglycerides, pH, rheumatoid factor, antinuclear antibodies, or complement levels)

   A simultaneous serum LDH, protein, and glucose should be drawn to compare with the results of the pleural fluid.
5. Order tube thoracostomy.

   If frequent taps are required for recurrent accumulation of fluid, such as in chylothorax, consider placement of a moderately sized (25–28 Fr) chest tube.

Pneumonia

1. Deliver oxygen as required.
2. Identify the organism.

   Perform a Gram stain on the sputum and send for culture. Obtain special stains as necessary (ZN stain, TB culture, and immunofluorescence staining for *Pneumocystis carinii* in human immunodeficiency virus–positive patients). Sputum may be induced with nasotracheal suction if a sample is difficult to obtain.
3. Order blood cultures × 2.

   Order CBC and differential.

4. Begin empirical antibiotic treatment if indicated (Table 28–6).
   Focus the therapy based on Gram stain and culture results when available.
5. Order chest physical therapy.
6. Order thoracentesis, if an effusion is present.
   Evaluate the pleural fluid as described above.

Aspiration of Gastric Contents

Patients with impaired mental status or who are vomiting are at risk for aspiration of gastric contents. This results in chemical

Table 28–6 □ EMPIRICAL TREATMENT FOR SUSPECTED PNEUMONIA

Community Acquired

Streptococcus pneumoniae Haemophilus influenzae	Penicillin G 1–2 million U IV every 4–6 hr or ampicillin 1 g PO or IV every 6 hr or 1st-generation cephalosporin
Mycoplasma pneumoniae Legionella pneumophila	Erythromycin 500 mg PO or IV* every 6 hr

COPD Associated

Streptococcus pneumoniae Haemophilus influenzae	Penicillin G 1–2 million U IV every 4–6 hr or ampicillin 1 g PO or IV every 6 hr or 1st-generation cephalosporin

Hospital Acquired or Elderly Patients

In addition to the community-acquired infection coverage, consider treatment for Gram-negative organisms.

Cefuroxime 750 mg IV every 8 hr
Ceftazidime 1 g IV or IM every 8–12 hr
Gentamicin 1.5–2 mg/kg IV loading dose followed by 1–1.5 mg/kg IV every 8 hr† or 5 mg/kg per day (follow 8-hr post-dose trough levels)

In the ICU or CCU, very virulent organisms such as *Pseudomonas* and *Acinetobacter* species are also present. They should be treated with combination therapy of a 3rd-generation cephalosporin and aminoglycoside according the specific sensitivities of the hospital flora.

Aspiration

Consider in patients who have decreased mental status or defective cough or gag reflex. Treat with antibiotics only if there are associated symptoms of bacterial disease (e.g., fever, leukocytosis, and purulent sputum)

Mouth anaerobes	Penicillin G 2 million U IV every 4 hr Clindamycin 300–600 mg PO or IV every 6 hr

Table 28–6 □ EMPIRICAL TREATMENT FOR SUSPECTED PNEUMONIA *Continued*

Alcoholic Associated

In addition to organisms associated with aspiration pneumonia, alcoholic patients also have a high incidence of *Klebsiella pneumoniae,* which is treated with double antibiotic therapy as listed above for ICU or CCU bacteria, according to the hospital flora sensitivities.

HIV Positive

Pneumocystis carinii‡	Trimethoprim-sulfamethoxazole (TMP-SMX) 15–20 mg/kg (based on TMP) IV every 6–8 hr Pentamidine isethionate§ 4 mg/kg IV or IM every day

*Administration of IV erythromycin is associated with severe venous burning and thrombophlebitis. Dilute the dose in 500 ml NS and run slowly over 6 hours.

†Gentamicin and other aminoglycoside medications are nephrotoxic and ototoxic. They should have their maintenance doses adjusted based on serum peak and trough levels, with special care with their use in patients with renal insufficiency.

‡If *Pneumocystis carinii* is suspected, then diagnosis should be made by bronchoscopy. Infectious disease consultation is advisable when managing the infections of HIV-positive patients.

§Pentamidine administration is associated with hypotension, tachycardia, nausea, vomiting, and hyperemia. Side effects may be limited by dilution in 500 ml 5% dextrose in water and by administration over 2 to 4 hours. Other associated derangements include hyperkalemia, hypocalcemia, megaloblastic anemia, leukopenia, thrombocytopenia, hyperglycemia or hypoglycemia, increased LFTs, and dose-related nephrotoxicity.

IV = intravenously; PO = orally; COPD = chronic obstructive pulmonary disease; IM = intramuscularly; ICU = intensive care unit; CCU = cardiac care unit; HIV = human immunodeficiency virus; NS = normal saline; LFT = liver function test.

pneumonitis as well as bacterial pneumonia. Treat as in pneumonia (above).

■ SPECIAL SURGICAL CONSIDERATIONS

Preoperative Considerations

- Severe SOB indicates the new onset or exacerbation of a problem that may affect a scheduled procedure.
- Steps that aid in the prevention of specific etiologies of SOB are as follows:

Pulmonary Embolism

1. All patients scheduled to undergo general anesthesia should have thigh-high support (TED) stockings and sequential compression devices in place before induction.

2. Patients with a history of thromboembolic phenomena may benefit from additional treatment with **low-dose heparin 5000 U SC every 8 hours before and after surgery.** Discuss this with the attending surgeon before ordering this therapy.

   As an alternative, low-dose warfarin may be given in doses sufficient to maintain the PT in the upper normal range (i.e., prolonged by 1–3 seconds) for 10 to 14 days before surgery. Immediately after surgery, the warfarin dose is doubled to maintain the PT in the 1.5 times normal range. This therapy decreases the incidence of postoperative thromboembolism and is not associated with a significantly increased risk of postoperative bleeding.

Atelectasis.   The most important preventive measure is patient education. Make sure the patient understands the importance of ambulation, incentive spirometry, and cough.

Reactive Airway Disease
1. Patients with known asthma or COPD must be stable and prepared for surgery. Review with the patient possible modalities for postoperative care such as nebulizer treatments, incentive spirometry, and medication use.
2. Patients who are on chronic steroid therapy will need stress doses of steroids perioperatively (see Table 28–3).
3. Preoperative pulmonary testing may be required in some patients with severely diminished pulmonary reserves.

Postoperative Considerations

Most susceptible to SOB are those patients who have undergone thoracic or abdominal procedures.

Thoracic Surgery
1. Think first of chest tube malfunction (see Chapter 30 for a complete discussion). If the chest tube was recently removed, evaluate the patient for possible replacement.
2. In patients after lung resection, think of a pulmonary staple line leak. This is mostly evident by a persistent air leak through the chest tube but may occur after chest tube removal.
3. Pneumothorax and hemothorax are frequent findings after thoracic surgery and are generally well controlled and monitored by tube thoracostomy. SOB will result from tube malfunction.
4. Chylothorax is an infrequent complication of thoracic surgery or penetrating chest trauma with injury to the thoracic duct. Findings include pleural effusion with high triglyceride content (generally right sided). This is controlled with

tube thoracostomy. Be mindful that much of the patient's nutrition is draining into the Pleur-Evac tube, and IV lipids may be required if the leak is prolonged.

Abdominal Surgery
1. Respirations are painful after abdominal surgery, so splinting with poor lung expansion is the rule. Incentive spirometry and frequent coughing help avoid atelectasis and postoperative pneumonia. Make sure that the patient is alert and has adequate pain control.
2. Abdominal distention secondary to bowel obstruction may decrease the diaphragmatic excursion and may lead to hypoventilation. NG decompression may aid in decreasing the distention.
3. Rarely, dehiscence of diaphragmatic hernia repairs may result in herniation of abdominal contents back into the thoracic cavity. This is evident on CXR and requires immediate surgical repair.

■ **RESPIRATORY FAILURE**

Respiratory failure is defined as inadequate effort to supply the existing oxygenation needs. It may result from any of the etiologies above and requires immediate treatment to correct hypoxia. Initial findings of hypoventilation may be RR of <12 breaths/ min and cyanosis, agitation, or lethargy. ABG results may show progressive hypoxia (PaO_2 of <60 mm Hg), hypercapnia (PCO_2 of >50 mm Hg), and acidosis (pH of <7.30). In settings of impaired gas exchange, such as adult respiratory distress syndrome, the RR may be >20. Correct the cause if it is immediately evident. If not, act immediately to ensure adequate oxygenation, as follows:
1. Reverse narcotic medication.
    Use **naloxone hydrochloride (Narcan) 0.2 to 2.0 mg IV** immediately. Pinpoint pupils may aid in the diagnosis of narcosis.
2. Ventilate the patient.
    Use bag-valve-mask ventilation to adequately oxygenate the patient until intubation may be performed. This is a **code** situation; notify the resident and get help immediately. Make sure the resuscitation cart is on hand and open.
3. Monitor oxygenation with pulse oximetry.
    Follow acidosis and hypercapnia with frequent ABGs.
4. Arrange for intubation of the patient and transfer to the ICU or CCU.
    Do not panic if you are not skilled at endotracheal intubation. Bag-valve-mask ventilation is often adequate to oxygenate and ventilate a patient for long periods of time until a skilled individual arrives.

29

SYNCOPE

Syncope is a brief loss of consciousness due to an interruption of cerebral blood flow. Causes range from benign processes such as vasovagal episodes to more serious conditions such as dysrhythmias. As the on-call physician, your job is to identify the cause of the syncopal episode, to stabilize the patient if necessary, and to identify any injuries resulting from falls secondary to the syncopal episode.

■ PHONE CALL

1. **Does the patient have a regular pulse and vital signs, and is there any history of syncope?**

   Patients who have a history of syncopal episode are more likely to have another syncopal event. These patients will often have had a prior syncopal workup, which makes it easier to identify the likely cause of the current syncopal event.

2. **Did the patient lose consciousness or just feel faint?**

   There is a difference between true syncope and presyncope. In presyncope, a patient feels on the verge of losing consciousness but actually does not.

3. **How long was the patient unconscious, and is the patient still unconscious?**

4. **Did the patient have a seizure before the loss of consciousness (LOC), and is there any history of epilepsy?**

   It is important to rule out seizures as a cause for LOC. If a patient had an unwitnessed seizure, it may be difficult to rule out seizure as a cause for an alteration in consciousness. Bites to the tongue, incontinence, and prolonged postictal period after regaining consciousness suggest seizure.

5. **What medical problems does the patient have?**

   Diabetes (hypoglycemia), cardiac disease (e.g., dysrhythmias, myocardial infarction [MI], aortic stenosis), and neurologic conditions (transient ischemic attacks [TIAs] and stroke) can cause syncope.

6. **Was the patient injured from a fall?**

   Elderly patients are most likely to have syncopal episodes. These patients are susceptible to fractures and soft-tissue injury.

Orders

If the patient is still unconscious or has any instability of vital signs, give the following orders to the RN:

1. Take vital signs.
2. Establish an intravenous (IV) line immediately. Run 5% dextrose in one-half normal saline to keep the vein open.
3. If the patient is still unconscious, turn the patient on the left side with the mouth in a slightly downward direction. This will minimize the risk of aspiration and will help the tongue move forward to avoid obstructing the airway.
4. Order 12-lead electrocardiogram (ECG) with rhythm strip immediately.
5. Repeat vital signs now.

Inform RN

"Will arrive at the bedside in . . . minutes."

Syncope associated with prolonged unconsciousness or instability requires assessment of the patient immediately. This is especially true in neurosurgical patients, whose postoperative or posttraumatic course is evaluated and followed by the state of consciousness or mental status examination.

■ ELEVATOR THOUGHTS

What are the causes of syncope?
- Cardiovascular causes
  1. Rate and rhythm problems
     Ventricular tachyarrhythmias
     Sinus bradycardia
     Atrioventricular block (secondary or tertiary)
     Sick sinus syndrome
     Pacemaker problems
  2. Mechanical problems
     Aortic stenosis
     Mitral stenosis
     Pulmonic stenosis
     MI
     Hypertrophic obstructive cardiomyopathy
     Pulmonary embolism
- Reflex-vagal causes
  1. Vasovagal episodes (fainting)
  2. Orthostatic hypotension
     Hypovolemia
     Drug related
  3. Carotid sinus syncope

- Neurologic causes
  1. TIAs
  2. Costovertebral angle (CVA)
  3. Seizure
  4. Cervical spondylosis
  5. Subclavian steal syndrome
- Psychiatric causes
  1. Anxiety disorder (hysteria and panic attack)
  2. Hyperventilation

■ MAJOR THREAT TO LIFE

- Dysrhythmia

  Dysrhythmias represent the most acute threat to life. Ventricular tachyarrhythmias often present with syncope. These rhythms may persist or deteriorate to ventricular fibrillation. If you believe that the patient has suffered a transient tachyarrhythmia, it is appropriate to transfer the patient to a monitored (ECG) hospital bed. A patient with ongoing tachyarrhythmia should be treated as outlined in Chapter 11.

- Aspiration

  It is important to protect an unconscious patient from airway obstruction and aspiration. When a patient is unconscious and supine, the tongue falls to the back of the oropharynx and may obstruct the airway. Furthermore, because emesis may be concurrent with syncope, it is important to minimize the risk of aspiration. Positioning of the patient in the left decubitus position, with the mouth turned slightly downward, helps maintain the open airway by moving the tongue anteriorly. If emesis occurs, this positioning allows vomitus to flow out of the mouth.

- Intracranial bleeding

  Neurosurgical or trauma patients who develop intracranial bleeding after craniotomy or trauma may have an LOC. They will often develop a deteriorating LOC that progresses to a state of unconsciousness. Although this is not true syncope, it may be mistaken as syncope. These patients usually do not recover rapidly from the LOC. Computed tomographic (CT) scanning may be required to assess intracerebral or extracerebral collections of blood.

■ BEDSIDE

Quick Look Test

Does the patient look well (comfortable), sick (uncomfortable or distressed), or critical (about to die)?

Patients who have had a brief syncopal episode and have regained consciousness will often look well. Patients who have ongoing dysrhythmias, poor cerebral perfusion, or unstable vital signs will look sick or critical.

Airway and Vital Signs

Airway

Patients who have regained consciousness from a short-lived syncopal episode will generally have control of their airway. However, patients who are still unconscious should be placed on the left side as described earlier. Proper positioning will diminish the risk of airway obstruction and aspiration.

Heart Rate

Symptomatic bradycardia should be treated with atropine as discussed in Chapter 11. Supraventricular or ventricular tachyarrhythmias causing syncope should be documented by ECG and treated as outlined in Chapter 11. Consider transferring a patient with significant dysrhythmia and hemodynamic instability to the cardiac care unit (CCU) or the intensive care unit (ICU).

Blood Pressure

Hypotension may result in syncope. Evaluate the patient for hypovolemia, bradycardia, and signs of shock. Orthostatic hypotension should be treated as outlined in Chapter 12. Hypertension may result in CVA or subarachnoid hemorrhage. Although these conditions may not result in an interruption of blood flow to the brain, they may first present with an episode of LOC.

Temperature

A fever in the presence of syncope may indicate an infectious process of the central nervous system. Evaluate the patient carefully for meningitis. LOC and fever may also be seen in septic processes.

Selective History and Chart Review

Does the patient have a history of syncopal episode?
    Patients who present with syncope frequently have had a prior syncopal episode. The cause of the prior episode may be known and documented in the medical record. If workup has been done previously, management will be much easier.

Does the patient have a history of heart disease?
    Look for a history of coronary artery disease, valvular stenoses (especially aortic stenosis), and dysrhythmias.

Does the patient have a history of seizure disorder?

A patient with a seizure disorder who has a reported syncopal episode is more likely to have had a seizure.

What does the patient recall just before losing consciousness?

A patient who recalls an aura (auditory, visual, or olfactory) is likely to have suffered a seizure. A patient who recalls that he or she suddenly changed position (supine or sitting position to standing position) just before losing consciousness may have had an orthostatic hypotensive syncopal episode. Chest pain or palpitations before syncope suggests a cardiac cause.

What medications or drugs is the patient taking?

Certain medications are known to increase the occurrence of syncope. Alpha blockers (e.g., prazosin), smooth-muscle relaxants (e.g., hydralazine), and angiotensin-converting enzyme inhibitors (e.g., enalapril) reduce afterload and may cause syncope in elderly or hypovolemic patients. Drugs that slow the heart rate, such as calcium channel blockers (e.g., nifedipine), digoxin, and beta blockers (e.g., propranolol), may cause bradycardia and result in syncope. Sympathetic stimulants such as tricyclic antidepressants (imipramine) and cocaine may cause tachyarrhythmias and syncope.

Selective Physical Examination

As you examine the patient, try to ascertain the cause of the syncopal episode. First, make sure that the patient is stable. Then try to identify the cause of the syncopal episode. Finally, make sure that the patient has not suffered any injuries related to a fall.

VS:	Repeat now.
HEENT:	Examine tongue, cheeks, and lips for lacerations or bite injuries (seizure). Neck stiffness suggests meningitis.
	Examine face and scalp for traumatic injuries.
Resp:	Listen for crackles or wheezes secondary to aspiration.
CVS:	Irregularly irregular rhythm suggests atrial fibrillation.
	Note murmurs consistent with a valvular stenosis. Look for presence of a pacemaker (look for subcutaneous pocket on upper chest).
	Note jugular venous distention (volume depletion).
GU:	Urinary incontinence suggests seizure.
GI:	Incontinence of stool suggests seizure.
MSS:	Examine patient for evidence of contusions or fractures.
Neuro:	Complete neurologic examination is required.

Look for focal findings suggestive of a distinct lesion. Focality suggests CVA, TIA, or space-occupying lesion.

■ MANAGEMENT

In many cases, it will be difficult to arrive at the cause of a syncopal episode. Many of the causes of syncope are transient events. It generally takes a fairly extensive workup to collect the information necessary to arrive at a likely cause. For this reason, definitive treatment for syncope is reserved for medical conditions that have been clearly defined and documented. As the on-call physician, your job is to assess the syncopal patient, to document the syncopal event, to stabilize the patient if necessary, and to arrange initial workup.

Syncope Due to Cardiac Events

1. Syncope can result from a dysrhythmia or a mechanical problem.

   Any patient who has a syncopal episode from a cardiac cause should be transferred to a continuous ECG monitored unit (transitional care unit, CCU, or ICU).
2. If dysrhythmia is likely, consider silent ischemia or MI as a possible cause of transient rhythm disturbances.

   Evaluate the 12-lead ECG carefully, and consider enzyme studies if indicated. Treat cardiac ischemia as outlined in Chapter 7.
3. If dysrhythmia is ongoing, treat specific rhythm disturbances as outlined in Chapter 11.
4. Holter monitoring may be helpful to evaluate the occurrence of transient rhythm disturbances in stable patients.
5. Pacemaker problems require cardiology consultation.
6. Mechanical problems such as aortic stenosis, obstructive cardiomyopathy, and pulmonic stenosis should be worked up with a nonemergent echocardiogram. Cardiology consultation is also advisable.

Syncope Due to Vagal Events

1. If the patient is bradycardic and symptomatic, consider **atropine 0.5 to 1.0 mg IV; the dose may be repeated every 5 minutes, for a maximum dose of 2 mg.**
2. If the syncopal episode is due to a simple vasovagal attack, place the patient supine with the legs elevated.

   Spontaneous resolution will generally occur. Vasovagal episodes are one of the most common causes of syncope.

Syncope Due to Orthostatic Hypotension

Syncope may occur in volume-depleted patients. Simple dehydration, inadequate fluid resuscitation after surgery or illness, or postoperative or posttraumatic bleeding will lead to states of volume depletion. These patients are susceptible to syncope when moving from supine to sitting or standing positions. Treatment consists of fluid resuscitation or transfusion as outlined in Chapter 12.

Orthostatic hypotension may also result from vasodilator drugs and autonomic dysfunction. When evaluating a patient with orthostatic hypotension, be sure to evaluate the medications a patient is taking. It is appropriate to hold medications that are vasodilators or antihypertensives.

Syncope Due to Psychiatric Factors

Patients can lose consciousness from sudden shock, anxiety, or stress. It is important to reassure anxious patients. Antianxiety medications may be appropriate (e.g., **diazepam [Valium] 5–10 mg orally)**. Remind the anxious patient not to hyperventilate. Hypocapnia, resulting from hyperventilation, can lead to syncope.

Syncope Due to Neurologic Events

1. A patient who is believed to have had a stroke or a brain stem TIA should have a CT scan of the head.

    The CT scan is best performed with contrast. Neurologic consultation should be obtained if workup suggests that the patient has had a stroke.

2. If a patient is believed to have had a subarachnoid hemorrhage (SAH), CT scan is appropriate.

    More than 90% of patients will show blood in the subarachnoid spaces of the sulci and the cisternae in the first 24 hours after SAH. CT scan may also show evidence of aneurysm. Lumbar puncture should be performed if the clinical impression leads strongly to SAH but CT scan is negative.

3. Intracerebral hemorrhage is diagnosed by CT scan.

    Treatment consists of supportive care and control of blood pressure. Neurosurgical consultation should be obtained for cerebral and cerebellar hematomas.

4. Seizures are managed as outlined in Chapter 27.

TUBES AND DRAINS

Many postoperative patients will have drainage devices to facilitate their care. The types used most often fall into the following broad categories:

- **Chest tubes**
- **Urinary drainage tubes** (urinary catheters)
- **Gastrointestinal (GI) tubes** (nasogastric [NG] or mercury-weighted tubes for decompression, feeding tubes, and gastrostomy and jejunostomy tubes)
- **Biliary drainage tubes** (T-tubes)
- **Wound drainage tubes** (Jackson-Pratt, Penrose, and other suction drains)

Problems with these tubes are frequent but generally straightforward. This section is organized by the type of tube. Intravenous lines are covered in Chapter 19.

Chest Tubes

Appropriate treatment of the problems associated with chest tubes begins with a fundamental knowledge of how the tubes work. The apparatus is a means to apply external suction to the pleural cavity to rid the space of unwanted air or fluid. The collection apparatus looks complicated but may be easily understood if the components are considered separately; the apparatus may be thought of as three separate interconnected bottles (Fig. 30–1), as follows:

1. Suction from the wall or from a vacuum device is connected to the suction control bottle (see Fig. 30–1*a*). The volume of water in this bottle (*f*) dictates the amount of suction that is transmitted to the patient. When suction is ordered, it is ordered in units of centimeters of water (cm H_2O).

2. The suction control bottle is connected to the underwater seal bottle (*b*). This bottle allows separation of the patient from the suction if desired, and is the site of indication of an air leak. Continued air evacuation is noted as persistent bubbling in this chamber.

3. The underwater seal bottle is connected to the collection bottle (*c*), which is the site of fluid collection. Fluid draining from the chest tube is stored in this chamber for measurement and testing if desired. The collection bottle is then

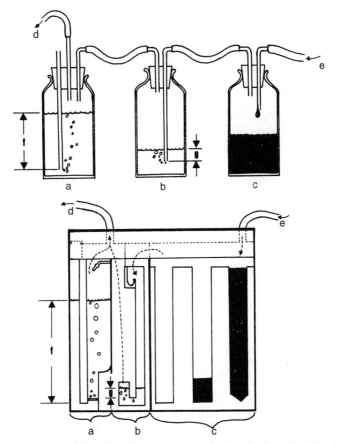

Figure 30–1 □ Chest tube apparatus. *a,* Suction control chamber. *b,* Underwater seal. *c,* Collection chamber. *d,* To suction. *e,* From patient. *f,* Height equals amount of suction in units of cm H_2O. *g,* Height equals underwater seal in units of cm H_2O. (From Marshall SA, Ruedy J: ON CALL: Principles and Protocols, 2nd ed. Philadelphia, WB Saunders Co, 1993, p 180.)

connected to the chest tube in the patient. These bottles may be combined into a single box-type drainage apparatus (Pleur-Evac).

Indications

1. Pneumothorax
2. Pyothorax

3. Hemothorax
4. Chylothorax
5. Persistent pleural effusion
6. Postoperative application after thoracic procedures

Placement

1. **Have all equipment ready.** You will need the following:
   - Skin preparation supplies (iodine, chlorhexidine, or alcohol)
   - Local anesthetic lidocaine hydrochloride or a lidocaine and bupivacaine hydrochloride (lidocaine–Marcaine HCl) mixture
   - Sedative medication as necessary
   - Pulse oximeter
   - Chest tube of appropriate diameter, i.e., thin for air removal (24–28 Fr) and thicker for fluid removal (28–32 Fr). The perforated end may be cut down to facilitate tube placement in a smaller patient. Placing a bevel on the end is not recommended. It may facilitate placement, but it is a perforation risk to the lung once inside the patient.
   - A chest tube insertion tray, including blades, gauze, hemostats, trocars, thick silk suture with needle, and drapes
   - Petroleum gauze dressing
   - Wide, gas-impermeable, occlusive tape
   - Suction device (i.e., wall suction or portable apparatus)
   - Chest tube suction apparatus (Pleur-Evac) prefilled with water and hooked up to the suction device
2. **Prepare the patient.**
   - Explain the procedure.
   - Explain the risks and the alternatives.
   - Answer any questions.
   - Have a consent form prepared and signed.
   - Position the patient supine.
3. **Premedicate the patient.**
   - The patient should have intravenous (IV) access.
   - A short-acting benzodiazepine such as **lorazepam (Ativan) 1 to 2 mg IV** is usually sufficient. As much as 4 mg may be required.
   - Opiate pain medication may also be beneficial in selected patients, but bear in mind the respiratory depressant effects.
   - Skip premedication if the patient is in distress or is at risk for respiratory depression.
4. **Prepare the skin.**
   - Use a sterile technique.
        Scrub your hands and don sterile gloves, mask, and gown.
   - Plan the incision.

The midaxillary line is generally used, with anterior direction of the chest tube to remove gas and with posterior direction of the chest tube to remove fluid. Plan to make the skin incision about 2 to 3 cm below the rib interspace to be entered so there is an oblique skin channel. This usually facilitates closure on removal of the tube. On occasion, the anterior midclavicular line is used to relieve pneumothorax.

- Perform local skin preparation and draping.
- Infiltrate locally with 1 to 2% lidocaine into the skin at the entry site and over the rib at the selected interspace.

   The periosteum of the top of the rib is very sensitive, so do not skimp on lidocaine. Infiltrate the subcutaneous tunnel as well while removing the needle.

5. **Place a purse-string suture.**

   When adequate local anesthesia has been obtained, place a purse-string suture at the site of skin entry. Position the tie such that the loose ends are inferior to the tube exit site, and place a single throw loosely (Fig. 30–2).

6. **Make the skin incision over a rib.**

   Cutting over the bone allows a clean, deep cut and avoids the neurovascular bundle that travels on the underside of each rib. The incision should be about 1.5 times the diameter of the chest tube and should be positioned inside the purse-string suture. (**Do not cut the purse-string su-**

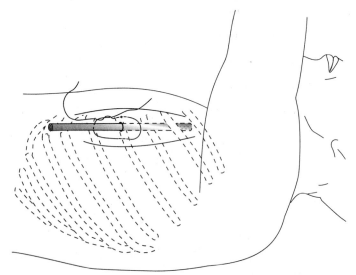

Figure 30–2 □ Purse-string ligature around chest tube site.

ture!) Control any bleeding with pressure. Reinject with lidocaine as necessary.

7. **Dissect bluntly toward the pleura.**
   - Using a hemostat, create a subcutaneous channel superiorly from the skin incision to over the top of the rib at the desired interspace.
   - Spread the hemostat to ensure room enough for the diameter of the chest tube.
   - Using a fair amount of pressure and with the hemostats closed, force the hemostats in between the ribs through the intercostal muscles; stay right on top of a rib to avoid the neurovascular bundle.
   - You may notice a "pop" when the pleural cavity has been entered; often there is also a noticeable gush of air through the wound.
   - Spread the hemostat tips to create enough space in the intercostal muscles to allow the tube to pass.
   - Remove the hemostat.

8. **Insert the chest tube.**
   Using the hemostat, grasp the perforated end of the chest tube and place the tube through the subcutaneous channel and the intercostal muscle opening. This is often a difficult maneuver; it may take several passes to refind the channel you created. It is often helpful to palpate the dissected tract with your sterile gloved finger. This allows you to have a good idea of the direction the tube will pass most easily. (With trocar insertion, the tube is placed over the trocar and forced into the pleural cavity without hemostat perforation of the intercostal muscles.)

9. **Position the chest tube.**
   Note that the chest tube has a mark below the last perforations. When the tube has been placed into the chest and directed in the appropriate direction, insert the tube until the mark is just visible at the skin incision line.

10. **Secure the tube.**
    - Pull the purse-string suture snugly around the tube without adding throws. Wrap the loose ends around the tube several times to hold it in place. Make sure that several inches of suture are wrapped around the tube, because this will be used to tie off the wound when the tube is removed. Once wrapped, the loose ends may be tied down securely.
    - Occasionally, it is necessary to place one or two 2–0 silk sutures in the incision site to close the wound around the tube.

11. **Connect the chest tube to the Pleur-Evac and to wall suction.**
    The suction pressure is defined by the volume of water

(in cm) in the suction control chamber of the Pleur-Evac. A bubbling in the underwater seal chamber will indicate adequate suction to remove gas and will continue for as long as there is an air leak. If fluid is to be removed, it will collect in the collection chamber (see Fig. 30–1*a*).

12. **Tape the chest tube site.**
    - Wrap the tubing at the skin site with petroleum gauze.
    - Apply occlusive tape in such a way that the tube site is relatively air-tight and that the tube is safe from being dislodged.
    - Further secure the tube by applying an umbilical tape such that unexpected pulls on the tube will pull on the tape umbilicus instead of the suture (Fig. 30–3).

13. **Confirm tube placement by bedside upright anterior–posterior (AP) and lateral chest x-rays (CXRs) immediately.**
    Reposition as necessary. This must be done in a sterile manner. Never push an unsterile chest tube farther into the chest. Daily CXRs are recommended to follow the course of therapy and to confirm continued adequate placement of the tube.

14. **Control pain.**
    The tube insertion site will remain uncomfortable until the tube is removed; make sure the patient has adequate pain relief.

15. **Pulmonary toilet is important in patients with chest tubes.**
    Make an incentive spirometer available, and instruct the patient as to its use and importance. Encourage coughing.

16. **Send fluid efflux from the chest tube to the laboratory.**
    The following studies may be indicated:
    - Gram stain
    - Cultures (aerobic and anaerobic bacterial, fungal, and mycoplasma)
    - Ziehl-Neelsen stain and TB culture
    - Cell count and differential
    - Lactate dehydrogenase (LDH)

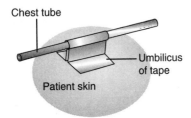

Chest tube

Umbilicus of tape

Patient skin

Figure 30–3 □ Tape umbilicus technique for securing chest tubes.

- Protein
- Glucose
- Cytology for malignant cells
- Other studies as appropriate (amylase, triglycerides, pH, rheumatoid factor, and antinuclear antibodies or complement levels)

A simultaneous serum LDH, protein, and glucose should be drawn to compare with the results of the pleural fluid.

Removal of the Tube Thoracostomy

This procedure is quick and easy but requires two individuals and patient cooperation, i.e., a conscious and alert patient.

1. **Confirm that the patient is ready to have the chest tube removed.**
   - There should be no persistent air leak, or the patient should have been stable for ≥24 hours on water seal alone.
   - Ongoing fluid leak or bleeding should have stopped.
   - The lung should be inflated on CXR.
   - There is no other reason to consider leaving the tube in place.
2. **Have all equipment ready.** You will need the following:
   - Blade or scissors to cut the knot from the purse-string suture
   - Petroleum gauze
   - Wide, gas-impermeable, occlusive tape
   - Dry gauze sponges (4 in. × 4 in.)
   - Pulse oximeter (as necessary)
3. **Explain the procedure.**
   Removal of the chest tube is painful and requires cooperation by the patient. Explain clearly what is to occur. Avoid excessive administration with opiate pain medication, as this may depress respiratory function and affect the patient's ability to cooperate.
4. **Position the patient upright or supine.**
5. **Remove existing tape.**
6. **Cut the purse-string knot.**
   Leave the long suture ends intact.
7. **Tighten the purse-string suture such that the skin closes tightly around the tube.**
   Confirm that the tube is free from the suture and tape.
8. **Confirm that the suction is turned off.**
9. **Remove the chest tube.**
   - Have the patient inhale completely and hold his or her breath at the peak of inhalation. This guarantees a positive pressure in the pleural cavity and does not allow an involuntary gasp by the patient when the tube is removed.

- While the breath is being held, the first person pulls the chest tube out. Immediately place the petroleum gauze over the skin site to avoid the influx of air.
- At the same time as the tube is being removed, the second person pulls the ends of the purse-string suture such that the skin seals tightly underneath the petroleum gauze bandage; tie the ends down.

10. **Apply dry gauze and occlusive tape to the site.**
11. **Obtain a CXR to assess for pneumothorax.**

    A small amount of air is common and may be treated with 100% O_2 therapy.

12. **Observe the patient over the next few hours for adequate breath sounds and oxygenation.**
13. **Examine the patient in 24 hours and obtain a follow-up CXR.**

    If at any time respiratory distress develops, evaluate the patient for replacement of the chest tube.

Complications of Tube Thoracostomy

1. Lack of resolution of the problem
2. Perforation of the lung
3. Perforation of abdominal viscera
4. Perforation of the heart

Problems with Chest Tubes

1. Persistent air leak
2. Persistent blood leak
3. Bleeding at the entry site
4. Loss of underwater seal fluctuation
5. Shortness of breath (SOB)
6. Subcutaneous emphysema
7. Discomfort at the tube entry site

■ PERSISTENT AIR LEAK

This is manifest by continuous bubbling in the underwater seal compartment of the drainage apparatus (see Fig. 30–1a). It may be present with or without the application of suction to the tube.

Phone Call

Questions

1. **Why was the chest tube inserted?**
2. **How long ago was the tube inserted?**
3. **Is the patient short of breath?**
4. **Has the patient undergone a surgical procedure, and if so, how long ago?**

5. **Are there any other symptoms?**
6. **Are there any changes in vital signs?**

Degree of Urgency

If there is a significant change in vital signs or symptoms, the patient must be evaluated immediately.

Elevator Thoughts

What causes persistent air leak?
1. Loose tubing or connectors
2. Air leaking into the chest
   - From the entrance wound
   - From a new bronchial or pulmonary injury
3. Persistent bronchopleural fistula
   - After thoracic surgery (lobectomy and open biopsy)
   - After a closed chest procedure (needle biopsy and thoracentesis)
   - Due to ruptured bleb (asthma and emphysema)

Major Threat to Life

- Hypoxia, if the air leak is new or if it is associated with SOB
- Pneumothorax

Bedside

Quick Look Test

If the air leak is small, the patient may look comfortable. A patient who has a new pneumothorax may look acutely distressed.

Selective History and Chart Review

- Review why the chest tube was placed.
- Discern if the air leak had ever resolved.

    If the patient is recovering from a thoracic procedure, the air leak may persist for 2 to 5 days. A new air leak may indicate a complication derived from the procedure or from placement of the chest tube.

Selective Physical Examination

VS:	Increased respiratory rate (RR) (hypoxia)
Resp:	Unilateral decrease in aeration, and hyperresonance (pneumothorax)
Tubes:	Connections secure
Special examination:	Some air leaks are small and will be noted only during increases in intrapleural pressure such as coughing

Additional tests:

1. Pulse ox-   Hypoxia
   imetry

Management

1. Check for hypoxia with a pulse oximeter.
2. Supply supplemental oxygen as required (see Chapter 28).
3. Check the tubing between the drainage apparatus and the patient for loose connections.
4. Untape the wound site and confirm that the chest tube is inserted properly.

   Each chest tube has a visible line a few centimeters away from the most distal holes. The tube must be inserted such that the line is at or inside the skin line.
5. If the entry site is not well closed or if a sucking sound is noted at the site, it may be necessary to close the site further with 2–0 silk sutures.

   Be sure to adequately prepare and anesthetize the area before repair.
6. Reposition the chest tube if necessary, and re-dress the site using petroleum gauze.
7. If the connections are intact and the site is dressed in an airtight manner, order a portable AP CXR to assess the patient's lungs and the tube position.
8. If the CXR shows lack of resolution of pneumothorax, consider placement of a second tube.

■ PERSISTENT BLOOD LEAK

Phone Call

Questions

1. **Why was the chest tube inserted?**
2. **How long ago was the tube inserted?**
3. **Is the patient short of breath?**
4. **Has the patient undergone a surgical procedure, and if so, how long ago was it performed?**
5. **Are there any other symptoms?**
6. **Are there any changes in vital signs?**

Orders

Order a hematocrit as a baseline if the bleeding is brisk.

Degree of Urgency

If there is a significant change in vital signs or symptoms, the patient must be evaluated immediately.

Elevator Thoughts

What causes excess blood efflux?
1. Erosion of the tube into a bronchial artery or vein
2. Coagulopathy
3. Injury to an intercostal neurovascular bundle

Major Threat to Life

- Hypotension and shock if the blood loss is great
- Disseminated intravascular coagulation (DIC)
- Hypoxia

Bedside

Quick Look Test

Massive blood loss may result in shock. The patient may be lethargic or comatose. Hypoxia will result in agitation.

Airway and Vital Signs

Severe fluid loss may lead to tachycardia and hypotension. Hypoxia may be associated with tachypnea.

Selective History and Chart Review

- Review why the chest tube was placed.
- Is the patient taking an anticoagulant such as warfarin or heparin?
   Can the medication be safely reversed?
- Determine the amount of blood lost and whether the current efflux rate is a change.

Management

1. Check for hypoxia with a pulse oximeter.
2. Supply supplemental oxygen as required (see Chapter 28).
3. If tachycardia or hypotension is present, begin fluid resuscitation with normal saline (NS) or lactated Ringer's (LR) (see Chapters 12 and 17).
   - Start a large-bore IV.
   - Give **500-ml NS or LR quickly.**
   - Send blood for a crossmatch for 4 to 6 units of packed red blood cells.
   - Order a portable AP CXR immediately.
4. If coagulopathy is present, correct with fresh frozen plasma or cryoprecipitate as per Chapter 26.
5. If the rate of loss is >500 ml over 6 to 8 hours, consider returning to the operating room (or consult a thoracic surgeon, if the patient is not a thoracic surgery patient).

Special Surgical Considerations

Postoperative Considerations

1. Bleeding is common after open thoracic procedures.
    This generally tapers off by 24 hours after the operation. If the bleeding does not abate, consider evaluating the patient for coagulopathy (prothrombin time, partial thromboplastin time, fibrinogen, fibrin degradation products, and platelets) or continued surgical bleeding.
2. New onset of blood in the chest tube may indicate a complication of the tube.

■ BLEEDING AT THE ENTRY SITE

Phone Call

Questions

1. Why was the chest tube inserted?
2. How long ago was the tube inserted?
3. Is the patient short of breath?
4. Has the patient undergone a surgical procedure, and if so, how long ago was it performed?
5. Are there any other symptoms?
6. Are there any changes in vital signs?

Degree of Urgency

Brisk bleeding in a patient is a serious finding, and the patient must be seen immediately. If there is a significant change in vital signs or symptoms, the patient must be evaluated immediately.

Elevator Thoughts

What causes bleeding around the entry site?
1. Inadequate hemostasis during insertion of the tube
2. Inadequate closure of the incision site after removal of the tube
3. Coagulation disorders
4. Trauma to intercostal vessels during insertion of the tube
5. Loss of patency of the chest tube
    Blood from the pleural space may drain around the tube.

Major Threat to Life

- Hypotension and shock if the blood loss is great
- DIC

Bedside

Quick Look Test

Most bleeding is mild and is not associated with changes in patient condition. Severe bleeding, however, may be associated with development of shock. The patient may be lethargic or comatose. Hypoxia will result in agitation.

Airway and Vital Signs

Severe fluid loss may lead to tachycardia and hypotension. Hypoxia may be associated with tachypnea.

Selective History and Chart Review

- Review why the chest tube was placed.
- Is the patient taking an anticoagulant such as warfarin or heparin?
    Can the medication be safely reversed?
- Determine the amount of blood lost and whether the current bleeding rate is a change.
    Note also the output through the chest tube lumen.

Management

1. Check for hypoxia with a pulse oximeter.
2. Supply supplemental oxygen as required (see Chapter 28).
3. Untape the wound site; inspect the wound.
    If the entry site is not well closed, it may be necessary to close the site further with 2–0 silk sutures. Be sure to adequately prepare and anesthetize the area before repair. Look for sites of active bleeding and ligate as necessary.
4. Re-dress the site using petroleum gauze.
    Apply a pressure dressing.
5. If the chest tube is clotted, milk the tube to attempt to clear it.
    Special chest tube stripper instruments are available for this purpose, or it may be accomplished by lubricating the tube with lotion and using your fingers to milk the tube toward the drainage apparatus. If you are unable to clear the tube or if the tube size is inadequate to manage the amount of drainage, consider replacement of the tube through a different site.

■ LOSS OF UNDERWATER SEAL FLUCTUATION

Phone Call

Questions

1. **Why was the chest tube inserted?**
2. **How long ago was the tube inserted?**

3. **Is the patient short of breath?**
4. **Has the patient undergone a surgical procedure, and if so, how long ago was it performed?**
5. **Are there any other symptoms?**
6. **Are there any changes in vital signs?**

Degree of Urgency

Loss of fluctuation of the underwater seal is a common but potentially serious problem. The patient should be seen fairly soon. If there is a significant change in vital signs or symptoms, the patient must be evaluated immediately.

Elevator Thoughts

What causes loss of underwater seal fluctuation?
1. Kink in the tubing
2. Occlusion of the tubing
3. Improper positioning of the chest tube within the pleural cavity

Major Threat to Life

- Tension pneumothorax
- Accumulation of fluid within the pleural space due to inadequate drainage

Bedside

Quick Look Test

A patient with a tension pneumothorax will appear acutely ill. Hypoxia, hypotension, and shock may follow.

Airway and Vital Signs

Hypotension and tachypnea are indications of pneumothorax.

Selective History and Chart Review

- Review why the chest tube was placed.
- How long has the tube been malfunctioning?
- What volume has been draining from the tube?

Management

1. Check for hypoxia with a pulse oximeter.
2. Supply supplemental oxygen as required (see Chapter 28).
3. Check the tubing between the drainage apparatus and the patient for loose connections. Look also for regions of clotting or kinking.

4. Confirm that the suction is appropriately applied.
5. Inspect the tube and drainage apparatus.

There are two regions that give clues to the function of a chest tube (Fig. 30–4). The underwater seal chamber (see Fig. 30–1a) is a low-pressure, one-way valve. Gas will bubble through this chamber if there is a continuous flow of air through the chest tube from the patient (such as a persistent air leak). Fluctuations may also be observed in the tubing itself between the patient and the drainage apparatus. Often fluid will collect in dependent regions of this tubing and will act as an additional underwater seal site. Fluctuations in this region indicate normal functioning of the chest tube between this site and the patient. Have the patient cough during your observation of this region.

6. Attempt to milk the tubing with strippers or your fingers to loosen a clot.

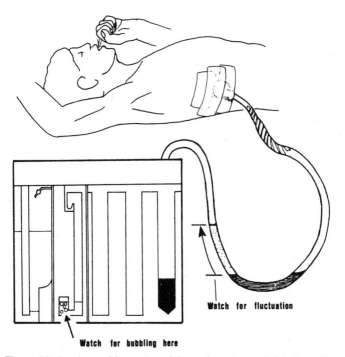

Watch for fluctuation

Watch for bubbling here

Figure 30–4 □ Loss of fluctuation of the underwater seal. Ask the patient to cough, and observe for any fluctuation or bubbling. (From Marshall SA, Ruedy J: On Call: Principles and Protocols, 2nd ed. Philadelphia, WB Saunders Co, 1993, p 187.)

7. If these measures do not reestablish normal chest tube function, obtain a portable AP CXR immediately.

Check for proper placement of the tube and for persistence or worsening of the intrapleural pathology. A new tube may need to be placed.

■ SHORTNESS OF BREATH

See also Chapter 28.

Phone Call

Questions

1. **Why was the chest tube inserted?**
2. **How long ago was the chest tube inserted?**
3. **Is the patient short of breath?**
4. **Has the patient undergone a surgical procedure, and if so, how long ago was it performed?**
5. **Are there any other symptoms?**
6. **Are there any changes in vital signs?**

Orders

1. Check for hypoxia with a pulse oximeter.
2. Supply supplemental oxygen as required (see Chapter 28).
3. Have a 16-gauge angiocatheter available at the bedside for use to diagnosis and to treat tension pneumothorax.

Degree of Urgency

The patient must be evaluated immediately.

Elevator Thoughts

What causes of shortness of breath are associated with chest tubes?

1. Tension pneumothorax
2. Increasing pneumothorax
   - Inadequate suction
   - Misplaced tube
   - Kinked or occluded tube
   - Bronchopleural fistula
3. Subcutaneous emphysema
   This may cause upper airway obstruction if the emphysema extends to the neck and displaces the trachea.
4. Increasing pleural effusion or hemothorax
5. Reexpansion pulmonary edema
   This may occur after rapid expansion of a pneumothorax or drainage of pleural effusion.

6. Non–chest tube–related causes (see Chapter 28)

Major Threat to Life

- Tension pneumothorax
- Upper airway obstruction

Bedside

Quick Look Test

Confirm the patency of the upper airway. Remove any oral obstruction such as dentures or foreign bodies. Tachypnea (RR >20 breaths/min) will be present if hypoxia, anxiety, pain, or acidosis is present. A drop in blood pressure may indicate a tension pneumothorax.

Selective History and Chart Review

- Review why the chest tube was placed.
- Was there a recent central line placement or thoracic surgery? Has a chest tube been recently clamped, placed to water seal, or removed? Is there a history of penetrating chest trauma or spontaneous pneumothorax?

Selective Physical Examination

VS: Repeat now; tachycardia, tachypnea, and hypotension (pneumothorax)
MS: Agitation (hypoxia) and lethargy (hypercapnia)
HEENT: Upper airway obstruction (foreign body and subcutaneous emphysema)
           Elevated jugular venous distention (pneumothorax)
           Deviated trachea (pneumothorax)
Resp: Decreased aeration, and unilateral hyperresonance (pneumothorax)
Tubes: Chest tube functioning normally
           Recent central venous line placement
Additional tests:
  1. CXR   Portable AP immediately.
  2. ABG   Assessment of serum arterial partial pressure of oxygen (Pa_{O_2}), partial pressure of carbon dioxide (P_{CO_2}), and pH and calculation of serum bicarbonate levels ($[HCO_3^-]$)

Management

1. If there is significant upper airway obstruction due to subcutaneous emphysema or other cause, do the following:

- Contact the resident.
- Prepare for possible intubation.
- Contact the intensive care unit (ICU) or cardiac care unit (CCU) for probable transfer.

2. For suspected pneumothorax, do the following:
   - Confirm the diagnosis.
       Findings may include decreased breath sounds and hyperresonance of the hemithorax, deviation of the trachea, hypoxia, and chest pain. In cases of tension pneumothorax, progressive cardiac outflow obstruction is apparent.
   - Immediately insert a 16-gauge needle into the second or third intercostal space anteriorly at the midclavicular line on the affected side.
       Enter 2 to 3 fingerbreadths below the clavicle to avoid the subclavian vessels. This will confirm the diagnosis and allow some relief of symptoms until adequate chest tube drainage can be reimplemented.
   - Reinsert the chest tube as necessary.
   - Confirm appropriate placement of the tube with a portable AP CXR immediately.
   - Pneumothoraces that do not respond to tube thoracostomy may require surgical repair.

■ SUBCUTANEOUS EMPHYSEMA

Phone Call

Questions

1. **Why was the chest tube inserted?**
2. **How long ago was the tube inserted?**
3. **Is the patient short of breath?**
4. **Has the patient undergone a surgical procedure, and if so, how long ago was it performed?**
5. **Are there any other symptoms?**
6. **Are there any changes in vital signs?**

Degree of Urgency

Subcutaneous emphysema is a potentially serious symptom and must be evaluated quickly. If there is a significant change in vital signs or symptoms, the patient must be evaluated immediately.

Elevator Thoughts

What causes subcutaneous emphysema?
1. Inadequate suction for the size of the pneumothorax

This may be a matter of too little suction or a tube size that is inadequate.

2. Misplacement of the tube, as in the chest wall or in the abdominal cavity
3. Gas-producing bacterial infection at the site of tube entry
4. A small amount of subcutaneous gas collection, not uncommon after chest tube placement

Major Threat to Life

- Upper airway obstruction due to accumulation of gas in the tissue around the trachea
- Necrotizing fasciitis

Bedside

Quick Look Test

Upper airway obstruction will cause distress and agitation. Early symptoms of local wound infection may be mild.

Airway and Vital Signs

Confirm that the airway is clear and that the subcutaneous gas has not impinged on the trachea. Tachypnea may indicate respiratory distress; also note symptoms of stridor. Fever may indicate infection.

Selective History and Chart Review

- Review why the chest tube was placed.

Management

1. If there is significant upper airway obstruction due to subcutaneous emphysema or other cause, do the following:
   - Contact the resident.
   - Prepare for possible intubation.
   - Contact the ICU/CCU for probable transfer.
2. Obtain a portable AP CXR immediately to confirm placement of the tube.
3. If there are continued symptoms of pneumothorax, do the following:
   - Increase the suction.
   - Consider repositioning the tube.
   - Consider replacing the tube with one of larger diameter.
4. Inspect the entry site, and confirm that all fenestrations are within the pleural cavity.

Remember

1. Never push an extruding chest tube back into the pleural cavity. If the fenestrations are not shown to be inside the chest cavity by CXR and additional drainage of fluid or air is required, insert a new tube through a fresh site.
2. Many cases require the placement of more than one tube for adequate resolution of the problem requiring the thoracotomy. The existing tube must be removed only if it no longer functions.
3. A tube that has been placed on water seal (no suction) too soon will allow reaccumulation of air or fluid within the pleural space. Remember that a simple solution to this problem is the reintroduction of suction.

Urinary Drainage Tubes

There are a variety of types of urinary drainage tubes. They fall into two basic placement approaches, transurethral and suprapubic. The transurethral approach may be used to place a long-term drainage tube or may be used simply to gain access to the bladder to obtain a sterile urine sample. Periodic in-and-out catheterization may be used if a patient cannot spontaneously void. The suprapubic approach is indicated in a patient whose urethra is not competent to drain urine, such as in a patient with perineal trauma or urethral surgery.

■ TRANSURETHRAL CATHETERS

Transurethral catheters come in single-, double-, or triple-lumen varieties. Their general shapes are shown in Figure 30–5.

Single-lumen tubes are used for sterile sample collection or acute relief of pressure. They are not meant to remain within the bladder for a long period of time. They include straight Robinson tubes (often called red Robinson tubes) and coudé tubes, which have a curved tip to facilitate passage through tight urethral obstructions.

Double-lumen tubes are the standard Foley catheters that allow urine drainage through the larger of the lumens. The smaller of the lumens leads to an intravesicular balloon that is filled with air or saline. This serves to anchor the tube within the bladder.

Triple-lumen catheters allow retrograde irrigation of the bladder to dilute active bleeding after urologic surgery. Each lumen is smaller in a triple-lumen catheter compared with a double-lumen tube. If large amounts of clots or sediment must be drained, a double-lumen tube may be preferable.

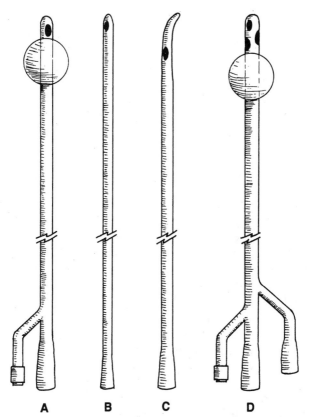

Figure 30–5 □ Urethral catheters. *A*, Foley catheter. *B*, Straight (Robinson) catheter. *C*, Coudé catheter. *D*, Three-way irrigation catheter. (From Marshall SA, Ruedy J: On Call: Principles and Protocols, 2nd ed. Philadelphia, WB Saunders Co, 1993, p 194.)

Indwelling catheters may also have stents passed through them that lead to individual ureters. These ureteral stents are placed cystoscopically or intraoperatively.

■ SUPRAPUBIC TUBES

Suprapubic tubes are placed in settings of urethral trauma or surgery or in any other case in which urethral drainage is undesirable. Placement is under local anesthesia by the Seldinger technique. Specific kits are available. Once in place, they may remain long term but are subject to the same complications as transurethral catheters. Additional complications include misplacement of the tube into the abdominal cavity, entry site infection, and vesiculocutaneous fistula formation.

Indications

1. Collection of accurate urine output data
2. Inability to spontaneously void
   Relief of acute distention
   Ongoing drainage
3. Collection of sterile urine, if a clean-catch specimen is inadequate
4. Maintenance of a lumen during the healing process after urethral trauma or surgery
5. Immobilized or incontinent patients

Complications of Urinary Drainage Tubes

1. Infection, especially with indwelling catheters of >3 days' duration
2. Misplacement of a catheter. Occasionally, false lumens may be created during the placement of a nonpliable tube.
3. Bladder or urethral trauma

Problems with Urinary Drainage Tubes

1. Blocked urethral catheter
2. Inability to place or replace catheter
3. Gross hematuria

■ BLOCKED URETHRAL CATHETER

Phone Call

Questions

1. **Why was the urinary drainage tube inserted?**
2. **How long ago was the tube inserted?**
3. **How long has the catheter been blocked?**
4. **Does the patient have suprapubic pain?**
   Differentiate whether this may be due to acute bladder distention or to postoperative pain.
5. **Has the patient undergone a surgical procedure, and if so, how long ago?**
6. **Are there any other symptoms?**
7. **Are there any changes in vital signs?**

Orders

Have a catheter insertion tray and sterile gloves available at the bedside.

If not already done, have the bedside caregiver flush the catheter gently with 30 to 40 ml sterile saline. If the patient is newly postoperative from a urologic procedure involving the bladder, prostate, or urethra, do this irrigation yourself. Clear this with the resident first.

Degree of Urgency

Patients with acute bladder distention with symptoms of pain must be seen immediately. Likewise, if there is a significant change in vital signs or symptoms, the patient must be evaluated immediately. If the patient is stable and without symptoms of acute pain or distention, the evaluation may wait for an hour or two.

Elevator Thoughts

What causes blockage of urinary catheters?
1. Blood clots
    - Postoperatively
        Early active bleeding is generally brisk, especially after transurethral resection of prostate procedures. This is treated by intraoperative placement of a triple-lumen catheter and bladder irrigation. This generally resolves within 24 to 48 hours.
    - Acute bladder trauma
        This is due to a misplaced tube or to attempted removal of the catheter before deflating the balloon.
2. Urinary sediment
    - Urinary tract infection
    - Lysis of bladder tumor
    - Urolithiasis
3. Catheter dysfunction, including clamped or kinked catheter
4. Improper placement, including urethral trauma or false passage formation

Major Threat to Life

- Bladder rupture
    This is preceded by very painful symptoms of increased bladder pressure in those patients who can identify and communicate these symptoms. Be careful with patients who are paraplegic or unconscious.
- Progressive renal failure
    This is secondary to long-term obstruction.

Bedside

Quick Look Test

Most patients will appear comfortable. If there are symptoms of acute distention, the patient will be in distress.

Airway and Vital Signs

Pain may be associated with tachypnea or tachycardia.

Selective History and Chart Review

- Review why the urinary drainage tube was placed and whether it is still necessary.
- Look for underlying causes (see Elevator Thoughts).

Selective Physical Examination

GU: Palpate the abdomen for bladder distention.

Tubes: Confirm that there are no kinks in or clamps on the tubing.

Confirm that the drainage bag is not full.

Examine the tubing for evidence of blood or sediment.

Additional tests:

1. UA   Rule out infection.

Management

1. Reattempt to flush the catheter.
   - Obtain a sterile irrigation tray or catheter insertion kit.
   - Wear sterile gloves.
   - Have someone immobilize the distal end of the catheter as you clean it with chlorhexidine or iodine.
   - Disconnect the catheter from the drainage bag, and have your assistant hold the bag end of the connection up, to maintain sterility.
   - Using a catheter tip syringe, aspirate vigorously, and remove any resultant clots or debris.
   - Gently flush the catheter with 30 to 40 ml sterile saline.
   - Repeat previous two steps if not initially successful.
   - Reconnect the catheter to the bag.
2. If not successful in restoring adequate drainage, replace the existing catheter with a new one.
   - Confirm that the patient still requires a catheter.
   - If the patient is freshly postoperative from a urologic procedure, check first with the resident.
   - If bladder irrigation will be required, replace the tube with a triple-lumen catheter. Otherwise, simply replacing the tube with a larger catheter may be sufficient.

■ INABILITY TO PLACE CATHETER

Phone Call

Questions

1. Why was the urinary drainage tube ordered?
2. Has one been in place previously?

3. **Does the patient have suprapubic pain?**
4. **How many attempts have been made to place the new catheter?**
5. **Has the patient undergone a surgical procedure, and if so, how long ago was it performed?**
6. **Are there any other symptoms?**
7. **Are there any changes in vital signs?**

Orders

Have a catheter insertion tray and sterile gloves available at the bedside.

Degree of Urgency

Patients with acute bladder distention with symptoms of pain must be seen immediately. Likewise, if there is a significant change in vital signs or symptoms, the patient must be evaluated immediately. If the patient is stable and without symptoms of acute pain or distention, the evaluation may wait for an hour or two.

Elevator Thoughts

What causes the inability to pass a catheter?
1. Urethral edema
   - Multiple insertion attempts
   - Urethral infection
   - Inadvertent removal of the old catheter without first deflating the balloon
2. Urethral obstruction
   - Benign prostatic hypertrophy
   - Carcinoma of the prostate
   - Urethral stricture
   - Other anatomic abnormality (diverticulum and false lumen)

Major Threat to Life

- Bladder rupture
  This is preceded by very painful symptoms of increased bladder pressure in those patients who can identify and communicate these symptoms. Be careful with those patients who are paraplegic or unconscious.
- Progressive renal failure
  This is secondary to long-term obstruction.

Bedside

Quick Look Test

Most patients will appear comfortable. If there are symptoms of acute distention, the patient will be in distress.

Airway and Vital Signs

Pain may be associated with tachypnea or tachycardia.

Selective History and Chart Review

- Review why the urinary drainage tube was ordered and whether it is still necessary.
- Is there a history of previous attempts to place a catheter?
- Is there a history of traumatic removal of a catheter?
- Is there evidence of obstruction? (see Elevator Thoughts)
    Look for a history of benign prostatic hypertrophy, carcinoma of the prostate, or anatomic abnormalities.

Selective Physical Examination

GU: Palpate the abdomen for bladder distention.

Management

1. Attempt to place the catheter.
2. If urethral swelling is the problem, consider using a tube with smaller diameter.
3. If obstruction is the problem, consider using a coudé catheter.
4. If the catheter cannot be placed by the transurethral approach, consider the suprapubic approach.
    Consult with your urology colleagues before attempting this procedure. They may have other transurethral options to try.

■ GROSS HEMATURIA

Hematuria is covered in Chapter 31.

Remember

1. Transurethral catheters in immediately postoperative urology patients require very gentle care; contact your resident before flushing, manipulating, or replacing them.
2. In patients who have perineal trauma, do not place a transurethral tube until the patency of the urethra is demonstrated with a retrograde contrast urethrogram.

Gastrointestinal Decompression Tubes

Adynamic ileus or intestinal obstruction can lead to accumulation of gases and liquids in the GI tract. Unless these are removed, a significant aspiration risk is present.

Indications

1. Adynamic ileus
2. Small-bowel or gastric outlet obstruction
3. Severe burns or polytrauma
4. After intestinal surgery with anastomosis
5. Gastric lavage for bleeding or poison ingestion

Placement

1. **Have all equipment ready.** You will need the following:
   - 16–18-Fr NG tube
   - Lubricant jelly
     K-Y jelly is sufficient, but lidocaine jelly may be used
   - Topical nasal vasoconstrictors such as phenylephrine or cocaine (optional)
   - Topical anesthetic such as benzocaine (Hurricaine spray) (optional)
   - Emesis basin
   - Catheter tip syringe
   - Suction apparatus (i.e., wall suction or portable apparatus) and tonsil tip suction tube
   - Gloves and eye protection
   - A small cup with water, with a straw for the patient to sip through
   - Benzoin and tape to secure the tube, once placed
2. **Prepare the patient.**
   - Explain the procedure.
   - Explain the risks and the alternatives.
   - Answer any questions.
   - Position the patient upright or decubitus, with the neck flexed.
3. **Estimate the tube length.**
   Measure the distance from the patient's ear to the umbilicus. This is a good estimate of the needed length.
4. **Premedicate the patient.**
   - Choose a nostril; select the most patent one.
   - Spray topical anesthetic to the back of the throat.
   - Apply vasoconstrictor and topical anesthetic to the nasal mucosa.
   - Apply lubricating jelly liberally to the tip of the tube and along the length of the tube.
5. **Have the suction apparatus turned on with the tonsil tip attached.**
6. **Insert the tube.**
   - With the patient's neck flexed (make sure there is no cervical spine injury), insert the tube into the nostril.
   - Aim straight back toward the occiput.
   - Apply firm constant pressure to the tube.

- Have the patient hold the cup of water; have the patient take small sips and swallow as you apply pressure (Fig. 30–6).
- Continue to advance the tube to the desired length.
- Anticipate some gagging during placement. This may be decreased by spraying additional topical anesthetic to the back of the throat.

7. **If the tube does not pass easily, do the following:**
   - If the tube coils in the mouth or esophagus, chill the tube in some ice to stiffen it.
   - If the tube does not pass at all, try the other nostril.
   - If, during advancement, the patient begins to cough, withdraw immediately. This indicates misplacement into the lung.

8. **Once the tube is advanced, do the following:**
   - Hold it firmly in place, close to the nostril, which often requires steadying your hand against the patient's nose.
   - Attach the catheter tip syringe to the tube and inject 30 to 60 ml of air into the tube. Listen over the epigastrium for the rumbling of the air into the stomach (Fig. 30–7).

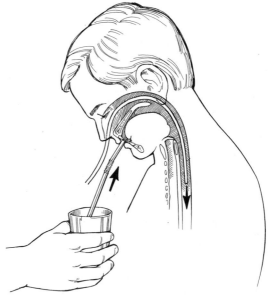

Figure 30–6 □ Position of patient while inserting a nasogastric tube. (From Rakel RR: Saunders Manual of Medical Practice. Philadelphia, WB Saunders Co, 1996, p 314.)

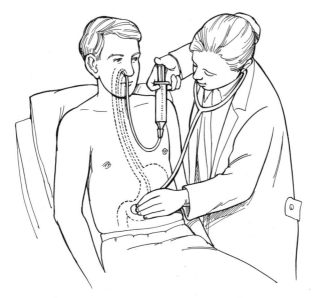

Figure 30–7 □ Technique for confirming nasogastric tube placement. (From Rakel RR: Saunders Manual of Medical Practice. Philadelphia, WB Saunders Co, 1996, p 314.)

- Aspirate back on the syringe to confirm the efflux of gastric fluid; pH should be <5.
- Secure the tube to the nose with benzoin and tape. Avoid taping the tube in such a way that pressure is applied to the nostril. This is a common cause of necrosis of the naris.
- Be sure to tape the tube down to a second site, such as the patient's forehead or shoulder, so that inadvertent traction on the tube does not dislodge it.
- Radiographic confirmation of the placement is often necessary. NG tubes have radio-opaque marker tape incorporated into their design so that they are visible on routine kidneys, ureter, and bladder (KUB) x-ray.
- Once radiographic evidence of adequate placement is available, the tube may be used for feeding. The tube may be placed to suction without radiographic verification.
- You may want to place a mark on the tube near the nose, to mark proper placement. A reasonable placement occurs if two lines are visible out of the nose, and the position at the nose is between the second and third lines.

9. **If duodenal placement is desired, do the following:**
   - Consider use of a weighted tube.

- Insert an additional 20 to 40 cm of length.
- Place the patient onto the right side for 8 to 12 hours.
- Fluid aspirates should have a pH of >7.
- Confirm placement by KUB x-ray.

10. **Routine care is as follows:**
    - Record suction output volume and character.
    - If the output is a large volume, consider replacement of NG output, as follows: 0.5 to 1 ml/ml of output with LR or 0.5 NS + 15 mEq KCl/L; replace each shift.
    - If the tube becomes blocked, attempt to irrigate it with 30 to 40 ml of saline. If the block does not resolve, reposition the tube. Check with the nursing staff to see if there are protocols regarding routine irrigation of NG tubes. If not, have the tube routinely irrigated at least every shift and as needed with 30 to 40 ml of NS.
    - Examine routine radiographs for placement of the tube, if possible.
    - An indwelling NG tube is often very uncomfortable. Make sure the patient has some throat lozenges at the bedside for use as needed.

Complications of Nasogastric Tubes

1. Aspiration pneumonia
2. Trauma to nasal mucosa or external nasal skin
3. Trauma to lung or esophagus
4. Sinusitis
   Indwelling catheters can cause trauma and swelling around sinus orifices, leading to acute sinusitis. Think of this as a possible cause of fever in a patient with an NG tube.

Problems with Nasogastric Tubes

1. Blocked tube
2. Dislodged tube

■ BLOCKED NASOGASTRIC TUBE

Phone Call

Questions

1. Why was the nasogastric tube inserted?
2. How long ago was the tube inserted?
3. What type of tube is in place?
4. How long has the tube been blocked?
5. Has the patient undergone a surgical procedure, and if so, how long ago was it performed?
6. Are there any other symptoms?
7. Are there any changes in vital signs?

Orders

Have a 60-ml catheter tip syringe, sterile NS, an emesis basin, gloves, and goggles at the bedside.

Degree of Urgency

Evaluating a patient with a nonfunctioning NG tube may be delayed for several hours if there are more urgent issues. If there is a significant change in vital signs or symptoms, the patient must be evaluated immediately.

Elevator Thoughts

What causes blockage of a nasogastric tube?
1. Debris within the tube lumen
    This includes food or medications. This generally results from failure to irrigate the tube routinely.
2. Clotted blood
3. Kinked tube
    A tube that is folded within the esophagus will appear clogged.

Major Threat to Life

- Aspiration pneumonia
    A nonfunctioning tube does not adequately empty the stomach, thus increasing the risk of aspiration of gastric contents.

Bedside

Quick Look Test

Nausea and vomiting may be present.

Airway and Vital Signs

Tachypnea with or without fever may indicate aspiration.

Management

1. Flush the tube with 30 to 40 ml sterile saline. Listen over the epigastrium to hear if the fluid is audible entering the stomach.
2. Remove the tape and reposition the tube a few centimeters in or out. Do not replace a guide wire into the tube for repositioning. This could cause perforation of the esophagus or the stomach.
3. If the above maneuvers are not effective in restoring function, replace the tube. The same tube may be used if it is

patent, or use a new one. Make sure that the indication for the tube still exists.

4. Confirm that the tube is being flushed routinely.

■ DISLODGED NASOGASTRIC TUBE

Phone Call

Questions

1. Why was the nasogastric tube inserted?
2. How long ago was the tube inserted?
3. What type of tube is in place?
4. Has the patient undergone a surgical procedure, and if so, how long ago was it performed?
5. Are there any other symptoms?
6. Are there any changes in vital signs?

Degree of Urgency

Evaluating a patient with a misplaced NG tube may be delayed for several hours if there are more urgent issues. If there is a significant change in vital signs or symptoms, the patient must be evaluated immediately.

Elevator Thoughts

What causes a dislodged nasogastric tube?
1. Inadvertent traction
   This may be caused accidentally by the medical staff or by a confused or uncooperative patient.
2. Failure to secure the tube appropriately

Major Threat to Life

- Aspiration pneumonia
  A nonfunctioning tube does not adequately empty the stomach, thus increasing the risk of aspiration of gastric contents.
- Hypoglycemia
  If the tube is used for feeding, be sure to arrange a way to deliver calories, especially in diabetic patients who have had their insulin administered.

Bedside

Quick Look Test

Nausea and vomiting may be present.

Airway and Vital Signs

Tachypnea with or without fever may indicate aspiration.

Management

1. Inspect the tube. Has the tube been marked to indicate proper placement? Has the tube moved from that position?
2. Flush the tube with 30 to 40 ml sterile saline. Listen over the epigastrium to hear if the fluid is audible entering the stomach.
3. Remove the tape and reposition the tube a few centimeters in or out. Do not replace a guide wire into the tube for repositioning. This could cause perforation of the esophagus or stomach.
4. If the above maneuvers are not effective in restoring function, replace the tube. The same tube may be used if it is patent, or use a new one. Make sure that the indication for the tube still exists.
5. Confirm that the tube is being routinely flushed.

Remember

1. NG tubes may be used for GI decompression or for enteral feeding. Generally, if a feeding tube is used, it is of smaller diameter and is made of softer material. Some feeding tubes are so flexible they require a guide wire for adequate placement.
2. Longer tubes with distal mercury weights are available for decompression of more distal aspects of the small bowel. These may take several days to pass into the desired region of the small bowel.
3. If a gastrostomy or a jejunostomy tube becomes dislodged, it may be safely replaced if the enterocutaneous tract is well healed, i.e., it is >6 weeks since the placement. Placement must take place within 12 to 24 hours of dislodgment and may be confirmed radiographically by injection of a small volume of water-soluble contrast material into the tube during the x-ray. More recently placed tubes must be reinserted with great care so as to not disturb the fistulizing tract. Use of a guide wire or repeat surgery may be necessary.

Biliary Drainage Tubes (T-Tubes)

T-tubes are placed intraoperatively into the common bile duct after reconstruction or exploration of the duct. They are also placed after procedures involving choledochoenteral anastomoses. The tube allows external drainage of bile while the bile duct heals. Seven to 10 days after a procedure, a contrast T-tube cholangiogram is performed to assess the patency of the bile duct. If it is normal, the T-tube is removed. If it is abnormal (because of stricture, retained stones, or occlusions), the T-tube is left in place. Normal outputs range from 300 to 750 ml/day.

Problems with Biliary Drainage Tubes

1. Blockage of the tube, i.e., loss of spontaneous flow
2. Dislodged tube

■ BLOCKED T-TUBE

Phone Call

Questions

1. **How long has the tube been blocked?**
2. **Has the tube been dislodged?**
3. **What was the surgical procedure, and how long ago was it performed?**
4. **What had the normal output been?**
5. **Are there any other symptoms?**
6. **Are there any changes in vital signs?**

Orders

Have a pair of sterile gloves, skin preparation supplies, and clean dressing materials available at the bedside.

Degree of Urgency

If the T-tube has not been displaced, the patient may be evaluated in 1 to 2 hours. If there is a significant change in vital signs or symptoms, the patient must be evaluated immediately.

Elevator Thoughts

What causes blockage of T-tubes?
1. Debris within the tube
2. Blood clots
3. Failure to irrigate the tube routinely
4. Inadvertent clamping

Major Threat to Life
- Sepsis from cholangitis
- Abscess formation

Bedside

Quick Look Test

Patients will tend to look well, unless their underlying condition is serious.

Airway and Vital Signs

No alteration is anticipated with blockage of T-tubes.

Management

1. Confirm that the tubing is not clamped or kinked, and confirm that the bag is not full.
2. Aspirate and irrigate the tubing as follows:
   - Ask an assistant to hold the distal end of the T-tube close to the connection with the drainage bag.
   - Using sterile technique, wearing sterile gloves, clean the connection site with chlorhexidine.
   - Disconnect the tubing from the drainage bag. Take care to maintain the sterility of both ends.
   - Using a 5-ml syringe, aspirate gently.
   - If aspiration is insufficient to dislodge the obstruction, fill a second 5-ml syringe with sterile saline and irrigate the tube gently.
3. If successful in dislodging the occlusion, reconnect the tube with the drainage bag.
4. If the aspiration and irrigation is not successful
   - Do not attempt to reirrigate.
   - Notify your resident.
   - Consider a contrast T-tube cholangiogram. If an intraluminal obstruction is noted in the tube, this often may be removed using a Fogarty balloon catheter.
   - Manipulation of the tube should be done only by someone familiar with the tube. For example, many operators remove the back wall of the top of the T to facilitate removal of the tube. This may make passage of a Fogarty catheter a potentially dangerous procedure.

■ DISLODGED T-TUBE

Phone Call

Questions

1. How long has the tube been dislodged?
2. What was the surgical procedure, and how long ago was it performed?

3. **What had the normal output been?**
4. **Are there any other symptoms?**
5. **Are there any changes in vital signs?**

Orders

Have sterile gloves, skin preparation supplies, and clean dressing materials available at the bedside.

Degree of Urgency

A patient with a dislodged T-tube needs to be evaluated immediately. Likewise, if there is a significant change in vital signs or symptoms, the patient must be evaluated immediately.

Elevator Thoughts

What causes a dislodged T-tube?
1. Failure to adequately secure the tube
2. Inadvertent traction on the tube
   - Accidentally by the medical staff
   - Accidentally by a confused or an uncooperative patient

Major Threat to Life

- Sepsis from cholangitis
- Abscess formation

Bedside

Quick Look Test

Patients will tend to look well, unless their underlying condition is serious.

Airway and Vital Signs

No alteration is anticipated with a dislodged T-tube.

Management

1. A T-tube cholangiogram should be obtained. If the cholangiogram demonstrates a dislodged tube in a newly postoperative patient, repeat surgery may be required. Contact your resident.
2. If the tract is fairly well healed and T-tube drainage is still required, interventional radiology can often place the T-tube or a similar drainage tube back into the common bile duct without subjecting the patient to another operation.
3. Check with your resident; occasionally, the T-tube may simply be left out.

Wound Drainage Tubes (Penrose, Jackson-Pratt, Blake, and Davol)

These drains are placed intraoperatively to facilitate drainage of fluids from a surgical site. This may include abscess material, serosanguineous fluid, or fluid resulting from anastomotic insufficiency. The output and character of the fluid draining from the wound should be monitored. The drains themselves usually exit from a site distal to the incision, but occasionally they exit through the incision. Removal of these drains is dependent on the output. Changes in output may indicate new infection, significant postoperative bleeding, or anastomotic leak. There are several types, as follows:

Penrose: This is a flat rubber tube of graded sizes that simply acts to keep a drainage tract open.

Closed suction: These include Jackson-Pratt, Blake, and Davol drains. These are placed in large spaces deep within a cavity. Drainage of these spaces postoperatively decreases the risk of abscess formation and seroma and facilitates healing.

Problems with Wound Drainage Tubes

1. Blockage of a drain
2. Dislodged drain

■ BLOCKED WOUND DRAINAGE TUBE

Phone Call

Questions

1. **What type of drain is in place?**
2. **How long has the drain been blocked?**
3. **Has the drain been dislodged?**
4. **What was the surgical procedure, and how long ago was it performed?**
5. **What has the normal output been?**
6. **Are there any other symptoms?**
7. **Are there any changes in vital signs?**

Orders

Have sterile gloves, skin preparation supplies, and clean dressing materials available at the bedside.

Degree of Urgency

If there is a significant change in vital signs or symptoms, the patient must be evaluated immediately.

Elevator Thoughts

What causes blockage of wound drains?
1. Debris within the tube
2. Blood clots

Major Threat to Life

- Sepsis
- Abscess formation

Bedside

Quick Look Test

Patients will tend to look well, unless their underlying condition is serious.

Airway and Vital Signs

No alteration is anticipated with blockage of wound drains.

Management

1. Confirm that the wound drain is still necessary.
2. Attempt to milk debris or clots into the collection chamber.
3. Do not attempt to reposition the drain, except to remove it if necessary. Advancement of the drain will introduce bacterial contamination into the surgical bed.
4. If these maneuvers are not sufficient to dislodge an obstruction, contact your resident to see if it is a reasonable time to remove the drain.

■ DISLODGED WOUND DRAINAGE TUBE

Phone Call

Questions

1. What type of drain is in place?
2. How long has the drain been dislodged?
3. What was the surgical procedure, and how long ago was it performed?
4. What has the normal output been?
5. Are there any other symptoms?
6. Are there any changes in vital signs?

Orders

Have sterile gloves, skin preparation supplies, and clean dressing materials available at the bedside.

Degree of Urgency

If there is a significant change in vital signs or symptoms, the patient must be evaluated immediately.

Elevator Thoughts

What causes a dislodged wound drain?
1. Failure to adequately secure the tube
2. Inadvertent traction on the tube
   - Accidentally by the medical staff
   - Accidentally by a confused or an uncooperative patient.

Major Threat to Life

- Sepsis
- Abscess formation

Bedside

Quick Look Test

Patients will tend to look well, unless their underlying condition is serious.

Airway and Vital Signs

No alteration is anticipated with a dislodged wound drain.

Management

1. Confirm that the wound drain is still necessary.
2. Do not attempt to reposition the drain, except to remove it if necessary. Advancement of the drain will introduce bacterial contamination into the surgical bed.
3. Secure the drain in its present position with silk suture.
4. Contact your resident to see if it is a reasonable time to remove the drain.

31

URINE OUTPUT CHANGES

Changes in urine output (UO) encompass a variety of complaints, the most common being a decrease in UO in a postoperative patient because of changes in intravascular volume. Also considered in this chapter are other causes of decreased UO, increased UO, and blood in the urine. Components of these evaluations are also covered in other chapters where indicated. The function of the kidney may be divided into two major categories, i.e., fluid management and solute management.

Decreased Urine Output

UO is considered one of the three major indicators of end-organ perfusion (remember from Chapter 12: UO, mental status, and skin temperature). In postoperative patients, a decreased UO must be considered a decrease in intravascular volume until proved otherwise because of the frequency of this occurrence and because of the seriousness of underestimating fluid resuscitation in a sick patient. Remember that the postoperative or gravely ill patient has undergone neuroendocrine changes that help to retain fluid and that third spacing of intravascular fluid is to be expected.

■ PHONE CALL

Questions

1. **How is the UO being measured?**
   Indwelling urinary catheters give the most reliable estimates of hourly output but are not always clinically appropriate. Routine intake and output (I/O) measurements without catheters can overestimate or underestimate UO volumes by a factor of close to 100%.
2. **What is the current trend, what is the trend over the last 2 to 3 hours, and what is it over the last 24 hours?**
   Oliguria is defined as <400 ml/day (<20 ml/hr). Anuria is defined as <50 ml/day. Great variances in hourly output suggest collection errors or postrenal obstruction.
3. **Have there been recent changes in laboratory studies**

including those for potassium, creatinine, blood urea nitrogen (BUN), and urinalysis (UA).
4. **Has the patient undergone a surgical procedure, and if so, how long ago was it performed?**
    Pay special attention to surgeries involving bladder, ureters, or kidneys, including renal transplants.
5. **Are there any other symptoms, including abdominal pain, fever, or dysuria?**
6. **Are there any changes in vital signs?**

Orders

1. If an indwelling urinary catheter (Foley) is present, it may be flushed gently with 20 to 30 ml normal saline (NS) to dislodge sediment or clots. Check with the chief resident or the attending physician before flushing a catheter in place after surgery on the bladder or urinary tract.
2. Take steps to evaluate the hydration status of the patient. Repeat taking the vital signs and order orthostatic blood pressure (BP) measurements.
3. If the patient is immediately postoperative, and fluid shifts out of the intravascular space are clinically apparent, a fluid bolus of 500 ml crystalloid is appropriate; note that the fluid status of a patient must be evaluated (see Chapter 12).

Degree of Urgency

If the patient is stable and comfortable, 30 to 60 minutes is appropriate. If there is a significant change in vital signs or symptoms, the patient must be evaluated immediately.

■ ELEVATOR THOUGHTS

What are the causes of decreased UO?

In the postoperative patient, intravascular fluid deficit is such a common cause of decreased UO that there is a tendency to believe that this is always the case. The fluid status should be quickly assessed, but do not forget to evaluate for other causes of oliguria. Decreased UO may be conveniently divided into three categories. Prerenal causes of oliguria are often due to poor kidney perfusion. Renal causes of oliguria include the major renal pathologies and result in poor kidney function (i.e., urine formation). Postrenal causes of oliguria are often due to external forces that block the flow of urine anywhere along the tract from the kidney to the outside world. These are listed in Table 31–1.

Remember that renal and prolonged prerenal and postrenal causes of oliguria can also lead to azotemia.

Table 31–1 □ COMMON CAUSES OF OLIGURIA

Prerenal	Renal	Postrenal
Volume depletion	Glomerular nephritides	Ureteral obstruction (must be bilateral)
Third spacing	Acute glomerulonephritis	Retroperitoneal mass
Hemorrhage	Vasculitis	Sloughed papillae
Gastrointestinal losses	Malignant hypertensive nephropathy	Strictures/valves
Renal losses	Renal thrombosis	Stones, clots
Poor cardiac output	Tubular interstitial	Bladder neck obstruction
Congestive heart failure	Pyelonephritis	Prostatic hypertrophy
Tamponade	Hypercalcemia	Tumor
Myocardial infarction	Multiple myeloma	Sphincter spasm
Pulmonary embolus	Acute interstitial nephritis	Strictures/valves
Shock/sepsis	Acute tubular necrosis	Urethral obstruction
Hepatorenal syndrome	Postischemic injury	Strictures/valves
	Prolonged vasopressor use	Bladder rupture
	Nephrotoxic agents	Blocked catheter
	Antibiotics	
	Contrast dye	
	Anesthetics	
	Nonsteroidal anti-inflammatory drugs	
	Chemotherapeutic agents	
	Vascular problems	
	Emboli	
	Renal vessel thrombosis	

■ MAJOR THREAT TO LIFE

- Hypotension and shock
- Acute renal failure
   This may require dialysis for treatment.
- Hyperkalemia

■ BEDSIDE

Quick Look Test

   Physical obstruction may be associated with abdominal discomfort, agitation, and sensation of needing to urinate. A serious deterioration of clinical status including neurologic changes or metabolic derangements may indicate hypotension or acute renal failure.

Airway and Vital Signs

   Look for evidence of dehydration. Resting tachycardia or postural changes in pulse rate (a drop of 15 beats/min) or BP (a drop in systolic BP [SBP] of 15 mm Hg or any fall in diastolic BP) indicate decreased intravascular volume. This is most likely due to underresuscitation, but be mindful of early sepsis or cardiogenic shock.

Initial Management

1. Support cardiac output and perfusion.
   A fluid bolus is indicated for patients who are intravascularly deplete.
2. Determine cause of decreased UO.
   Once this is determined, the management is more clear.

Selective History and Chart Review

- Is there a condition that would predispose a patient to decreased UO? (see Elevator Thoughts)
- Review trends in UO and I/Os, and review changes in weight.
- Review recent laboratory studies trends.

Selective Physical Examination

VS:	Tachycardia or postural BP changes (dehydration)
MS:	Decreased mental status (decreased perfusion)

HEENT:	Dry or sticky mucous membranes and flat neck veins (dehydration)
	Full neck veins (tamponade)
Resp:	Rales and decreased aeration (fluid overload and congestive heart failure [CHF])
Abd:	Pain and distention (obstruction of urinary tract and urinary tract infection [UTI])
GU:	Dysuria (UTI)
Skin:	Decrease in warmth or turgor, and dry axillae (dehydration)
	Itching (azotemia)
Rectal:	Enlarged prostate or mass
Tubes:	Blocked urinary catheter
Additional tests:	
1. UA:	White blood cells (WBCs) indicate UTI, high specific gravity supports dehydration, and red blood cells (RBCs) indicate UTI or urolithiasis
2. Electrolytes:	To assess for metabolic derangement, elevations in BUN, and creatinine
3. Urine Na^+:	Assessment of renal function (Table 31–2)
4. ECG:	Assess for peaked T waves, indicating hyperkalemia

■ MANAGEMENT

Prerenal

This is the most common etiology.

Fluid Deficit

1. Confirm with physical examination and laboratory studies.
2. Fluid bolus with 500 ml crystalloid; may repeat if not effective.

   If after two fluid boluses no effect is noted, reevaluate fluid status. Add invasive monitoring (central venous pressure, indwelling urinary catheter, and Swan-Ganz catheter) as necessary.
3. Monitor rehydration as needed with frequent vital signs checks and electrolyte evaluations.
4. Order daily weights and strict I/O measurements.

Normal or Increased Fluid Status

1. Rule out myocardial infarction as necessary.
2. If CHF, evaluate as directed in Chapter 28; evaluate oxygen status, and begin diuresis, as follows:

Table 31–2 □ COMPARISON OF LABORATORY FINDINGS IN VARIOUS URINE OUTPUT CHANGE CONDITIONS

| | Blood | | | Urine | | |
	Na	BUN	BUN/Cr	Output	SG	Urine Na
Prerenal	—	Incr.	>10:1	Decr.	Incr.	<40
ATN	—	Incr.	<10:1	—	<1.020	>40
SIADH	Decr.	Decr.	>50:1	Decr.	Incr.	>100
DI	Incr.	Incr.	<5:1	Incr.	Decr.	<10

Na = sodium; BUN = blood urea nitrogen; Cr = creatinine; SG = serum glucose; Incr. = increased; Decr. = decreased; ATN = acute tubular necrosis; SIADH = syndrome of inappropriate antidiuretic hormone secretion; DI = diabetes insipidus.

- **Furosemide (Lasix) 20 to 80 mg intravenously (IV) over 2 to 5 minutes.**

    The **dose may be doubled and administered every 1 hour as needed to a total dose of 400 mg** if no response is noted. Doses of >100 mg should be given slowly (<4 mg/min) to avoid ototoxicity. Also use caution when used in conjunction with aminoglycoside antibiotics.
- **Hydrochlorothiazide 25 to 50 mg orally (PO)** (a thiazide diuretic)

    or
- **Metolazone (Zaroxolyn) 5 to 10 mg PO** may be added **once or twice a day** to furosemide therapy (a loop diuretic) for more effective diuresis.

    If furosemide therapy is ineffective consider use of
- **Ethacrynic acid (Edecrin) 50 mg IV every hour × 2 doses**

    or
- **Bumetanide (Bumex) 1 to 10 mg IV over 1 to 2 minutes.**

3. Monitor diuresis as needed with frequent checks of vital signs and evaluations of electrolytes.

    Supplemental K^+ may be necessary with massive or prolonged diuresis.

Postrenal

This is most likely if UO is absent or is fluctuating widely.

1. Place a urinary catheter if one is not already in place.

    Note the postvoid residual. If the residual volume is >400 ml and the discomfort is relieved, leave the catheter in place and reassess in 1 to 2 days. This will give the distended bladder muscles a chance to recover function. Always consider subacute bacterial endocarditis prophylaxis when inserting a urinary catheter in a patient with a cardiac murmur. Current recommendations include treatment of patients with valvular abnormalities such as mitral valve prolapse with a persistent systolic murmur. Acceptable antibiotics include **ampicillin 2 g intramuscularly (IM)** or **vancomycin 1 g IV over 1 hour, plus gentamicin 1.5 mg/kg IM** or **IV 30 minutes before a urinary procedure and repeat in 8 hours.**

2. If a urinary catheter is already in place, flush with 20 to 30 ml sterile NS.

    This must be done with **extreme** caution in the setting of recent bladder or kidney surgery. If the catheter will not flush, replace with a new catheter.

3. Look for nonbladder causes of postrenal oliguria such as stones or mass externally obstructing the urinary tract.

4. Order daily weights and strict I/O measurements.

Renal

1. Confirm with physical examination and laboratory studies.
2. Consult specialists as necessary.
3. Order daily weights and strict I/O measurements.
4. Manage associated problems.
   a. **Hyperkalemia**

   Limit exogenous K^+. Place on continuous cardiac monitoring. Treat severe hyperkalemia as outlined in Chapter 12.

   - **Calcium gluconate 5 to 10 ml of a 10% solution IV over 2 minutes.**

     This is symptomatic relief only to stabilize neuromuscular and cardiac effects of hyperkalemia and does not alter the concentration of potassium in the serum. Its effects last only 1 hour.

   - **50% dextrose in water, 50 ml IV followed by regular insulin 5 to 10 U,** effects a shift of the extracellular potassium to intracellular. Its effects last 1 to 2 hours.

   - **Sodium bicarbonate 1 ampule (44.6 mmol) IV** also effects a shift of potassium from the extracellular to the intracellular space.

     The glucose/insulin/bicarbonate therapies, as follows, may be combined in an IV bag.

   - **1000 ml 10% dextrose in water + 3 ampules of sodium bicarbonate + 20 U regular insulin to run at 75 ml/hr** until the desired K^+ level is reached.

   - **Sodium polystyrene sulfonate (Kayexalate) 15 to 30 g (4–8 tsp) in 50 to 100 ml of 20% sorbitol PO every 3 to 4 hours or in 200 ml 20% sorbitol of 20% dextrose in water rectally (PR) by retention enema for 30 to 60 minutes every 4 hours.**

     This is chelation therapy and is the only treatment listed here that will remove potassium from the body. In the absence of functioning kidneys, the only other option is hemodialysis, which can remove up to 25 to 30 mEq/hr.

   b. **Metabolic acidosis**

   Evaluate with arterial blood gas and serum bicarbonate levels ($[HCO_3^-]$) and treat as necessary (see Chapter 12), as follows:

Mild	pH = 7.30 to 7.35
Moderate	pH = 7.20 to 7.29
Severe	pH = <7.20

   Mild and moderate acidosis generally requires no specific therapy short of reversal of the underlying cause. Severe acidosis that results in decreased mental status, hyperventilation, cardiac abnormalities, and hypotension is treated with sodium bicarbonate as determined by the following formula:

Bicarbonate required (in mmol) =
$$(\text{wt in kg}) (0.4) (\text{desired } [HCO_3^-]) - (\text{measured } [HCO_3^-])$$

Replace bicarbonate slowly, over 24 hours; i.e., one-half to one-third of the deficit in the first 6 to 12 hours with the remaining deficit replaced in the remaining 12 to 18 hours. The usual desired $[HCO_3^-]$ is generally 15. Remember that the goal of bicarbonate therapy is not to normalize the pH but rather to reverse the physiologic effects of acidosis. This usually occurs when the pH is at >7.20. Remember also that severe acidosis is also associated with hyperkalemia, as intracellular K^+ is exchanged with extracellular hydrogen ions.

c. **Fluid overload**

Treat with diuretics as listed above. If the kidneys are not sufficiently excreting free water despite diuretic therapy, there are only two ways to decrease the total body water:

1. Decrease the input by restricting oral and IV intake of fluid to minimums
2. Fluid reduction by dialysis

Make sure the patient is oxygenating well. Treat symptoms of CHF as outlined in Chapter 28.

- Sit the patient up to allow maximum aeration of the lungs.
- **Morphine sulfate (MSO_4) 2 to 4 mg IV every 5 to 10 minutes up to 10 to 12 mg** will pool the blood in the splanchnic circulation and decrease pulmonary edema.

   Hold MSO_4 treatment if symptoms of decreased respiratory drive or hypotension are apparent. Reverse the effects of MSO_4 as necessary with **naloxone hydrochloride 0.2 to 2.0 mg IV, IM, or subcutaneously (SC) to a total of 10 mg.** Note that the half-life of naloxone effect is shorter than that of most narcotics and that repeat doses may be necessary.
- **Nitroglycerin ointment 2.5 to 5.0 cm topically every 4 hours.**

   Nitroglycerin tablets 0.3 to 0.6 µg sublingually (SL) every 5 minutes or nitroglycerin spray 1 puff every 15 minutes may be used if ointment is not available. Hold nitroglycerin for SBP of <90 mm Hg. Adequate function of nitroglycerin is generally confirmed by a headache that usually responds to **acetaminophen (Tylenol and others) 350 to 1000**

mg PO every 4 hours as needed. Diuretic therapy as outlined above.

   d. **Uremia**

This is manifest by elevated BUN with symptoms of decreased mental status, pericarditis, or seizures. It is treated with hemodialysis.

5. Stop any nephrotoxic medications (nonsteroidal anti-inflammatory drugs and aminoglycosides), and adjust the doses of renally excreted medications.
6. Limit magnesium- and aluminum-containing medications.
7. Determine if the patient requires dialysis. The following are indications for dialysis:

   ▪ Fluid overload unresponsive to diuretics and resulting in CHF or edema
   ▪ Hyperkalemia, severe and symptomatic, with serum K^+ at 6 to 8 mmol/L
   ▪ Metabolic acidosis, severe, acute, and symptomatic, pH of <7.20
   ▪ Uremia, severe with symptoms of decreased mental status, pericarditis, or seizure, and BUN at >35 mmol/L

   A nephrologist should be consulted to confirm the need for dialysis and to arrange the therapy.

▪ SPECIAL SURGICAL CONSIDERATIONS

Preoperative Considerations

A serious decrease in UO in a preoperative patient is an indication of a serious problem and may require changing plans for a scheduled procedure.

Postoperative Considerations

1. The most common cause in immediately postoperative patients is insufficient resuscitation with intravascular volume deficit.
2. Expect low UO in patients with prolonged procedures.

   Postoperative IV fluid rates should routinely be at 100 to 150 ml/hr until adequate fluid hydration is ensured and UO is normal.
3. The syndrome of inappropriate antidiuretic hormone (SIADH) secretion is the condition of high ADH secretion in the absence of the normal stimulus of high serum osmolarity.

   It is generally considered pathologic, but it is common after significant surgical procedures or major stresses. It is diagnosed as outlined in Table 31–2 and treated initially with maintenance of intravascular volume, and then with fluid restriction until physiologic diuresis ensues.

Remember

1. Azotemia may present with oliguria, but it may also have normal or increased UO.
2. Review all medications in oliguric patients, and adjust doses as necessary.

Increased Urine Output

■ PHONE CALL

Questions

1. **How is the urine output measured?**
   Indwelling urinary catheters give the most reliable estimates of hourly output but are not always clinically appropriate. Routine I/O measurements without catheters can overestimate or underestimate UO volumes by a factor of close to 100%.
2. **What is the current trend, what is the trend over the last 2 to 3 hours, and what is it over the last 24 hours?**
   Polyuria is defined as >3 L/day. Great variances in hourly output suggest collection errors or resolution of an obstruction. Make sure that the volume is reported and not just the patient's sensation of frequency or urgency.
3. **Have there been recent changes in laboratory studies, including serum glucose, potassium, creatinine, BUN, and UA?**
4. **Has the patient undergone a surgical procedure, and if so, how long ago was it performed?**
   This concerns especially neurosurgical or renal procedures.
5. **Are there any other symptoms?**
   A change in mental status may indicate decreased intravascular volume or a primary intracranial problem.
6. **Are there any changes in vital signs?**

Orders

1. Establish an IV to replace ongoing fluid losses if necessary.
2. Serum and urine electrolytes may be ordered at this time if indicated.
3. If the patient is becoming more ill, order an indwelling urinary catheter if not already in place.
   Avoid this measure if the major complaint is that of incontinence.

Degree of Urgency

A stable patient may be evaluated in an hour or so. If there is a significant change in vital signs, mental status changes, or symptoms of dehydration, the patient must be evaluated immediately.

■ ELEVATOR THOUGHTS

What are the causes of increased UO?

1. Diabetes mellitus

    New-onset or undertreated diabetes mellitus results in increased blood sugar. When the glucose concentration is >300 mg/dl, the kidney's ability to reabsorb sugar may be overwhelmed and glucose is passed into the urine, causing an osmotic diuresis.

2. Diabetes insipidus (DI)

    This is a loss of normal secretion of ADH (or vasopressin) from either neurologic or nephrogenic causes. This occurs in settings of head trauma, cerebral edema (a late finding), pituitary tumors, and occasionally after neurosurgical procedures. Symptoms include massive UO at 5 to 10 L/day, polydipsia, and progressive dehydration. It is differentiated from other diuretic states by analysis of urine electrolytes. As listed in Table 31–2, the urinary sodium in DI is very low, as is the specific gravity because the kidney is unable to reabsorb water from the distal tubule. It is treated with intranasal **vasopressin 5 to 10 U three times per day** and treatment of fluid deficits.

3. High-output renal failure

4. Diuretic therapy

    This includes treatments for CHF or therapies to treat increased intracranial pressure.

5. Postobstructive diuresis

6. Diuretic phase of acute tubular necrosis

7. Salt-wasting nephritis

8. Physiologic diuresis

    This results from increased PO or IV intake during the resolution phase of a major illness or during recovery from major surgery.

■ MAJOR THREAT TO LIFE

- Dehydration leading to hypovolemic shock
- Cerebral edema resulting in DI
- High-output renal failure

■ BEDSIDE

Quick Look Test

Patients tend to look well, unless significant dehydration is present. If a serious illness is present, such as new-onset diabetes mellitus, other problems (e.g., ketoacidosis) may be present.

Airway and Vital Signs

Look for evidence of dehydration. Resting tachycardia or postural changes in pulse rate (a drop of 15 beats/min) or BP (a drop in SBP of 15 mm Hg or any fall in diastolic BP) indicate decreased intravascular volume.

Initial Management

1. Support cardiac output and perfusion.
   A fluid bolus is indicated for patients who are intravascularly deplete.
2. Determine cause of increased UO.
   Once this is determined, the management is more clear.

Selective History and Chart Review

- Is there a condition that would predispose a patient to increased UO? (see Elevator Thoughts)
- Review trends in UO and I/Os, and review changes in weight, which is a good indicator of whole body fluid status.
- Review recent laboratory studies trends, especially BUN, creatinine, and Na^+.
- Review current medications and whether the patient is taking diuretics.

Selective Physical Examination

VS:	Tachycardia, or postural BP changes (dehydration)
MS:	Decreased mental status (decreased perfusion and intracranial problem)
HEENT:	Dry, sticky mucous membranes and flat neck veins (dehydration)
	Visual field defects (pituitary tumor)
	Papilledema (increased intracranial pressure)
Resp:	Rales and decreased aeration (fluid overload and CHF)
	Kussmaul's respirations (rate of 25 to 30 per minute, continuous and sonorous, an indication of acidosis, i.e., in diabetic ketoacidosis)
	Fruity breath (diabetic ketoacidosis)

Abd:	Pain (an occasional finding in diabetes mellitus)
Skin:	Decrease in warmth or turgor, and dry axillae (dehydration)
	Itching (azotemia)
Neuro:	Any change, especially lateralizing signs (intracranial process)
Tubes:	Presence of urinary catheter

Additional tests:

1. UA:	High specific gravity supports dehydration; low specific gravity supports DI.
	RBCs indicate UTI or urolithiasis
2. Electrolytes:	To assess for metabolic derangement and elevations in BUN and creatinine
3. Urine Na$^+$:	Assessment of renal function (see Table 31–2)

■ MANAGEMENT

1. Major management is directed at correcting the cause.
2. Replace depleted intravascular volume with crystalloid (see Chapter 12).
3. Maintain ongoing losses with crystalloid by supplying insensible losses (400–800 ml/day in addition to replacement of urinary and other measurable losses, e.g., nasogastric [NG] suction and drain output).

   The usual rate is 0.5 to 1.0 ml/ml of measurable output. Make sure to replace the type of fluid lost (see Chapter 12). When replacing ongoing losses of fluids, it is advisable to check electrolytes frequently to assess electrolyte balance.
4. Order daily weights and strict I/O measurements.
5. Stop or alter the dose of all diuretic medications.

■ SPECIAL SURGICAL CONSIDERATIONS

Preoperative Considerations

1. A serious decrease in UO in a preoperative patient is an indication of a serious problem and may require changing plans for a scheduled procedure.
2. In a patient with increased intracranial pressure, DI is a very late finding, and a patient with this manifestation is likely to die soon.

Postoperative Considerations

1. There is a normal diuresis of third-spaced fluid 3 to 4 days after an uncomplicated procedure or during the resolution phase of a serious illness.

Be mindful of the patient's preoperative weight, and do not be alarmed if the patient who is well or improving, and is still above the preoperative weight, begins a normal diuresis.

2. Massive increases in UO in a postoperative neurosurgical patient are an indication for a computed tomographic scan immediately.

Hematuria

Blood in the urine is always abnormal. When it is brought to your attention on call, it generally represents gross hematuria or that noticeable without a microscope. A volume as small as 1 ml of blood/L of urine is noticeable as red. Although it is infrequent for hematuria to cause significant blood loss, occasionally an ill or unstable patient will be further stressed by what small blood loss is present. After a urologic procedure, urinary bleeding with clot formation is common and may be a cause of urinary obstruction.

■ PHONE CALL

Questions

1. **When did the hematuria start?**
   Has there been prolonged blood loss?
2. **What is the urine output?**
   Make sure that clots have not stopped the flow of urine.
3. **Is there a urinary catheter in place?**
   This is a common cause of microscopic hematuria but is also an avenue through which the bladder may be irrigated to treat occlusion caused by clots.
4. **Is the patient anticoagulated?**
   These patients must be evaluated immediately and have their anticoagulation reversed as necessary.
5. **Has the patient undergone a surgical procedure, and if so, how long ago was it performed?**
   Procedures on the bladder or the kidney are associated with some transient bleeding but not generally with prolonged symptoms.
6. **Are there any other signs and symptoms?**
   Signs and symptoms such as fever, dysuria, or flank pain may suggest a diagnosis.
7. **Are there any changes in vital signs?**
   Significant loss of blood may be associated with tachycardia, tachypnea, and hypovolemic shock.

Orders

For Significant Bleeding

1. Order a hematocrit and UA.
2. Make sure IV access is in place for fluid replacement if necessary.
3. If the last hematocrit was low or if clinical symptoms of anemia are present, make sure blood is available for this patient.

If Urinary Obstruction Is Present

See Decreased UO section above.

Degree of Urgency

Loss of small amounts of blood does not require immediate attention. However, if the bleeding is severe, if urinary obstruction is evident, or if there is evidence of symptomatic anemia, the patient must be seen immediately. Likewise, if there is a significant change in vital signs or symptoms, the patient must be evaluated immediately.

■ ELEVATOR THOUGHTS

What are the causes of hematuria?
1. Trauma to the urinary tract
    This is usually from the presence of a urinary catheter. Improper or traumatic placement can cause transient bleeding, as can attempted removal before the balloon is completely deflated. A large indwelling catheter occasionally causes some bladder or urethral irritation and may result in small amounts of blood in the urine or at the meatus.
2. Coagulation abnormalities
    If the patient is anticoagulated and symptomatically anemic, reversal of the anticoagulation is indicated. Primary bleeding diatheses such as disseminated intravascular coagulation (DIC), thrombocytopenia, or hemophilia can also cause hematuria.
3. Infection
    Cystitis, prostatitis, or pyelonephritis is a frequent cause of hematuria, if an indwelling catheter is in place. Look for the presence of WBCs with bacteria to make a diagnosis, as catheters in place for ≥3 days are often chronically colonized with bacteria.
4. Medications
    These include anticoagulants such as heparin or warfarin; thrombolytics such as streptokinase, urokinase, and tissue plasminogen activator; and chemotherapeutic agents such as cyclophosphamide.

5. Genitourinary (GU) surgery

   Postoperative bleeding is common after bladder and prostate surgery, such as transurethral resection of the prostate and transurethral resection of a bladder tumor, and is generally treated preemptively with bladder irrigation. This bleeding is often associated with passage of blood clots and may be obstructing.

6. Renal calculi

   Stones may be present anywhere in the urinary tract. They irritate the lumen wall and cause bleeding. This is usually associated with renal colic when flow is obstructed.

7. GU cancer

   This is commonly of the bladder or the kidney. Hematuria may be a presenting symptom.

8. Abdominal trauma

   Blunt or penetrating injuries to the abdomen may cause hematuria. Gross hematuria must be evaluated immediately with an IV pyelogram (IVP). Microscopic hematuria may be present after a renal contusion.

9. Other kidney disease, such as glomerulonephritis, severe hypertension, or benign familial hematuria.

■ MAJOR THREAT TO LIFE

- Anemia with associated hypoxemia
- Hypovolemic shock
- Urinary obstruction and bladder rupture

■ BEDSIDE

Quick Look Test

Patients tend to look well but are distressed about the symptoms. They may be agitated if urinary obstruction is present.

Airway and Vital Signs

Hypovolemia is associated with tachycardia and hypotension. Hypoxia is associated with tachypnea and agitation. Elevated temperature may indicate an infectious cause.

Initial Management

1. Take steps to ensure the comfort of the patient and to reassure the patient.
2. Evaluate the severity.

   If urine is slightly pink and flowing well, identification of the problem and vigilance may be all that is required.

3. If symptoms are more severe
   - Support hemodynamics as necessary.
   - Treat hypoxia with O_2.
   - Relieve urinary obstruction.
   - Reverse anticoagulation if necessary (check with resident first).

Selective History and Chart Review

- Causes of hematuria (see Elevator Thoughts)
- History of bleeding diathesis
    Does the patient have a history or a family history of bleeding problems? Have there been any recent bleeding symptoms? Note that while bleeding disorders may indeed be present and contributing to the hematuria, in more than one-third the cases, an additional coexistent cause for bleeding will also be found.
- History of renal stones
    Risk factors include dehydration, hypercalcemia, hypercalcuria, hyperoxaluria, cystinuria, and recent UTI (especially with urease-producing bacteria such as *Proteus, Klebsiella, Serratia,* and *Pseudomonas* spp.). Loss of the normal diurnal pH variances in the urine can also cause stones. Consistent acid pH supports formation of uric acid stones, and persistent alkali conditions support precipitation of calcium phosphate salt.
- Risk factors for GU neoplasm
    These include occupational exposure to aniline dyes or rubber compounds, cigarette smoking, history of analgesic abuse, or prior pelvic irradiation.
- Evaluation of the need for a urinary catheter if present
    If it was recently inserted, look for evidence of trauma. If it has been in place for >3 days, consider infection. Catheters often get pulled or misplaced during their use; the resultant trauma often causes bleeding, but it is usually transient. If use of the catheter is unnecessary, consider discontinuing it.
- Review of recent laboratory studies and UO trends
    How stable has the hematocrit been? Are the platelets adequate?

Selective Physical Examination

VS:	Repeat now if evidence of hypovolemia or hypoxia
MS:	Confusion or delirium (hypoxia and early urosepsis)
CVS:	Tachycardia and orthostatic hypotension (hypovolemia)

Resp:	Tachypnea (hypoxia and early urosepsis)
Abd:	Bladder distention or discomfort to palpation (obstruction)
GU:	Flank pain (pyelonephritis and renal stone)
Skin:	Pale (anemia); clammy and cool (hypovolemia)
Tubes:	Urinary catheter in place, and if so, length of time
Special examinations:	Other sites of bleeding, e.g., wounds, gingival, and IV sites

Additional tests:

1. Urinalysis:	If not already done
2. Urine culture and sensitivities:	If fever or pyuria present
3. Urinary protein:	May indicate a primary kidney disease
4. Hematocrit and coagulation studies:	As clinically indicated
5. IVP:	If obstruction is suspected, IVP may be ordered to visualize the renal collecting system; except for acute traumas, this is a nonurgent test. If IVP is normal, future tests may include cystoscopy and urine cytology to rule out neoplastic cells

■ MANAGEMENT

1. Management is directed at correcting the underlying cause.
2. Replace depleted intravascular volume with crystalloid (see Chapter 12).
3. Evaluate carefully the need for blood replacement.
   This is rarely necessary. Always consult the resident before transfusing, and check to see if the patient has autologous blood available.
4. Recheck UA in the morning, hematocrit as necessary.

■ SPECIAL SURGICAL CONSIDERATIONS

Preoperative Considerations

1. Gross hematuria noted on the initial acute trauma evaluation requires an IVP to assess patency of the urinary tract. Do

not place a urinary catheter until the patency of the urethra has been documented with a retrograde urethrogram.

2. Significant hematuria or hypotension indicates an underlying condition that would affect a scheduled procedure. Check with the attending physician or chief resident to see if the case should be canceled.

Postoperative Considerations

Postoperative urologic patients often have transient bleeding with clot formation. Prophylactic treatment often includes continuous bladder irrigation with NS through a multilumen urinary catheter. The efflux of NS generally clears with time. If the efflux does not begin clearing within one shift, further evaluation is warranted. These patients are likely to form clots and are at the greatest risk for significant blood loss. Many, especially after radical prostatectomy, start off with a significant intraoperative blood loss and may be anemic as a baseline. Transfusions are not infrequent. If clots obstruct the urinary tract or catheter, first try to unplug the catheter by flushing gently with 20 to 30 ml NS. If this is ineffective, replacement of the urinary catheter is often necessary. Err toward a larger catheter if possible, as these are less likely to become clogged. Triple-lumen catheters add the advantage of being able to irrigate with NS but do not have as large a drainage tube as double-lumen catheters of the same outer diameter. Always consult with a resident or attending physician before replacing the catheter in a recent postoperative urology patient.

Remember

1. In crush injury patients, it is important to differentiate between rhabdomyolysis and RBCs in the urine.

   Both read positive on the orthotoluidine test of a urine dipstick, which does not differentiate between RBCs (hematuria), free hemoglobin (hemolysis), and myoglobin (rhabdomyolysis). Rhabdomyolysis and hemolysis may also be rapidly differentiated by looking at a spun vial of blood; clear plasma supports rhabdomyolysis, and red plasma suggests hemolysis. In cases where muscle breakdown is present
   - Maintain UO with adequate hydration and furosemide.
   - Confirm the diagnosis by checking urine for myoglobin.
   - Check serial creatine phosphokinase levels.
2. Any bleeding in a very ill patient may indicate DIC.
   Look for other sites of bleeding.

32

WOUNDS

The on-call physician for a surgical service should feel comfortable managing wound problems. Usually, most of these problems are routine and straightforward. However, some calls about wound problems lead to the diagnosis of a serious problem. For this reason, it is important that you examine the patient. What may appear as a benign process to the patient or the RN may appear as a more significant process to you.

■ PHONE CALL

Questions

1. **What operation did the patient have, and when was the operation performed?**

    It is important to consider the nature of the operation performed and the important anatomy in the surgical region. This helps you think about the possible causes of the wound problem. For example, consider a draining abdominal wound. If the patient had a small-bowel resection, you may consider a draining enteric fistula. On the other hand, if the patient had an operation limited to the abdominal skin and the fascia, you would probably consider a draining seroma.

    The number of days a patient is postoperative is also an important piece of information. For example, if you are asked to evaluate a wound with erythema, recall that early streptococcus and anaerobic infections may present at postoperative days 1 and 2. Typical wound infections with *Staphylococcus aureus* and other flora are most common between postoperative days 4 and 5.

2. **What are the vital signs?**

    It is important to know if the patient is hypotensive, tachycardic, or febrile.

3. **What is the presenting problem, e.g., is there pain, fever, swelling, drainage, or bleeding?**

4. **What medical problems does the patient have?**

    A patient who has wound healing problems due to steroids, diabetes, malnutrition, advanced malignancy, or chronic disease is more likely to have wound dehiscence and infection. Diabetic patients and patients taking steroids are immunosuppressed and often have few symptoms until they present with a serious wound problem.

5. What medications is the patient taking, e.g., anticoagulants, antibiotics, or steroids?

It is key to know if a patient is anticoagulated. You should be careful when manipulating a wound in an anticoagulated patient. If the patient has significant bleeding from the wound and is anticoagulated, platelets or fresh frozen plasma may be indicated. If a patient is taking intravenous (IV) antibiotics and develops a wound infection, consider the possible organisms responsible and adjust antibiotic therapy accordingly.

Orders

1. Have dressing supplies, sterile gloves, and proper lighting and suction available at the bedside.
2. If the patient has significant bleeding from the wound or evidence of hematoma, have the RN draw a hematocrit immediately.

Inform RN

"Will arrive at the bedside in . . . minutes."

Wound problems represent a variety of postsurgical complications, ranging from benign to life-threatening processes. Examine the patient expeditiously.

■ ELEVATOR THOUGHTS

What causes wound problems?

For common causes of wound problems, see Table 32–1.

■ MAJOR THREAT TO LIFE

- Sepsis secondary to wound infection
- Necrotizing fasciitis
- Postsurgical bleeding
- Intracranial hematoma

An unrecognized or an untreated wound infection can rapidly become a life-threatening process. In addition, bleeding from a wound may indicate that there may be bleeding into an undrained portion of the wound or bleeding into a body cavity. A patient can easily bleed to death if postsurgical or posttraumatic wounds bleed internally into large body cavities such as the pleural space, the abdomen, the retroperitoneum, or the deep compartment of the thigh. Intracranial bleeding after a neurosur-

Table 32–1 □ COMMON CAUSES OF WOUND PROBLEMS

Presenting Sign or Symptom	Potential Process
Wound erythema	Posttraumatic inflammation
	Cellulitis
	Fasciitis
	Abscess
Wound drainage (clear or cloudy)	Seroma
	Draining abscess
	Fistula (enteric, salivary, or urinary)
Wound drainage (bloody)	Draining hematoma (darker red)
	Active bleeding (lighter red)
Wound opening	Wound dehiscence
	Evisceration
Foul odor	Anaerobic wound infection
	Wound abscess
	Necrotic tissue
Wound swelling	Postsurgical inflammation
	Seroma
	Hematoma

gical procedure or a traumatic injury may lead to brain herniation and death.

■ BEDSIDE

Quick Look Test

Does the patient look well (comfortable), sick (uncomfortable or distressed), or critical (about to die)?

Most patients with small fluid collections in wounds look well. These collections may represent seromas or hematomas. When these collections become infected or represent an ongoing bleeding problem, the patient appears sick. Patients with cellulitis, abscess, or early fasciitis often present with fever and pain in the area of the wound. These patients are often uncomfortable and distressed. Patients with a rapidly progressive infection of a wound may present with fever, hypotension, and sepsis. These patients may look critically ill.

Airway and Vital Signs

What is the temperature?

Fever associated with a wound problem may represent infection. However, recall that the most common cause of fever in a postoperative patient is atelectasis, not infection.

What is the blood pressure and heart rate?

Hypotension, tachycardia, and fever may represent sepsis. In the presence of wound erythema, tenderness, or purulent drainage, suspect the wound as the source of infection.

Selective History and Chart Review

1. **Ask the patient when he or she noticed that the wound had changed.**

   When did the wound begin to swell, drain, hurt, or become erythematous? Understanding when the problem began helps you think about how to best manage the wound.

2. **Ask the patient if the wound problem is new, recent, or chronic.**

   A patient who has been having drainage from a wound for days may have a fistula or a chronic draining infection or an abscess. A patient who has just developed drainage from a wound may have a more benign problem, such as a draining seroma. A sudden-onset, rapidly spreading erythema extending from a wound may represent a *Streptococcus* or *Clostridium* infection, whereas a chronically erythematous wound often represents a chronic infection and a less emergent problem.

3. **Ask the patient if he or she has wound healing problems.**

   Patients who have had past problems with wounds are likely to have similar problems when you are on call. Learn about the past management by asking the patient how the wounds were treated and what the outcome was.

4. **Ask the patient if he or she is diabetic or if he or she has other medical problems.**

   Although the RN may have told you that the patient was diabetic or had other medical problems, it is wise to ask the patient about his or her medical history yourself.

5. **Review the chart briefly, paying special attention to medical history, current drugs, and recent surgical procedures.**

   A thorough evaluation of the medical record and of the patient is indicated to provide the best diagnosis and the best treatment.

Selective Physical Examination

VS: Repeat now. Note any change in temperature.

HEENT: Evaluate scalp and facial wounds with the aid of gauze (to blot bleeding) and adequate lighting. Note the deepest layer exposed (fat, muscle, or bone). Look for drainage or bleeding.

Look at oral wounds carefully with the aid of a

tongue retractor and light. Note the deepest structures exposed.

Evaluate any wounds in the ear canal with the aid of fine suction and an otoscope.

Chest: Evaluate midline sternotomy wounds. Note skin redness, bleeding, drainage, and dehiscence. Check for sternal stability.

Evaluate thoracotomy wounds. Note skin redness, bleeding, air leak, or dehiscence.

Abd: Evaluate abdominal wounds. If the wound is closed, note skin redness, drainage (serous, sanguineous, purulent, or fecal), swelling or fullness, and tenderness. If the wound is open, consider removing the dressing. Note the deepest closed layer (fascia, muscle, or fat), the presence of any granulation tissue, evidence of fascial dehiscence, evidence of early evisceration, and drainage from the abdominal cavity. Inspect any suction drains for the amount and the quality of fluid in the drainage system.

MSS: Examine wounds of the extremities carefully. Note any skin redness, bleeding, and drainage. Note the type of drainage (serous, serosanguineous, bloody, or purulent). Look for the deepest layer of tissue exposed at the base of the wound (fat, muscle, or bone). Note any nerves, vessels, or tendons exposed.

■ MANAGEMENT

Erythematous Wounds

Closed wounds that are erythematous outside the immediate edges of the wound may be infected. The skin may appear brawny red or reddish brown. These areas are usually indurated and tender. Wound cellulitis is best treated with elevation of the infected area, bed rest, and IV antibiotics. Common organisms include *S. aureus* and streptococci species. The classic antibiotics used for simple cellulitis are **cefazolin 1 g IV every 8 hours** or **nafcillin 1 to 2 g IV every 4 hours.** If the patient is already taking IV antibiotics and develops cellulitis, the organisms responsible for the infection may not be covered adequately by the antibiotic or the organisms are resistant to the antibiotic. Discuss adding a second drug or changing the primary antibiotic with the chief resident or the attending physician.

Rapid-Onset Cellulitis

Streptococci species or *Clostridium* may produce cellulitis in a wound within 12 to 24 hours. **Penicillin G potassium 2 to 4 million U IV every 4 hours** is usually effective if the infection is limited to the skin. If there is crepitus of the wound, skin discoloration (brown, blue, or black), and odor, the process may represent a severe infection involving mixed flora or clostridia. These infections require wound exploration and emergent surgical debridement. If you suspect a rapid, necrotizing process, call the chief resident or the attending physician before either opening the wound or arranging an emergent trip to the operating room (OR). In fulminant streptococcal infections such as those that can lead to toxic shock, clindamycin is a better antibiotic choice, as it is more active against the bacteria during a relatively penicillin-resistant growth phase.

Invasive or Gangrenous Wound Infection

These soft-tissue infections are usually caused by *Clostridium* species. The infection that may appear initially as a rapid-onset cellulitis, however, becomes rapidly progressive and invasive. Organisms initially invade superficial to the deep fascia but may move deeper into the muscle plane. Infected muscle tissue becomes necrotic. The skin appears discolored, edematous, and crepitant. A brown seropurulent exudate containing bubbles may drain from the wound or the involved area. The patient generally has significant pain, fever, and signs of toxemia. Treatment involves wide wound debridement, fascial compartment release if there are signs of compartmental syndrome, local wound care, and IV antibiotics. **Penicillin G potassium 20 to 40 million U/ day divided into every-4-hour dosing** is used. In patients allergic to penicillin or in whom double coverage is desired, consider **clindamycin 450 to 600 mg IV every 6 hours** or **metronidazole 1-g loading dose followed by 500 mg IV every 6 hours.**

Necrotizing Fasciitis

This is an invasive infection of the fascia caused by a mixed infection. Infection begins in proximity to a wound. Organisms may include streptococci, staphylococci, Gram-negative organisms, bacteroides, and clostridia. The skin adjacent to the wound first shows hemorrhagic bullae, followed by skin death. Crepitus of the involved skin is common as well as fever, tachycardia, and toxemia. At surgery, necrotic skin, fascia, and fat are seen. Thrombosis of blood vessels also occurs. Necrotizing fasciitis usually begins in an extremity or in the perineal area and is more common in diabetic and immunocompromised patients. If you suspect that a patient may have necrotizing fasciitis, call the chief resident or the attending physician immediately. Arrange for emergent surgical debridement in the OR. Type and cross-match the patient for 2 units of packed red blood cells and order IV antibiotics. Triple IV antibiotics are appropriate. Commonly used combinations include penicillin, metronidazole (Flagyl), and gentamicin. Give IV antibiotics after cultures are taken in the OR. Remember that management of these patients includes both surgical debridement and IV antibiotics.

Wound Swelling

Wounds tend to swell postoperatively. However, closed wounds should not generally "bulge" or be fluctuant. A closed wound that appears abnormally swollen may have a trapped fluid collection. The fluid may be serum and lymph (seroma), blood (hematoma), or another bodily fluid. If the suspicion is high that the swelling represents a fluid collection, it is often appropriate to aspirate with a 20-gauge needle and syringe using sterile technique. However, it is safe to aspirate the wound only if you know that there is no vital structure or organ below the skin surface. Discuss the case with a supervising surgical resident or the attending physician before proceeding with aspiration. He or she will generally be familiar with the surgical anatomy of that patient. For example, a swelling under an abdominal wound could represent a hernia. Aspiration of such a wound could lead to perforation of the bowel or another abdominal organ.

Draining Wounds

A draining wound could represent wound infection, seroma, hematoma, or fistula. Carefully examine the patient and the wound. Does the drainage appear serous, serosanguineous, bloody, or purulent? Does the drainage have an odor (infection or fistula)? If you suspect infection, obtain a wound culture and Gram stain using a sterile culture swab. These wounds may need to be opened to allow adequate drainage. If the wound appears to be draining a serous or a serosanguineous drainage and there is no sign of infection, either reinforcing the wound with sterile gauze or gently packing any open area of the wound with sterile Nu-Gauze is appropriate. If you suspect a fistula, gently and superficially packing the fistulous tract with a sterile swab and Nu-Gauze is often appropriate. Consult the supervising resident or the attending physician in cases of significant wound drainage.

Wounds with Exposed Deep Structures

If called to evaluate a wound that has exposed deep structures, it is important to keep these deep structures moist. Deep wounds may have bone, muscle, fascia, nerve, or other structures exposed. These tissues are best kept viable by placing sterile gauze moistened with saline on the structure. Use sterile technique and make sure that the moist gauze is in gentle contact with the deep structure. Remember that when tissues dessicate, they die. Contact the appropriate surgical resident or the attending physician who can help with wound evaluation and closure.

Wound Dehiscence or Evisceration

Wounds may dehisce at any point in the postoperative period. You will likely be called to evaluate a wound that is opening spontaneously. Sutures may or may not still be in place. Usually, wounds dehisce because the fascial closure of a deep wound has broken down. The wound may have been closed with tension, or the tissues may be of poor quality. There may be a wound infection or a fluid collection. If the fascia and the skin breaks down, evisceration of abdominal organs may occur. The small bowel is the most common structure to eviscerate. In cases of wound dehiscence or evisceration, cover the wound and any exposed structures with sterile gauze moistened with saline. Place a sterile OR towel over the area. Call the supervising resident or the attending physician. These wound problems are best dealt with in the OR.

Superficial Wounds

Fresh wounds involving the skin may be easy to repair at the bedside. If a patient falls out of bed and suffers a simple laceration without other injury, you can clean the wound and repair it yourself. After anesthetizing the wound with a lidocaine 1% injection, clean the wound with large volumes of sterile saline. Use sterile technique. Wounds contaminated with dirt or debris will need some mechanical debridement with a sterile iris scissors, a scalpel, and a forceps. One-half strength hydrogen peroxide is often helpful in mechanically cleaning wounds. Prepare the skin adjacent to the wound with povidone-iodine (Betadine). Using sterile technique, place interrupted sutures of nylon or Prolene to approximate the skin edges. For the face, use 6–0 sutures. For the extremities or the trunk, usually 3–0 or 4–0 sutures are appropriate. Closure of the superficial fascia is often not necessary and may lead to increased risk of infection.

Actively Bleeding Wounds

Wounds that demonstrate bleeding may be difficult to manage. If the bleeding is from a superficial structure or from the wound edge, the bleeding structure can be seen and controlled. Have sterile gloves, adequate lighting, and gauze or suction available. Carefully visualize the bleeding structure. Frequently, you will see a small blood vessel in the wound or at the edge of the wound that is causing bleeding. Apply pressure to the area for 5 to 10 minutes. If bleeding persists, you can use silver nitrate sticks (for very small vessels or bleeding granulation tissue), bedside cautery, or carefully placed suture ligature (for almost any bleeding structure) to stop the bleeding. If there is significant or massive bleeding from a wound, obtain a hematocrit immediately, type and crossmatch the patient for 2 units of blood, and apply pressure to the bleeding area if possible. Use IV fluids to maintain hemodynamic stability. Call for help. You may need an emergent trip to the OR to explore the wound and to control the bleeding.

APPENDICES

APPENDIX A

READING X-RAYS, READING ECGs, CARDIAC ARREST PROTOCOLS

READING X-RAYS

1. Clavicles
2. Trachea
3. Right mainstem bronchus
4. Left mainstem bronchus
5. Aortic knuckle
6. Superior vena cava
7. Right pulmonary artery
8. Left pulmonary artery
9. Left atrium
10. Right atrium
11. Left ventricle
12. Aortic stripe
13. Costophrenic angles
14. Gastric bubble

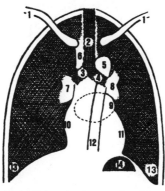

Figure A–1 □ Posteroanterior chest x-ray. (Reprinted from Marshall SA, Ruedy J: On Call: Principles and Protocols, 2nd ed. Philadelphia, WB Saunders Co, 1993, p 332.)

1. Trachea
2. Left mainstem bronchus
3. Right pulmonary artery
4. Left pulmonary artery
5. Aortic arch
6. Manubrium
7. Sternum
8. Breast shadow
9. Retrosternal space
10. Retrocardiac space
11. Left atrium
12. Right ventricle
13. Left ventricle
14. Inferior vena cava
15. Gastric air bubble
16. Left hemidiaphragm
17. Right hemidiaphragm
18. Costophrenic angle
19. Scapular shadows

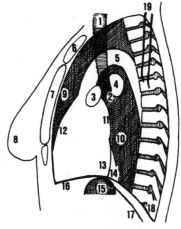

Figure A–2 □ Lateral chest x-ray. (Reprinted from Marshall SA, Ruedy J: On Call: Principles and Protocols, 2nd ed. Philadelphia, WB Saunders Co, 1993, p 333.)

READING ECGs

Rate

Multiply the number of QRS complexes in a 6-second period (30 large squares) (between the two large dots) by 10 = beats/min (Fig. A–3).
- Normal = 60 to 100 beats/min
- Tachycardia = >100 beats/min
- Bradycardia = <60 beats/min

Rhythm

Is the rhythm regular?

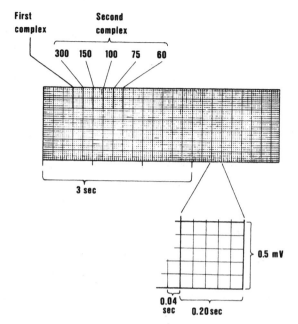

Figure A–3 □ Reading ECGs. Rate. (Reprinted from Marshall SA, Ruedy J: On Call: Principles and Protocols, 2nd ed. Philadelphia, WB Saunders Co, 1993, p 328.)

Is there a P wave preceding every QRS complex? Is there a QRS complex following every P wave?
1. Yes = sinus rhythm.
2. No P waves with irregular rhythm = atrial fibrillation.
3. No P waves with regular rhythm = junctional rhythm. Look for retrograde P waves in all leads.

Axis

See Figure A–4.

P Wave Configuration

Normal P wave. Look at all leads (Fig. A–5*A*).

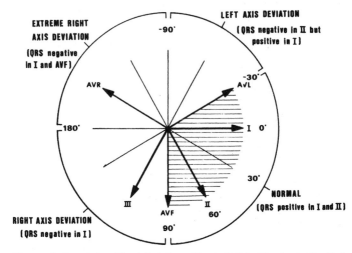

Figure A–4 □ Axis. (Reprinted from Marshall SA, Ruedy J: On Call: Principles and Protocols, 2nd ed. Philadelphia, WB Saunders Co, 1993, p 329.)

Left Atrial Enlargement (Fig. A–5B)

- Duration: 120 msec (three small squares in lead II). Often notched = P mitrale.
- Amplitude: Negative terminal P wave in lead V_1 >1 mm in depth *and* >40 msec (one small square).

Right Atrial Enlargement (Fig. A–5C)

- Amplitude: 2.5 mm in leads II, III, or aVF (i.e., tall, peaked P

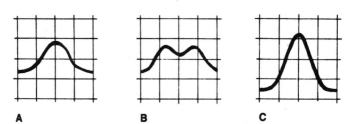

Figure A–5 □ Reading ECGs. P wave configuration in lead II. *A,* Normal P wave. *B,* Left atrial enlargement. *C,* Right atrial enlargement. (Reprinted from Marshall SA, Ruedy J: On Call: Principles and Protocols, 2nd ed. Philadelphia, WB Saunders Co, 1993, p 329.)

wave of P pulmonale); 1.5 mm in the initial positive deflection of the P wave in lead V_1 or V_2.

QRS Configuration

Left Ventricular Hypertrophy

1. Increased QRS voltage (S in V_1 or V_2 plus R in V_5 >35 mm or R in aVL $\geq$11 mm)
2. Left atrial enlargement
3. ST segment depression and negative T wave in left lateral leads

Right Ventricular Hypertrophy

1. R >S in V_1
2. Right axis deviation (> + 90°)
3. ST segment depression and negative T wave in right precordial leads

Conduction Abnormalities

First-Degree Block

- PR interval $\geq$0.20 second ($\geq$1 large square)

Second-Degree Block

Occasional absence of QRS and T after a P of sinus origin.
1. Type I (Wenckebach): Progressive prolongation of the PR interval before the missed QRS complex
2. Type II: Absence of progressive prolongation of the PR interval before the missed QRS complex

Third-Degree Block

Absence of any relationship between P waves of sinus origin and QRS complexes

Left Anterior Hemiblock

Left axis deviation, Q in I and aVL; a small R in III, in the absence of left ventricular hypertrophy.

Left Posterior Hemiblock

Right axis deviation, a small R in I and a small Q in III, in the absence of right ventricular hypertrophy.

Complete Right Bundle Branch Block

See Figure A–6*A*.

Complete Left Bundle Branch Block

See Figure A–6*B*.

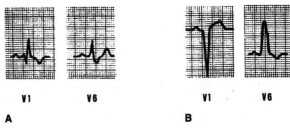

Figure A–6 □ Reading ECGs. QRS configuration. *A,* Complete right bundle branch block. *B,* Complete left bundle branch block. (Reprinted from Marshall SA, Ruedy J: On Call: Principles and Protocols, 2nd ed. Philadelphia, WB Saunders Co, 1993, p 331.)

Ventricular Preexcitation

1. PR interval <0.11 second with widened QRS (>0.12 second) due to a delta wave = Wolff-Parkinson-White syndrome.
2. PR interval <0.11 second with a normal QRS complex = Lown-Ganong-Levine syndrome.

MYOCARDIAL INFARCTION PATTERNS

Type of Infarct	Patterns of Changes (Q Waves, ST Elevation or Depression, T Wave Inversion)*
Inferior	Q in II, III, aVF
Inferoposterior	Q in II, III, aVF, and V_6
	R > S and positive T in V_1
Anteroseptal	V_1 to V_4
Anterolateral to posterolateral	V_1 to V_5; Q in I, aVL, and V_6
Posterior	R > S in V_1, positive T, and Q in V_6

*A significant Q wave is >40 msec wide or > one-third of the QRS height. ST segment or T wave changes in the absence of significant Q waves may represent a non–Q wave infarct.

CARDIAC ARREST PROTOCOLS*

Treatment Algorithm for Ventricular Fibrillation (VF) and Pulseless Ventricular Tachycardia (Fig. A–7). The pulse and rhythm should be checked after each electric shock. If VF recurs after transient conversion, the previously successful energy level

*Text and algorithms from AHA Standards and Guidelines for CPR and Emergency Care, JAMA 255(21): p. 2915. Copyright 1986, American Medical Association.

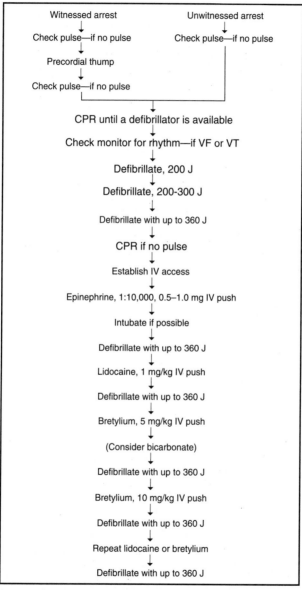

Figure A–7 □ Treatment algorithm for ventricular fibrillation (VF) and pulseless ventricular tachycardia.

should be used for defibrillation. If intubation can be performed simultaneously with other interventions, the patient should be intubated as early in the sequence as possible. However, defibrillation and epinephrine are more important initially if the patient can be ventilated without intubation. Epinephrine (in the indicated doses) should be administered every 5 minutes. Lidocaine hydrochloride 0.5 mg/kg every 8 minutes for a total dose of 3 mg/kg is an acceptable alternative to bretylium tosylate 5 mg/kg or 10 mg/kg. If sodium bicarbonate is given, a dose of 1 mmol/L followed by 0.5 mg/kg every 10 minutes may be used.

Treatment Algorithm for Sustained Ventricular Tachycardia (VT) with Pulse (Fig. A–8).   The unstable arm of the algorithm should be followed for stable patients who become unstable. Sedation before cardioversion should be considered for all patients except those with hemodynamic instability (e.g., hypotension, pulmonary edema, unconsciousness). For patients who are hemodynamically unstable, unsynchronized cardioversion is indicated to avoid delays associated with synchronization. A precor-

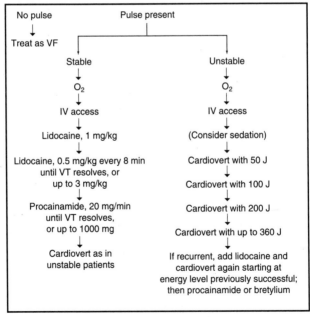

Figure A–8 □ Treatment algorithm for sustained ventricular tachycardia (VT) with pulse.

dial thump may be used before cardioversion in hemodynamically stable patients.

Treatment Algorithm for Asystole (Fig. A–9).   Intubation is recommended early in the sequence if it can be accomplished simultaneously with other interventions. However, CPR and epinephrine are more important initially if the patient can be ventilated without intubation. Epinephrine should be given every 5 minutes. The endotracheal route may be used. The value of sodium bicarbonate in this sequence is unproved, and routine use is not recommended. If sodium bicarbonate is given, a dose of 1 mmol/L followed by 0.5 mmol/L every 10 minutes may be used.

Treatment Algorithm for Electromechanical Dissociation (Fig. A–10).   Intubation is recommended early in the sequence if it can be accomplished simultaneously with other interventions. However, epinephrine is more important initially if the patient can be ventilated without intubation. Epinephrine should be administered every 5 minutes. The value of sodium bicarbonate in this sequence is unproved, and routine use is not recommended. If sodium bicarbonate is given, a dose of 1 mmol/L followed by 0.5 mmol/L every 10 minutes may be used.

Treatment Algorithm for Paroxysmal Supraventricular Tachycardia (PSVT) (Fig. A–11).   If PSVT recurs after successful cardioversion, repeated electric cardioversion is not indicated. Sedation should be used as time permits.

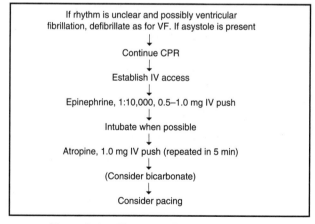

Figure A–9 □ Treatment algorithm for asystole.

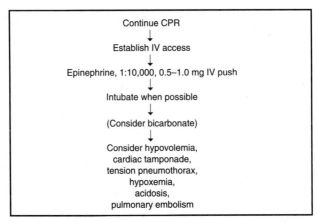

Figure A–10 □ Treatment algorithm for electromechanical dissociation.

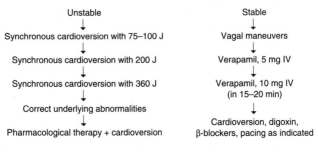

Figure A–11 □ Treatment algorithm for paroxysmal supraventricular tachycardia (PSVT).

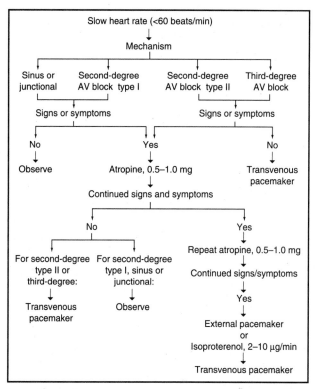

Figure A–12 □ Treatment algorithm for bradycardia.

Treatment Algorithm for Bradycardia (Fig. A–12).   A single chest thump or cough may stimulate cardiac electrical activity and improve cardiac output. These maneuvers may be tried initially. Use of isoproterenol or an external pacemaker for patients who do not respond to atropine is a temporizing measure.

Treatment Algorithm for Ventricular Ectopy: Acute Suppressive Therapy (Fig. A–13).   If ventricular ectopy persists following correction of treatable causes, an antidysrhythmic, such as lidocaine, procainamide, or bretylium, may be required.

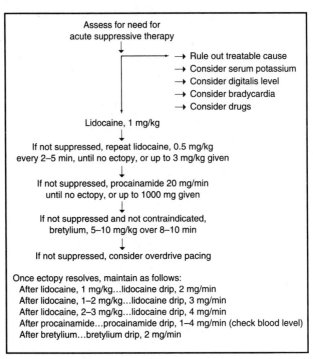

Assess for need for
acute suppressive therapy

→ Rule out treatable cause
→ Consider serum potassium
→ Consider digitalis level
→ Consider bradycardia
→ Consider drugs

Lidocaine, 1 mg/kg

If not suppressed, repeat lidocaine, 0.5 mg/kg
every 2–5 min, until no ectopy, or up to 3 mg/kg given

If not suppressed, procainamide 20 mg/min
until no ectopy, or up to 1000 mg given

If not suppressed and not contraindicated,
bretylium, 5–10 mg/kg over 8–10 min

If not suppressed, consider overdrive pacing

Once ectopy resolves, maintain as follows:
  After lidocaine, 1 mg/kg...lidocaine drip, 2 mg/min
  After lidocaine, 1–2 mg/kg...lidocaine drip, 3 mg/min
  After lidocaine, 2–3 mg/kg...lidocaine drip, 4 mg/min
  After procainamide...procainamide drip, 1–4 mg/min (check blood level)
  After bretylium...bretylium drip, 2 mg/min

Figure A–13 □ Treatment algorithm for ventricular ectopy: acute suppressive therapy.

APPENDIX B

OUTLINES OF COMMON SURGICAL NOTES

PREOP NOTE*
 Date and time:
 Preop diagnosis:
 Procedure planned:
 Staff surgeon:
 Preop examination:
 Preoperative laboratory studies:
 List of routine medications/therapies:
 Blood products available:
  (confirm availability with a phone call to the blood bank the night before surgery)
Bowel preparation (if any):
"On call to OR" instructions:
 Void:
 Preop antibiotics:
 SBE prophylaxis:
 Steroid preparation:
 Other special therapies needed:
PAR statement (a brief statement that the procedure has been discussed with the patient):
 e.g., "Procedure, alternatives, and risks, both foreseen and unforeseen, described in detail to the patient; questions were answered to his/her satisfaction. He/She elects to proceed as planned."
Consent signed and witnessed:

BRIEF OP NOTE

 Date and time:
 Preop diagnosis:
 Postop diagnosis:
 Procedure:
 Staff surgeon:
 Assistants:
 Anesthesia:
 Indications:
 Findings:
  (drawings are often useful to describe resultant anatomy)
 Specimens:
  (including results of frozen sections, if any)

---

*See also Chapter 24.

Drains:
Cultures:
Estimated blood loss:
Urine output:
Fluids received:
Complications:
   ("Returned to PAR/SICU in _____ condition")

POSTOP CHECK

Date and time:
Date of procedure:
Procedure:
Staff surgeon:
Postop examination:
   VS:
   Mental status:
   Cardiovascular:
   Lungs:
   Abdomen:
   Extremities/skin:
   Wound/dressing:
   Specific surgical site:
Postop laboratory studies:
Urine output:
Drain output and character of fluid draining:
Pain control:
Patient status:
Time until reassessment:

ON CALL/CROSS-COVERAGE NOTE

Date and time:
Contacted by:
Patient identification:
Operation:
   (date and type of procedure, staff surgeon, complications)
Brief summary of course since the operation:
Current problem:
History of problem:
Examination (problem oriented):
   VS:
   Mental status:
   Cardiovascular:
   Lungs:
   Abdomen:
   Extremities/skin:
   Wound/dressing:
   Specific surgical site:
   Specific problem site:

Recent laboratory studies:
Urine output:
Drain output and character of fluid draining:
Assessment:
Plans:
Persons contacted:
  (resident, attending, bedside care giver, family, consulting services, etc.)
Time until reassessment:

APPENDIX C

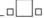

ON-CALL FORMULAE

FLUIDS AND ELECTROLYTES

1. Determination of serum osmolality (mOsm)

$$\text{Serum osmolality} = 2[\text{Na}] + \frac{[\text{glucose}]}{[18]} + \frac{[\text{BUN}]}{[2.8]}$$

Na	Serum sodium concentration (in mEq/L)
Glucose	Serum glucose concentration (in mg/dl)
BUN	Blood urea nitrogen concentration (in mg/dl)
Normal range	280–295 mOsm

2. Determination of free water deficit (in L) in settings of hypernatremia

$$\text{Water deficit} = \frac{[\text{Na (observed)} - \text{Na (desired)}]\,[0.6]\,[\text{Wt}]}{[\text{Na (desired)}]}$$

Na (observed)	Serum sodium concentration (in mEq/L)
Na (desired)	Assume 140 mEq/L
0.6	Volume of distribution of sodium
Wt	Weight (in kg)

3. Determination of actual serum sodium in settings of hyperglycemia

$$\text{Na (corrected)} = \frac{[\text{glucose (observed)} - \text{glucose (normal)}]\,[1.4]}{[\text{glucose (normal)}]} + \text{Na (observed)}$$

Na (corrected)	Actual serum concentration of sodium (in mEq/L)
Na (observed)	Serum sodium concentration (in mEq/L)
Glucose (observed)	Serum glucose concentration (in mg/dl)
Glucose (normal)	Assume 200 mg/dl
1.4	Correction factor, which considers the shift of water that follows glucose into the interstitial space

4. Determination of sodium deficit in settings of hyponatremia

$$\text{Na deficit} = [\text{Na (desired)} - \text{Na (observed)}]\,[0.6]\,[\text{Wt}]$$

Na (desired)	Assume 135 mEq/L
Na (observed)	Serum sodium concentration (in mEq/L)
0.6	Volume of distribution of sodium
Wt	Weight (in kg)

5. Determination of bicarbonate (HCO₃) deficit (in mEq/L)

$$\text{HCO}_3 \text{ deficit} = [\text{Wt}]\,[0.4]\,[\text{HCO}_3 \text{ (desired)} - \text{HCO}_3 \text{ (actual)}]$$

HCO$_3$ (desired)	Assume 15–20 mEq/L
HCO$_3$ (observed)	Serum concentration of bicarbonate (in mEq/L)

Wt   Weight (in kg)
0.4   Correction factor, which considers intracellular buff-
                       ering of bicarbonate
Goal of therapy   Serum pH >7.2

6. Determination of bicarbonate (HCO₃) deficit (in mEq/L) by using base deficit

$$HCO_3 \text{ deficit} = \frac{[\text{Base deficit}] \, [\text{Wt in kg}] \, [0.4]}{2}$$

7. Determination of anion gap (in mEq/L)

$$\text{Anion gap} = (Na + K) - (Cl + HCO_3)$$

Na   Serum sodium concentration (in mEq)
K   Serum potassium concentration (in mEq)
Cl   Serum chloride concentration (in mEq)
HCO₃   Serum bicarbonate ion concentration (in mEq)

8. Henderson-Hasselbalch equation

$$pH = 6.1 + \log \left(\frac{HCO_3}{0.03 \times P_{CO_2}} \right)$$

6.1   pH of the bicarbonate buffer system
HCO₃   Serum bicarbonate ion concentration (in mEq)
0.03   Solubility constant of CO_2 in arterial blood
P_{CO_2} Partial pressure of CO_2 in serum (in mm Hg)

9. Nitrogen balance (in g/day, may be a positive or a negative value)

$$N_2 \text{ balance} = \frac{24\text{-hour protein intake}}{6.25} - [(24\text{-hour UUN}) + (4)]$$

24-hour UUN   Urinary urea nitrogen excretion (in g/day)
4   Obligatory loss (in g/day)
6.25   The number of grams of protein that yield 1 g N_2
Goal of therapy +4 g/day balance

CARDIAC PHYSIOLOGY

1. Determination of cardiac output (CO)

$$CO = [HR] \, [SV]$$

CO   Cardiac output (in L/min)
HR   Heart rate (in beats/min)
SV   Stroke volume (in L/beat)

Normal CO = 3.5–8.5 L/min
Cardiac index (CI) = CO/patient surface area

2. Determination of blood pressure (BP)

$$BP = [CO] \, [SVR]$$

BP   Blood pressure (in mm Hg)

CO   Cardiac output (in L/min) $\left(\dfrac{\text{in dyne-sec}}{\text{cm}^5} \right)$
SVR   Systemic vascular resistance

3. Determination of mean arterial blood pressure (MAP)

$$MAP = \frac{DBP + [SBP - DBP]}{[3]}$$

MAP   Mean arterial pressure (in mm Hg)
DBP   Diastolic blood pressure (in mm Hg)
SBP   Systolic blood pressure (in mm Hg)

4. Determination of systemic vascular resistance (SVR)

$$SVR = \frac{[MAP - CVP] [80]}{[CO]}$$

SVR   Systemic vascular resistance $\left(\dfrac{\text{in dyne-sec}}{\text{cm}^5} \right)$

MAP   Mean arterial pressure (in mm Hg)
CVP   Central venous pressure (in mm Hg)
CO   Cardiac output (in L/min)

5. Conversion of pressure in millimeters of mercury (mmHg) to pressure in centimeters of water (cm H_2O)

$$mm\ Hg = \frac{cm\ H_2O}{1.36}$$

RESPIRATORY PHYSIOLOGY

1. The Fick law for transfer of gases

$$V_{gas} = \frac{(A)}{0.5} (k) (P_1 - P_2)$$

V_{gas} Rate of gas transfer across a membrane
A Tissue area
0.5   Thickness of the pulmonary membrane (in μm)
k Solubility coefficient of the gas
$P_1 - P_2$ Partial pressure gradient of the gas across the membrane (in mm Hg)

CO_2 diffuses 20 times faster than O_2 due to differences in their solubility coefficients.

2. Calculation of the alveolar oxygen partial pressure (PAO_2)

$$PAO_2 = (713) (FiO_2) - \frac{PaCO_2}{0.8}$$

PAO_2 Alveolar oxygen partial pressure (in mm Hg)
713   Sea level barometric pressure (760 mm Hg) minus the partial pressure of water vapor (PH_2O, 47 mm Hg)
FiO_2 Fractional concentration of inspired oxygen
$PaCO_2$ Partial pressure of CO_2 (in mm Hg, from arterial blood gas data)
0.8   Respiratory quotient

3. Calculation of the alveolar-arterial oxygen gradient (P[A-a]O$_2$)

$$P[A\text{-}a]O_2 = PA_{O_2} - Pa_{O_2}$$

P[A-a]O$_2$ Alveolar-arterial oxygen gradient (in mm Hg)
PA$_{O_2}$ Alveolar oxygen partial pressure (in mm Hg)
Pa$_{O_2}$ Arterial oxygen partial pressure (in mm Hg, from arterial blood gas data)

Normal P[A-a]O$_2$ is 12 mm Hg in young adults and increases to 20 mm Hg by the age of 70 years. In failure of ventilation, the P[A-a]O$_2$ will stay at 12–20 mm Hg. In failure of oxygenation, the P[A-a]O$_2$ will increase.

RENAL PHYSIOLOGY

1. Creatinine clearance (CrCl)

$$CrCl = \frac{(140 - \text{age})\,(\text{wt})}{(72)\,(Cr)}$$

CrCl   Creatinine clearance (in ml/min)
Age   Patient's age (in years)
Wt   Patient's weight (in kg)
Cr   Serum creatinine concentration (in mg/dl)
Normal CrCl   90–150 ml/min

APPENDIX D

ON-CALL FORMULARY

This formulary includes medications which are commonly encountered while on call. Dosages listed are for adults, and generic names are listed. Antibiotic dosages are listed in Appendix E. Always be mindful of the renal and hepatic function of the patient before administration of medications, and be aware that many medications require individualization of medications, and be aware that many medications require individualization of dose. For further information, consult the pharmacy or the medication insert instructions.

Acetaminophen

Proprietary name(s)	Tylenol and others
Therapeutic class	Analgesic and antipyretic
Indications	Pain and fever
Actions	Diminishes pain response and has direct action on hypothalamus temperature regulation centers
Metabolism	Hepatic
Excretion	Renal
Side effects	Uncommon; rash, drug fever, mucosal ulcerations, leukopenia, pancytopenia, and hepatic toxicity
Dose	325–1000 mg PO/PR every 4–6 hr as needed, to 4000 mg/24 hr.
Notes	Little to no anti-inflammatory action. Does not affect the aggregation of platelets. Does not interact with anticoagulants. Antidote for overdose is N-acetylcysteine.

Albuterol

Proprietary name(s)	Proventil and Ventolin
Therapeutic class	β_2-Adrenergic agonist
Indications	Bronchospasm due to asthma, bronchitis, or chronic obstructive pulmonary disease (COPD)
Actions	β_2-Adrenergic agonist
Metabolism	Hepatic; less than 20% of the inhaled dose is absorbed systemically.

Excretion	Renal
Side effects	Headache, tachycardia, lightheadedness, dizziness, tremor, palpitations, and nausea
Dose	2.5–5 mg in 3 ml normal saline (NS) by nebulizer every 4 hr as needed. Severe acute bronchospasm may require doses every 3–5 min initially.
Notes	May alternate with metaproterenol.

Allopurinol

Proprietary name(s)	Lopurin and Zyloprim
Therapeutic class	Xanthine oxidase inhibitor
Indications	Symptomatic gout, uric acid nephropathy, and lysis of tumor
Actions	Inhibits formation of uric acid
Metabolism	Metabolite oxipurinol is also active
Excretion	Renal
Side effects	Rash, fever, gastrointestinal (GI) upset, cataracts, renal toxicity, and hepatotoxicity
Dose	100–300 mg PO every day after meals. Severe cases may require doses up to 800 mg/day.
Notes	Reduce the dose in renal or hepatic insufficiency. Acute gout episodes may follow initiation of therapy. Aminophylline, mercaptopurine, and azathioprine levels may be increased by allopurinol. Nonsteroidal anti-inflammatory drugs (NSAIDs) are the first-line therapy for acute gout.

Aluminum hydroxide

Proprietary name(s)	Amphojel and ALternaGEL
Therapeutic class	Antacid
Indications	Epigastric pain due to peptic ulcer disease or gastritis. Prophylaxis for stress ulcers. Reduction of urinary phosphate in patients with phosphate-containing renal stones.
Actions	Buffers gastric acid; binds to phosphate in the GI tract
Side effects	Constipation, anorexia, nausea, hypophosphatemia and aluminum toxicity in patients with renal failure
Dose	For acute symptoms, 30–60 ml PO every 1–2 hr as needed. For maintenance therapy, 30–60 ml PO every 1 to 3 hr when symptomatic and before bedtime as needed.

| Notes | May bind to and reduce the absorption of tetracycline, thyroxine, and other medications. |

Aluminum hydroxide/magnesium hydroxide

Proprietary name(s)	Gelusil, Maalox, and Mylanta
Therapeutic class	Antacid
Indications	Pain due to peptic ulcer disease, reflux esophagitis, and prophylaxis of stress ulcers
Actions	Buffers gastric acidity
Side effects	Diarrhea, hypermagnesemia, or aluminum toxicity in patients with renal failure
Dose	For acute symptoms, 30–60 ml PO every 1–2 hr as needed. For maintenance therapy, 30–60 ml PO every 1 to 3 hr when symptomatic and before bedtime as needed.
Notes	Aluminum salts cause constipation. Magnesium salts cause diarrhea. The mixture of the salts tends to balance the effects. May bind to and reduce the absorption of tetracycline, thyroxine, and other medications.

Amikacin — See antibiotic listing in Appendix E

Aminocaproic acid

Proprietary name(s)	Amicar
Therapeutic class	Plasminogen activator inhibitor
Indications	Hemorrhage due to fibrinolysis
Actions	Inhibits plasminogen activator; also has antiplasmin activity
Metabolism	65% of drug is excreted unchanged
Excretion	Renal
Side effects	Increased risk of deep venous thrombosis (DVT), cerebral embolism, and pulmonary embolism. Nausea, abdominal cramps, dizziness, rash, and headaches.
Dose	Loading dose of 4–5 IV g over 1 hr, followed by maintenance infusion of 1–1.25 g/hr to achieve plasma levels of 0.13 mg/ml or until clinical bleeding stops. Maximum dose, 30 g/24 hr. Loading dose may be given PO.
Notes	Rule out disseminated intravascular coagulation (DIC) before administration.

Aminophylline

Therapeutic class	Bronchodilator
Indications	Bronchospasm due to asthma
Actions	Methylxanthine; inhibits phosphodiesterase activity resulting in smooth muscle relaxation and bronchodilation. Also activates respiratory centers.
Metabolism	Hepatic (90%)
Excretion	Renal
Side effects	Tachycardia, increased ventricular ectopy, nausea, vomiting, headaches, seizures, insomnia, and nightmares
Dose	Loading dose of 6 mg/kg IV, followed by maintenance infusion of 0.5–0.7 mg/kg/hr. Use 0.5 loading dose if the patient is already taking theophylline.
Notes	May follow plasma level, but patient side effects generally limit therapeutic usefulness. Decrease the dose in patients with congestive heart failure (CHF), liver disease and elderly patients. Aminophylline clearance is decreased by erythromycin, cimetidine, propranolol, allopurinol, and a number of other medications.

Amoxicillin — See antibiotic listing in Appendix E

Amphotericin B

Proprietary name(s)	Fungizone
Therapeutic class	Polyene antifungal
Indications	Systemic fungal infections
Actions	Disruption of fungal cell membrane
Excretion	Renal
Side effects	Fever, chills, nausea, vomiting, diarrhea, hypotension, nephrotoxicity, hypokalemia, hypomagnesemia, and thrombophlebitis
Dose	Initial test dose: 0.1 mg/kg in 100 ml 50% dextrose in water IV over 2 hr. If tolerated, further doses of 10 mg may be given on the first day. Daily dose then may be increased by 0.25 mg/kg/day until the desired dose of 0.5–1.0 mg/kg/day is achieved. Administer IV over 4–6 hr.

It is more important to administer a complete total course than it is to achieve the desirable daily dose. If the patient does not tolerate that high a concentration, simply lower the daily dose and extend the length of therapy.

Notes	Patients vary with respect to how well they tolerate amphotericin B therapy. Premedicate before each dose with antipyretics, antihistamines, antiemetics, and corticosteroids to reduce side effects. Follow serial potassium and magnesium levels during therapy and watch for renal insufficiency.

Ampicillin	**See antibiotic listing in Appendix E**

Aspirin (acetylsalicylic acid)

Therapeutic class	Analgesic, antipyretic, and anti-inflammatory
Indications	Pain due to inflammation, fever, and anti-platelet aggregation agent in coronary syndromes
Actions	Acts peripherally by interfering with the production of prostaglandins, thus reducing pain and inflammation Acts centrally to reduce pain perception and reduce temperature by increasing heat loss
Side effects	Gastric erosion and bleeding, tinnitus, fever, thirst, and diaphoresis Severe allergic reactions can occur, including asthma-like symptoms
Dose	For mild pain or fever, 325–650 mg PO every 4–6 hr. For chest pain due to pericarditis, 650 mg PO 4 times per day. For angina and antiplatelet effects, 30–325 mg PO every day or every other day. For treatment of rheumatoid arthritis, 2.6–5.2 g/day in divided doses.

Aztreonam	**See antibiotic listing in Appendix E**

Beclomethasone

Proprietary name(s)	Beclovent and Vanceril
Therapeutic class	Inhaled corticosteroid
Indications	Bronchial asthma and long-term therapy

Actions	Topical anti-inflammatory
Excretion	Fecal
Side effects	Oral and pharyngeal candidiasis, laryngeal myopathy
Dose	2 inhalations 2–4 times per day. May be more effective if administered 3–5 min after a bronchodilator dose.
Notes	Not indicated for acute bronchospasm.

Bisacodyl

Proprietary name(s)	Dulcolax
Therapeutic class	Laxative
Indications	Constipation
Action	Stimulates peristalsis
Metabolism	Poorly absorbed
Side effects	Abdominal cramping, nausea, rectal burning or bleeding
Dose	10–15 mg PO every night as needed. 10-mg suppository PR every night as needed.
Notes	Avoid in pregnancy or after a myocardial infarction (MI). May worsen orthostatic hypotension, weakness, and incoordination in elderly patients. Avoid in acute abdomen, intestinal obstruction, or with recent intestinal anastomoses. Onset of action is 6–10 hr after PO dose, 15–60 min after a PR dose.

Bumetanide

Proprietary name(s)	Bumex
Therapeutic class	Loop diuretic; rapid onset, short duration of action
Indications	Edema associated with CHF, cirrhosis, renal disease, or nephrotic syndrome
Actions	Inhibits the reabsorption of Na^+ and Cl^- in the ascending limb of the loop of Henle. Increases potassium excretion.
Excretion	Renal (80%)
Side effects	Electrolyte depletion, rash, hyperuricemia, and reversible deafness
Dose	0.5–1.0 mg PO/IV per day in a single dose. May repeat every 20 min, if necessary, to a maximum of 3 mg.
Notes	1 mg bumetanide is equivalent to 40 mg furosemide.

Calcium gluconate

Therapeutic class	Calcium supplement
Indications	Symptomatic hypocalcemia, and hyperkalemia. Adjunct therapy in cardiopulmonary resuscitation (CPR)
Actions	Replacement. Decreases cardiac automaticity and raises cardiac cell resting potential.
Side effects	Administration to patients concurrently on digoxin therapy may precipitate ventricular dysrhythmias due to combined effects of digoxin and Ca^{2+}
Dose	For control of hypocalcemia, 1–15 g PO every day. For more rapid response, 5–10 ml of 10% solution IV.
Notes	500 mg of calcium gluconate = 2.3 mmol ionized Ca^{2+}. 10% solution contains 0.45 mmol ionized Ca^{2+}/ml.

Captopril

Proprietary name(s)	Capoten
Therapeutic class	Angiotensin-converting enzyme (ACE) inhibitor
Indications	Hypertension, CHF, and prophylaxis against diabetic nephropathy
Actions	Inhibits the enzyme responsible for pulmonary conversion of angiotensin I to angiotensin II
Excretion	Renal (59%)
Side effects	Hypotension, impaired taste, cough, rash, angioedema, neutropenia, proteinuria, and renal insufficiency
Dose	Begin with a test dose of 6.25 mg PO and monitor blood pressure (BP) for 4 hr. For hypertension, titrate to 25–50 mg PO 2–3 times per day. For CHF, titrate to 25–50 mg PO 3 times per day.
Notes	May cause hyperkalemia if used in patients receiving potassium-sparing diuretics or receiving potassium supplementation.

Cefazolin	**See antibiotic listing in Appendix E**
Cefotaxime	**See antibiotic listing in Appendix E**

Cefoxitin	**See antibiotic listing in Appendix E**
Ceftazidime	**See antibiotic listing in Appendix E**
Ceftriaxone	**See antibiotic listing in Appendix E**
Cefuroxime	**See antibiotic listing in Appendix E**

Chloral hydrate

Proprietary name(s)	Noctec and others
Therapeutic class	Alcohol hypnotic
Indications	Insomnia
Actions	Hypnotic
Side effects	Gastric irritation, rash, paradoxical agitation
Dose	0.5–1.0 g PO/PR every night as needed.
Notes	Avoid in patients with liver or kidney disease.

Chlordiazepoxide

Proprietary name(s)	Librium and others
Therapeutic class	Benzodiazepine
Indications	Anxiety and alcohol withdrawal
Actions	Benzodiazepine sedative, and anxiolytic agent
Metabolism	Hepatic
Excretion	Renal
Side effects	Central nervous system (CNS) depression, drowsiness, ataxia, confusion, and pruritic rash
Dose	For anxiety, 5–25 mg PO 3–4 times per day. For alcohol withdrawal, 50–100 mg intramuscularly (IM)/IV every 2–6 hr as needed, maximum dose of 500 mg in the first 24 hr.
Notes	Dose must be individualized. Unpredictable absorption after IM injection. Antidote is flumazenil.

Chlorpromazine

Proprietary name(s)	Thorazine
Therapeutic class	Phenothiazine antipsychotic and antiemetic

Indications	Agitation, nausea, vomiting, and hiccoughs
Actions	Antagonist of dopamine, histamine, muscarine, and α_1-adrenergic responses
Side effects	CNS depression, hypotension, extrapyramidal effects, and jaundice
Dose	For mild agitation, 25–75 mg PO every day. For more severe cases, 150 mg PO or every day 25–50 mg IM with repeated doses every 3–4 hr, as needed. For hiccoughs, nausea, and vomiting, 10–15 mg PO/IM every 6–8 hr.
Notes	For acute agitation, haloperidol may be a more appropriate choice as it has less effect on BP.

Chlorpropamide

Proprietary name(s)	Diabinese and others
Therapeutic class	Oral hypoglycemic agent
Indications	Non–insulin-dependent diabetes mellitus (NIDDM)
Actions	Sulfonylurea. Stimulates insulin secretion, and increases the effects of insulin on the liver to increase gluconeogenesis and on the muscle to increase glucose use.
Metabolism	Renal excretion
Side effects	Hypoglycemia, rash, blood dyscrasias, jaundice, hyponatremia, and edema
Dose	100–500 mg PO every day in 1 or 2 doses.
Notes	Has a long duration of action (20–60 hr). Hypoglycemic reactions may be prolonged in elderly patients and in those patients with renal impairment. Drug associations causing hypoglycemia: NSAIDs, salicylates, sulfonamides, chloramphenicol, cimetidine, ranitidine, probenecid, warfarin, monoamine oxidase (MAO) inhibitors, β-blockers, and metformin. Drug associations causing hyperglycemia: Thiazides, diuretics, corticosteroids, phenothiazines, thyroid hormone replacement agents, oral contraceptive agents, phenytoin, sympathomimetics, calcium channel blockers, and isoniazid.

Cimetidine

Proprietary name(s)	Tagamet
Therapeutic class	Histamine$_2$ antagonist
Indications	Peptic ulcer disease and gastroesophageal reflux
Actions	Inhibits histamine-induced secretion of gastric acid
Metabolism	Hepatic
Excretion	Renal
Side effects	Gynecomastia, impotence, confusion, diarrhea, leukopenia, thrombocytopenia, and increased serum creatinine
Dose	For peptic ulcer, 300 mg PO or IV every 6–8 hr, or 800 mg PO every night. For reflux, 400 mg PO 2 times per day.
Notes	Reduces, microsomal enzyme metabolism of medications, including oral anticoagulants, phenytoin, and theophylline.

Ciprofloxacin	**See antibiotic listing in Appendix E**

Clindamycin	**See antibiotic listing in Appendix E**

Codeine

Therapeutic class	Narcotic analgesic
Indications	Pain, cough, and diarrhea
Actions	Narcotic analgesic, depresses the medullary cough center, and decreases propulsive contractions of the small bowel
Metabolism	Hepatic
Excretion	Renal (90%)
Side Effects	Dysphoria, agitation, pruritus, constipation, lightheadedness, and sedation
Dose	For analgesia, 30–60 mg PO/subcutaneously (SC)/IM every 4–6 hr, as needed. For cough or diarrhea, 8–30 mg PO/SC/IM every 4 hr, as needed.
Notes	Useful for mild to moderate pain. May be habit forming.

Clotrimazole

Proprietary name(s)	Lotrimin and Mycelex
Therapeutic class	Antifungal
Indications	Esophageal, vaginal, and intertrigonal candidiasis
Actions	Damages fungal cell membranes
Side effects	Local irritation
Dose	For esophageal candidiasis, 10-mg troche PO 4 times per day. For vaginal candidiasis, 100 mg intravaginally every night × 7 nights. For intertrigonal candidiasis, 1% cream or solution applied 2 times per day.

Diazepam

Proprietary name(s)	Valium and others
Therapeutic class	Benzodiazepine
Indications	Anxiety, seizures, and alcohol withdrawal
Actions	Benzodiazepine sedative and anxiolytic agent
Metabolism	Hepatic (to active metabolites)
Excretion	Renal
Side effects	Sedation, hypotension, respiratory depression, and paradoxical agitation
Dose	For anxiety, 2–10 mg PO/IM/IV 2–4 times per day. For status epilepticus, 2 mg/min IV until the seizure ceases or to a total dose of 20 mg. For alcohol withdrawal, 5–10 mg IV at a rate of 2–5 mg/min every 30–60 min until the patient is sedated, then maintain on 10–20 mg PO 4 times per day.
Notes	Dose must be individualized. Unpredictable absorption after IM injection. Rectal and endotracheal tube (ET) administration possible in emergency situations. Antidote is flumazenil.

Digoxin

Proprietary name(s)	Lanoxin
Therapeutic class	Digitalis glycoside
Indications	Supraventricular tachycardia and CHF

Actions	Slows atrioventricular (AV) conduction, increases the force of cardiac contraction, and Na^+/K^+-ATPase inhibitor
Metabolism	Hepatic (<10%)
Excretion	Renal (80%)
Side effects	Dysrhythmias, nausea, vomiting, and neuropsychiatric disturbances
Dose	Load with 0.125–0.5 mg IV every 6 hr to a total dose of 1 mg, or load with 0.125–0.5 mg PO every 6 hr to a total dose of 1.5 mg, then maintain on 0.125–0.25 mg PO/IV every day. Some supraventricular tachycardias may require higher doses.
Notes	Reduce dose in elderly patients and in those patients with renal impairment. May cause arrhythmias in settings of hypokalemia or hypercalcemia.

Diltiazem

Proprietary name(s)	Cardizem
Therapeutic class	Calcium channel blocker
Indications	Angina pectoris, coronary spasm, and hypertension
Actions	Calcium channel blocker and vasodilator
Metabolism	Hepatic
Excretion	Renal and biliary
Side effects	First-degree AV block, bradycardia, flushing, dizziness, headache, peripheral edema, nausea, rash, and asthenia
Dose	Initial dose, 30 mg PO 3–4 times per day, with titration to 180–360 mg/day administered in divided doses.
Notes	Maximum antihypertensive effect is seen at 14 days. Sustained release forms are available.

Diphenhydramine

Proprietary name(s)	Benadryl
Therapeutic class	Antihistamine
Indications	Allergic reactions
Actions	Antihistamine and anticholinergic
Metabolism	Hepatic
Excretion	Renal

Side effects	Drowsiness, dizziness, dry mouth, and urinary retention
Dose	25–50 mg PO/IV/IM every 6–8 hr as needed.
Notes	Anticholinergic effects may be additive to those noted with other medications such as tricyclic antidepressants.

Docusate

Proprietary name(s)	Colace and Dialose
Therapeutic class	Laxative
Indications	Prevention of constipation
Actions	Stool softener and lowers surface tension
Side effects	Nausea and bitter taste
Dose	100 mg PO 3 times per day.
Notes	Effects not immediate, may not be noticeable for 1–2 days.

Enalapril

Proprietary name(s)	Vasotec
Therapeutic class	ACE inhibitor
Indications	Hypertension and CHF
Actions	Inhibits the enzyme responsible for conversion of angiotensin I to angiotensin II
Metabolism	Hepatic (to active metabolite, enalaprilat)
Excretion	Renal
Side effects	Hypotension, headache, nausea, and diarrhea
Dose	Begin with a test dose of 2.5 mg PO and monitor BP for 4 hr. For hypertension, titrate to 2.5–40 mg PO every day. For CHF, titrate to 10–25 mg PO 2 times per day.
Notes	May cause hyperkalemia if used in patients receiving potassium-sparing diuretics or receiving potassium supplementation.

Erythromycin   See antibiotic listing in Appendix E

Ethacrynic acid

Proprietary name(s)	Edecrin

Therapeutic class	Loop diuretic
Indications	CHF and edema
Actions	Inhibition of the reabsorption of Na^+ and Cl^- in the ascending limb of the loop of Henle
Side effects	Electrolyte depletion, hyperuricemia, hyperglycemia, anorexia, nausea, vomiting, diarrhea, and sensorineural hearing loss
Dose	50 mg IV × 1 or 2 doses.
Notes	May have more side effects than other loop diuretics. Onset is rapid, within 30 min of a PO dose or within 5 min of an IV dose.

Famotidine

Proprietary name(s)	Pepcid
Therapeutic class	Histamine$_2$ antagonist
Indications	Peptic ulcer disease and gastroesophageal reflux
Actions	Inhibits histamine-induced secretion of gastric acid
Metabolism	Hepatic (to inactive metabolite)
Excretion	Renal (70%)
Side effects	Headache, dizziness, constipation, diarrhea, GI upset, and rash
Dose	For acute disease, 40 mg PO every day or 20 mg IV 2 times per day. For maintenance, 20 mg PO every night.
Notes	Less effect on microsomal enzymes or androgen blocking than cimetidine.

Ferrous sulfate

Therapeutic class	Iron supplement
Indications	Iron deficiency
Actions	Replaces iron stores
Side effects	Constipation, nausea, diarrhea, and abdominal cramping
Dose	325 mg PO 3 times per day.
Notes	300 mg ferrous sulfate = 60 mg elemental iron. Stool may turn black. GI absorption enhanced on an empty stomach with concomitant vitamin C

administration (200 mg vitamin C/30 mg iron).

Iron stores will not be completely replaced for up to 4–6 mo of therapy after normalization of the hematocrit.

Fluconazole

Proprietary name(s)	Diflucan
Therapeutic class	Antifungal
Indications	Orthopharyngeal, esophageal, and systemic candidiasis; cryptococcal meningitis
Actions	Inhibition of cell membranes of yeasts and fungi
Excretion	Renal
Side effects	Nausea, vomiting, headache, rash, abdominal pain, diarrhea, and hepatic necrosis
Dose	For oral or esophageal disease, initial dose of 200 mg PO followed by 100 mg PO every day. For systemic candidiasis and cryptococcal meningitis, 200–400 mg PO every day. Reduce the dose in those patients with renal impairment.
Notes	Many drug interactions due to the microsomal enzyme inhibition, including sulfonylureas, phenytoin, warfarin, and cyclophosphamide.

Flumazenil

Proprietary name(s)	Romazicon
Therapeutic class	Benzodiazepine antagonist
Indications	Reversal of benzodiazepine-induced sedation
Actions	Benzodiazepine receptor antagonist
Metabolism	Hepatic
Excretion	Renal
Side effects	Seizures, headache, vasodilation, nausea, vomiting, agitation, dizziness, abnormal vision, and paresthesias
Dose	For reversal of sedation, 0.2 mg IV over 15 sec. Repeat as necessary in increments of 0.2 mg every 60 sec, to a maximum dose of 1 mg.

For treatment of benzodiazepine overdose, 0.2 mg IV over 30 sec.
An additional 0.3 mg IV may be administered after 30 sec, if necessary.
Further doses of 0.5 mg may be given IV every 30 sec as needed to a maximum of 3 mg.

Notes | Avoid in patients with evidence of cyclic antidepressant overdose.
Does not reverse benzodiazepine-induced respiratory depression.
Monitor for return of benzodiazepine-related symptoms of sedation and respiratory depression.

Furosemide

Proprietary name(s)	Lasix
Therapeutic class	Loop diuretic
Indications	CHF, edema, hyperkalemia, and hypercalcemia
Actions	Inhibition of the reabsorption of Na^+ and Cl^- in the ascending limb of the loop of Henle
Metabolism	Hepatic
Excretion	Renal
Side effects	Electrolyte depletion, hyperuricemia, hyperglycemia, and reversible deafness
Dose	For acute pulmonary edema, 20–40 mg PO/IV with repeat doses every 60–90 min as needed, to a maximum of 600 mg/day. Higher doses may be required in patients with severe disease or renal failure.
Notes	Loop diuretics are well absorbed orally with rapid onset of action.

Gentamicin   See antibiotic listing in Appendix E

Haloperidol

Proprietary name(s)	Haldol
Therapeutic class	Antipsychotic
Indications	Psychotic disorders and acute agitation
Actions	Antipsychotic neuroleptic butyrophenone
Side effects	Extrapyramidal reactions, postural hypotension, sedation, galactorrhea, jaundice, blurred vision, bronchospasm, and neuroleptic malignant syndrome
Dose	0.5–2.0 mg PO 3 times per day.

For acute psychotic crises, 2–10 mg IM every 1 hr as needed.

Notes	Extrapyramidal side effects are more pronounced, but hypotension is less frequent than with phenothiazines.

Heparin sodium

Therapeutic class	Anticoagulant
Indications	Prophylaxis and treatment of DVT, pulmonary embolism, embolic costovertebral angle (CVA). Adjunct in treatment of unstable angina, and thrombolytic therapy.
Actions	Acts in conjunction with antithrombin III, which neutralizes several activated clotting factors. Antithrombin effect.
Metabolism	Hepatic
Excretion	Renal
Side effects	Hemorrhage and thrombocytopenia
Dose	For DVT or pulmonary embolus, load IV with 5000–10,000 U followed by continuous infusion of 1000–2000 U/hr IV. Low-dose SC: 5000 U every 8–12 hr. High-dose SC: 10,000–12,500 U every 8–12 hr. Titrate to desired partial thromboplastin time (PTT) (generally 1.5–2 × control).
Notes	Monitor PTT closely. Also prolongs prothrombin time (PT). Overheparinization is treated with protamine sulfate. Usual dose is 1 mg protamine/100 U heparin given slowly IV.

Hydralazine

Proprietary name(s)	Apresoline
Therapeutic class	Arterial vasodilator
Indications	Hypertension
Actions	Arterial vasodilator
Metabolism	Hepatic
Side effects	Tachycardia, headache, blood dyscrasias, nausea, vomiting, diarrhea, systemic lupus erythematosus (SLE) reaction at higher doses (>200 mg/day)
Dose	10–25 mg PO every 6 hr. 20–40 mg IV/IM every 3–6 hr as needed.

| Notes | Very limited effect on veins, so minimal postural hypotension.
Monitor carefully in patients with coronary artery disease. |

Hydrochlorothiazide

Proprietary name(s)	Esidrix and HydroDIURIL
Therapeutic class	Thiazide diuretic
Indications	Hypertension, CHF, and edema
Actions	Blocks Na^+ and Cl^- reabsorption in the cortical diluting segment of the loop of Henle
Excretion	Renal
Side effects	Electrolyte depletion, hyperuricemia, hyperglycemia, hypercalcemia, pancreatitis, jaundice, nausea, vomiting, and diarrhea
Dose	12.5–50 mg PO every day.
Notes	Adequate potassium replacement necessary with long-term therapy.

Hydrocortisone

Therapeutic class	Corticosteroid
Indications	Severe bronchospasm, anaphylaxis, hypercalcemia, and adrenal insufficiency
Actions	Anti-inflammatory
Side effects	Na^+ retention, hyperglycemia, and K^+ loss. Behavioral disturbances.
Dose	250 mg IV followed by 100 mg IV every 6 hr.
Notes	Contraindicated in settings of systemic fungal infections.

Hydroxyzine

Proprietary name(s)	Atarax and Vistaril
Therapeutic class	Antihistamine and antiemetic
Indications	Anxiety, pruritus, nausea, and vomiting
Actions	Suppression of activity in subcortical CNS sites
Metabolism	Hepatic
Side effects	Drowsiness, dry mouth, and tremor
Dose	For anxiety, 50–100 mg PO/IM 4 times per day.
For pruritus or nausea, 25–100 mg PO/IM 3–4 times per day.

Notes	May potentiate the sedation effects of other CNS depressants.

Ibuprofen

Proprietary name(s)	Motrin and others
Therapeutic class	NSAID
Indications	Inflammation due to arthritis, soft-tissue injuries, and analgesia
Actions	Propionic acid derivative. Interferes with the production of prostaglandins.
Metabolism	Hepatic
Excretion	Renal
Side effects	Nausea, diarrhea, gastric pain, gastric erosions, dizziness, headache, tinnitus, and vision changes. May compromise renal function in patients with renal impairment. Contraindicated in the syndrome of aspirin sensitivity, nasal polyps, and bronchospasm.
Dose	For analgesia, 200 mg PO 3–4 times per day. For anti-inflammatory effects, 200–400 mg PO 3–4 times per day. Maximum dose: 3200 mg/day.
Notes	Available in many over-the-counter preparations. Should be used with caution in patients receiving anticoagulant medications.

Imipenem   See antibiotic listing in Appendix E

Indomethacin

Proprietary name(s)	Indocin
Therapeutic class	NSAID
Indications	Inflammation due to arthritis, acute gout, soft-tissue injury, and pericarditis
Actions	Indole acetic acid derivative. Interferes with the production of prostaglandins.
Metabolism	Hepatic
Excretion	Renal
Side effects	Headache, dizziness and lightheadedness, and epigastric pain. May compromise renal function in patients with renal impairment. Contraindicated in the syndrome of aspirin sensitivity, nasal polyps, and bronchospasm.

Dose	25–50 mg PO 3 times per day. Maximum daily dose: 150–200 mg/day.
Notes	May increase the risk of bleeding in patients receiving anticoagulants. Take with food to minimize GI upset.

Insulin

Therapeutic class	Hypoglycemic
Indications	Diabetes mellitus
Actions	Enhances hepatic glycogen storage, enhances entry of glucose and potassium into cells, and inhibits the breakdown of protein and fat
Side effects	Hypoglycemia, local skin reactions, and lipohypertrophy
Dose	Must be individualized. See Chapter 14.
Notes	Less immunogenicity is seen with recombinant human insulin than with insulins from animal sources.

Isosorbide dinitrate

Proprietary name(s)	Isordil and Sorbitrate
Therapeutic class	Vasodilator
Indications	Angina pectoris and CHF
Actions	Venous, coronary, and arterial vasodilator
Side effects	Headache, hypotension, and flushing
Dose	5–30 mg PO 4 times per day.
Notes	Nitrate tolerance may develop with prolonged continuous administration.

Ketoconazole

Proprietary name(s)	Nizoral
Therapeutic class	Imidazole antifungal
Indications	Esophageal candidiasis, pulmonary histoplasmosis
Actions	Inhibition of yeast and fungal cell growth
Metabolism	Hepatic
Excretion	Biliary (>80%)
Side effects	Nausea, anorexia, vomiting, rash, pruritus, gynecomastia, and impotence. Inhibits microsomal enzymes, so may interfere with the metabolism of warfarin, cyclophosphamide, and other medications.
Dose	200–400 mg PO every day.

Notes   Absorption is impaired in patients
                         receiving medications that reduce gastric
                         acidity.

Labetalol

Proprietary name(s)   Normodyne and Trandate

Therapeutic class α_1- and β-blocker

Indications   Hypertensive emergencies

Actions α_1-blocking action is predominant in acute
                         use but is accompanied by nonspecific β-
                         blockade

Metabolism   Hepatic

Excretion   Renal

Side effects   Postural hypotension, bronchospasm,
                         jaundice, bradycardia, and negative
                         inotropic effect. Avoid in patients with
                         asthma or with severe bradycardia.

Dose   20 mg IV every 10–15 min.
                         Increase the dose incrementally (e.g., 20
                         mg, 20 mg, 40 mg, 40 mg . . .) every 10
                         min until the desired supine BP is
                         achieved.
                         Alternatively, a continuous drip may be
                         started at 2 mg/min with titration to
                         desired BP response, with a maximum
                         daily dose of 2400 mg.

Notes   Contraindicated in patients in whom β-
                         blockade is undesirable.

Levodopa–Carbidopa

Proprietary name(s)   Sinemet

Therapeutic class   Dopamine agonist

Indications   Parkinson's disease

Actions   Levodopa is converted to dopamine in the
                         basal ganglia.
                         Carbidopa inhibits the peripheral
                         destruction of levodopa.

Side effects   Anorexia, nausea, vomiting, abdominal
                         pain, dysrhythmias, behavioral changes,
                         orthostatic hypotension, and involuntary
                         motions

Dose   Begin with 1 tablet (100 mg/10 mg) PO 2
                         times per day.
                         Increase the dose until the desired
                         response is obtained, with a maximum
                         daily dose of 8 tablets (800 mg/8 mg).

| Notes | Side effects are common. |

Lidocaine

Proprietary name(s)	Xylocaine
Therapeutic class	Class IB antiarrhythmic
Indications	Ventricular arrhythmias, prophylaxis, and treatment
Actions	Lengthens the effective refractory period in the ventricular conduction system. Decreases ventricular automaticity.
Metabolism	Hepatic
Excretion	Renal
Side effects	Nausea, vomiting, hypotension, confusion, seizures, perioral paresthesias, drowsiness, and dizziness
Dose	Load with 1 mg/kg IV over 2–3 min. Further doses of 50 mg IV may be given at 5–10-min intervals to a total dose of 300 mg. Maintain with 1–4 mg/min continuous IV infusion. For prophylaxis, a loading dose of 200 mg given in 50-mg increments every 5 min, followed by maintenance IV infusion of 3 mg/min.
Notes	Lower maintenance doses are required in elderly patients or in those with CHF, hepatic failure, or hypotension.

Lorazepam

Proprietary name(s)	Ativan
Therapeutic class	Benzodiazepine
Indications	Insomnia and anxiety
Actions	Benzodiazepine sedative-hypnotic
Metabolism	Hepatic
Excretion	Renal
Side effects	Sedation and respiratory depression
Dose	For sleep, 0.5–1.0 mg PO/IM every night. For anxiety, 1 mg PO/IM 2 times per day. Maximum dose: 4 mg/dose.
Notes	Peak effect in 1–6 hr. Antidote is flumazenil.

Mannitol

Proprietary name(s)	Osmitrol

Therapeutic class	Osmotic diuretic
Indications	Peripheral edema, cerebral edema, and hemolytic transfusion reactions
Actions	Osmotic diuresis
Excretion	Renal
Side effects	Volume overload, hyperosmolality, hyponatremia, nausea, and headache
Dose	Test dose of 12.5 g over 3–5 min. Effects should be noted within 2 hr. 25–100 g IV over 15–30 min every 2–3 hr as needed.
Notes	Requires functioning kidneys to work, contraindicated in renal failure. Monitor electrolytes.

Meperidine

Proprietary name(s)	Demerol
Therapeutic class	Narcotic analgesic
Indications	Moderate to severe pain
Actions	Narcotic analgesic
Metabolism	Hepatic
Excretion	Renal
Side effects	Respiratory depression, hypotension, nausea, vomiting, constipation, agitation, and rash
Dose	50–150 mg SC/IM/PO every 4 hr.
Notes	60–80 mg meperidine (SC/IM/PO) is equivalent to 10 mg morphine (SC/IV). Often administered with concomitant antinausea medication. Antidote is naloxone. May be habit forming.

Metaproterenol

Proprietary name(s)	Alupent and Metaprel
Therapeutic class	β_2-adrenergic agonist
Indications	Bronchospasm due to asthma, bronchitis, or COPD
Actions	β_2-adrenergic agonist
Metabolism	Hepatic. 3% of aerosol dose is systemically absorbed.
Side effects	Headache, tachycardia, hypertension, lightheadedness, dizziness, tremor, palpitations, nausea, and vomiting

Dose	0.2–0.3 mg in 3 ml NS by nebulizer every 4 hr as needed. Severe acute bronchospasm may require doses every 3–5 min initially.
Notes	May alternate with albuterol.

Metformin

Proprietary name(s)	Glucophage
Therapeutic class	Antihyperglycemic agent
Indications	NIDDM as monotherapy or in conjunction with sulfonylureas.
Actions	Decreases hepatic glucose production, decreases intestinal absorption of glucose, and increases peripheral glucose uptake and utilization
Excretion	Renal
Side effects	Lactic acidosis, diarrhea, nausea, vomiting, abdominal bloating, flatulence, and anorexia
Dose	Dose must be individualized. Start with 500 mg PO 2 times per day and increase to desired blood glucose effect, to a maximum daily dose of 2500 mg. Decrease dose in renal failure.
Notes	Hypoglycemic reactions are not seen as with sulfonylureas.

Metolazone

Proprietary name(s)	Zaroxolyn
Therapeutic class	Quinazoline diuretic
Indications	Hypertension, CHF, edema, and some types of renal failure
Actions	Blocks Na^+ and Cl^- reabsorption in the cortical diluting segment of the loop of Henle
Excretion	Renal
Side effects	Electrolyte depletion, hyperuricemia, hyperglycemia, and hypomagnesemia. Do not use in anuric patients.
Dose	2.5–10 mg PO every day.
Notes	Similar properties to thiazide diuretics but longer acting than hydrochlorothiazide. Monitor electrolytes. Additive effects when administered with furosemide.

Metronidazole	**See antibiotic listing in Appendix E**

Midazolam

Proprietary name(s)	Versed
Therapeutic class	Benzodiazepine
Indications	Sedation before surgery or diagnostic procedure
Actions	Benzodiazepine sedative-hypnotic
Side effects	Sedation, paradoxical agitation, respiratory depression
Dose	Induction dose, 0.20–0.35 mg/kg IV as needed over 20–30 sec. Reduce dose in elderly patients and in those already receiving other sedative medications.
Notes	Inject slowly to avoid complications of respiratory depression and hypotension. Should be used with appropriate monitoring for respiratory complications. Antidote is flumazenil.

Misoprostol

Proprietary name(s)	Cytotec
Therapeutic class	Synthetic prostaglandin E_1 analogue
Indications	Prophylaxis of NSAID-related gastric ulcers
Actions	Inhibits gastric acid secretion and protects mucosal cells
Excretion	Renal (80%)
Side effects	Diarrhea, abdominal pain, nausea, headache, flatulence, and dyspepsia
Dose	0.1–0.2 mg PO 4 times per day with food.
Notes	Do not administer to pregnant women.

Morphine sulfate

Therapeutic class	Narcotic analgesic
Indications	Moderate to severe pain and pulmonary edema
Actions	Narcotic analgesic and splanchnic venodilation
Metabolism	Hepatic
Excretion	Renal (90%) and biliary (7–10%)
Side effects	Respiratory depression, hypotension, sedation, nausea, vomiting, and constipation
Dose	For pulmonary edema or chest pain due to

coronary ischemia, 2–4 mg IV every 5–10 min to a maximum dose of 10–12 mg.
For pain, 2–15 mg IV/IM/SC every 4 hr as needed.

Notes	10 mg morphine (IM/SC) is equivalent to 60–80 mg meperidine (IM/SC/PO). Often administered with concomitant antinausea medication. May be habit forming. Antidote is naloxone.

Naloxone hydrochloride

Proprietary name(s)	Narcan
Therapeutic class	Narcotic antagonist
Indications	Reversal of narcotic-induced effects
Actions	Narcotic receptor antagonist
Metabolism	Hepatic
Excretion	Renal
Side effects	Nausea, vomiting, and may precipitate withdrawal in narcotic abusers
Dose	0.2–2.0 mg IV/IM, SC every 5 min to a maximum dose of 10 mg.
Notes	Effects are shorter than most narcotics. Monitor for return of narcotic-induced symptoms, and repeat naloxone dose as necessary. May be administered via ET in emergency situations.

Naproxen

Proprietary name(s)	Naprosyn
Therapeutic class	NSAID
Indications	Inflammation due to arthritis, soft-tissue injury, and pericarditis.
Actions	Propionic acid derivative; interferes with production of prostaglandins
Metabolism	Hepatic
Excretion	Renal
Side effects	Headaches, dizziness and lightheadedness, and epigastric pain. May compromise renal function in patients with renal impairment. Contraindicated in the syndrome of aspirin sensitivity, nasal polyps, and bronchospasm.

Dose	250 mg PO 2 times per day. Maximum dose: 1250 mg/day.
Notes	Should be used with caution in patients receiving anticoagulant medications.

Nifedipine

Proprietary name(s)	Adalat and Procardia
Therapeutic class	Calcium channel blocker
Indications	Angina pectoris, coronary spasm, and hypertension
Actions	Calcium channel blocker and vasodilator
Metabolism	Hepatic
Excretion	Renal (80%)
Side effects	Hypotension, flushing, dizziness, headache, and peripheral edema
Dose	10–30 mg PO 3 times per day. Maximum dose: 180 mg/day.
Notes	The edema due to nifedipine is due to vasodilation and does not respond to diuretics. Hypotension is often difficult to treat with fluids alone and may require vasopressor agent administration. Nifedipine has a greater effect than verapamil and diltiazem in peripheral vasculature.

Nitroglycerin

Therapeutic class	Vasodilator
Indications	Angina pectoris and CHF
Actions	Venous, coronary, and arterial vasodilation
Metabolism	Hepatic
Excretion	Renal
Side effects	Headache, hypotension, and flushing
Dose	Sublingual (SL) 0.15–0.6 mg every 3–5 min. Lingual aerosol 1–2 sprays onto or under the tongue every 3–5 min to a maximun dose of 3 sprays/15 min. Transdermal patch 0.2 mg/hr, increasing to 0.4 mg/hr. Patch should be left on for 10–12 hr then removed for 12–14 hr to avoid tolerance. Transdermal paste 0.5–4 inches every 4–8 hr. Rotate sites.

Oral (sustained-release) 2–9 mg PO 2–3
times per day.
IV 0–3 µg/kg/min. Titrate to desired BP.

Notes | Nitrate tolerance may develop with
prolonged continuous administration.
Dose must be individualized.

Nystatin

Proprietary name(s)	Mycostatin and Nilstat
Therapeutic class	Antifungal
Indications	Oral and esophageal candidiasis
Actions	Disruption of fungal cell membranes
Excretion	Fecal for a PO dose
Side effects	Minimal; nausea and vomiting
Dose	400,000–600,000 U PO swish and swallow 4 times per day.
Notes	Not absorbed orally.

Omeprazole

Proprietary name(s)	Prilosec
Therapeutic class	H^+/K^+-ATPase inhibitor
Indications	Active peptic ulcer disease, gastroesophageal reflux, severe erosive esophagitis, gastric acid hypersecretion
Actions	Gastric acid pump inhibitor
Excretion	Renal (77%), remainder biliary
Side effects	Headache, diarrhea, abdominal pain, nausea, vomiting, rash, dizziness
Dose	For ulcer, reflux and esophagitis, 20 mg PO every day. For hypersecretion syndromes, start with 60 mg PO every day, increase to 120 mg 3 times per day as required to achieve desired results.
Notes	Not recommended for long-term maintenance therapy.

Oxazepam

Proprietary name(s)	Serax
Therapeutic class	Benzodiazepine
Indications	Insomnia and anxiety
Actions	Benzodiazepine sedative-hypnotic
Side effects	Sedation, respiratory depression, and confusion

Dose	For sleep, 10–30 mg PO every night as needed. For anxiety, 30–100 mg PO every day in divided doses.
Notes	Peak effect in 1–4 hr. Relatively short duration. Antidote is flumazenil.

Penicillin	**See antibiotic listing in Appendix E**

Pentamidine isethionate

Proprietary name(s)	Pentam
Therapeutic class	Anti-PCP agent
Indications	*Pneumocystis carinii* pneumonia (PCP)
Actions	Unknown
Excretion	Renal
Side effects	Hypotension, renal failure, cardiac arrhythmias, hypoglycemia, and pancreatitis
Dose	4 mg/kg/day in 50–250 ml 5% dextrose in water IV over 2 hr. Reduce dose in renal-impaired patients.

Phenazopyridine

Proprietary name(s)	Pyridium
Therapeutic class	Urinary analgesic
Indications	Cystitis and urethritis
Actions	Analgesic effect on inflamed urinary tract mucosa
Excretion	Renal
Side effects	Orange discoloration of secretions including urine, tears, and semen; nausea, headache, rash, and pruritus
Dose	200 mg PO 3 times per day after meals, as needed.
Notes	No antibacterial effects. May stain contact lenses.

Phenytoin

Proprietary name(s)	Dilantin
Therapeutic class	Anticonvulsant
Indications	Seizure disorders, prophylaxis, and treatment
Actions	Anticonvulsant and reduces Na^+ transport across cerebral cell membranes

Metabolism	At therapeutic doses, phenytoin is metabolized by the liver in zero-order kinetics (a fixed amount of drug is metabolized per unit time). Relatively small changes in the dose can cause major changes in serum concentrations in the long term. Serum levels are greatly affected by medications altering microsomal enzyme activity.
Excretion	Renal
Side effects	Hypotension, cardiac dysrhythmias, ataxia, nystagmus, dysarthria, hepatotoxicity, gingival hypertrophy, hirsutism, megaloblastic anemia, lymphadenopathy, fever, and rash
Dose	For status epilepticus, 18 mg/kg IV in NS loading dose at a rate of 25–50 mg/min, followed by a maintenance dose of 300 mg PO/IV every day.
Notes	Dose must be individualized. Follow serum levels. IM administration is erratically absorbed. Abrupt withdrawal may precipitate seizure activity.

Phytonadione (vitamin K₁)

Proprietary name(s)	AquaMEPHYTON
Therapeutic class	Vitamin replacement
Indications	Replacement in vitamin K deficiency and reversal of warfarin effects
Actions	Vitamin K is essential for hepatic synthesis of clotting factors II, VII, IX, and X
Side effects	Hematoma formation with SC/IM administration
Dose	For reversal of overcoumarinization: 2.5–5.0 mg PO/SC/IM. For vitamin supplementation in total parenteral nutrition (TPN): 2.5 mg IM weekly.
Notes	Avoid IV administration because of hypotension and anaphylaxis. Severe hemorrhage due to warfarin therapy is best treated with fresh frozen plasma. The effects of vitamin K take several days to overcome with continuous warfarin therapy.

Piperacillin	**See antibiotic listing in Appendix E**

Potassium

Proprietary name(s)	Slow K, Micro-K, and Kay Ciel
Therapeutic class	Potassium supplement
Indications	Hypokalemia
Actions	Potassium supplement
Side effects	Nausea, vomiting, diarrhea, abdominal discomfort, and hyperkalemia
Dose	For prevention, 24–40 mEq/day. For treatment, 60–120 mEq/day.
Notes	Danger of hyperkalemia in patients with renal impairment, patients receiving potassium-sparing diuretics, and in those on ACE inhibitors.

Procainamide

Proprietary name(s)	Procan
Therapeutic class	Class IA antiarrhythmic
Indications	Atrial and ventricular arrhythmias
Actions	Reduces the maximum rate of depolarization in atrial and ventricular conducting tissues
Metabolism	Hepatic
Excretion	Renal
Side effects	Hypotension, anorexia, nausea, vomiting, heart block, proarrhythmia, rash, fever, SLE-like syndrome, and arthralgias
Dose	Load with 1 g PO followed by 250–500 mg PO every 3 hr. Delayed-release formulations may be given every 6 hr. For life-threatening tachydysrhythmias, 100 mg IV over 2 min, repeating the dose until the arrhythmia abates or to a maximum dose of 1 g. Follow with a maintenance infusion of 2–4 mg/min.
Notes	Actions are similar to quinidine except no atropinic effect. Cross-allergic with procaine.

Prochlorperazine

Proprietary name(s)	Compazine
Therapeutic class	Phenothiazine
Indications	Agitation, nausea, and vomiting
Actions	Antagonist of dopamine, histamine, muscarine, and α_1-adrenergic responses

Metabolism	Hepatic, with enterohepatic recirculation
Excretion	Renal
Side effects	Drowsiness, dizziness, amenorrhea, blurred vision, skin reactions, hypotension, extrapyramidal effects, jaundice, tardive dyskinesia, and neuroleptic malignant syndrome
Dose	For nausea, 5–10 mg PO/IM every 6–8 hr, as needed, or 2.5–10 mg IV every 6–8 hr, as needed.
Notes	Extrapyramidal symptoms may be treated with diphenhydramine.

Promethazine

Proprietary name(s)	Phenergan
Therapeutic class	Phenothiazine
Indications	Sedation, antianxiety, nausea, and vomiting
Actions	Antihistamine and anticholinergic
Metabolism	Hepatic
Excretion	Renal and fecal
Side effects	Extrapyramidal symptoms, drowsiness, dizziness, constipation, dry mouth, and urinary retention
Dose	25–50 mg PO/PR/IM every 4–6 hr, as needed. 12.5–25 mg IV every 4–6 hr, as needed.
Notes	Anticholinergic effects are additive with those of other medications such as tricyclic antidepressants.

Propranolol

Proprietary name(s)	Inderal
Therapeutic class	Nonspecific β-blocker
Indications	Angina pectoris, post-MI treatment of supraventricular tachycardia (SVT), hypertension, and thyrotoxicosis
Actions	Nonspecific β-blockade
Metabolism	Hepatic
Excretion	Renal (<1%)
Side effects	Hypotension, bradycardia, bronchospasm, CHF, nausea, vomiting, fatigue, nightmares, and may mask symptoms of hypoglycemia
Dose	10–80 mg PO 2–4 times per day.

| | Begin with a low dose and adjust to desired effect. |
| Notes | Abrupt withdrawal may precipitate symptoms of angina in patients with coronary artery disease. Dose must be individualized. |

Protamine sulfate

Therapeutic class	Heparin antagonist
Indications	Reversal of heparin-induced anticoagulation
Actions	Binds to and inactivates heparin
Side effects	Hypotension, bradycardia, and flushing
Dose	1 mg/100 mg heparin. Administer by slow IV push, no more than 50 mg in a 10-min period.
Notes	Overdosage may paradoxically worsen hemorrhage as protamine also possesses anticoagulant properties. Effects may be transient.

Quinine sulfate

Proprietary name(s)	Quinamm
Therapeutic class	Antimalarial
Indications	Nocturnal leg cramps
Actions	Increases muscular refractory period, decreases motor endplate excitability, and affects the distribution of calcium within the muscle fiber
Side effects	Nausea, visual disturbances, hemolytic anemia, and thrombocytopenia
Dose	300 mg PO every night as needed.
Notes	Side effects are unusual at this dose, which is $\frac{1}{10}$ that used to treat malaria.

Ranitidine

Proprietary name(s)	Zantac
Therapeutic class	Histamine$_2$ antagonist
Indications	Peptic ulcer disease and gastroesophageal reflux
Actions	Inhibits histamine-induced secretion of gastric acid
Metabolism	Hepatic
Excretion	Renal (30% of PO dose, 70% of IV dose)

Side effects	Jaundice, gynecomastia, headache, confusion, and leukopenia
Dose	For acute symptoms, 50 mg IV every 8 hr or 150 mg PO 2 times per day or 300 mg PO every night. For maintenance therapy, 150 mg PO every night.
Notes	Generally well tolerated. Does not have the same effect as cimetidine on microsomal enzymes or androgen blocking.

Retinol (vitamin A)

Proprietary name(s)	Aquasol A
Therapeutic class	Vitamin replacement
Indications	Replacement in vitamin A deficiency
Actions	Vitamin A is essential in the production of rhodopsin in the eye and preserves the integrity of epithelial cells
Metabolism	Fat-soluble vitamin, stored in liver and excreted in feces
Side effects	Due to overdose. Fatigue, malaise, lethargy, abdominal discomfort, anorexia, nausea, irritability, headache, and skin changes.
Dose	100,000–500,000 U every day $\times$ 3 days PO/IM, followed by 50,000 U PO/IM every day $\times$ 2 mo.
Notes	May facilitate wound healing in steroid-dependent patients.

Sodium polystyrene sulfonate

Proprietary name(s)	Kayexalate
Therapeutic class	Cation exchange resin
Indications	Hyperkalemia
Actions	Nonabsorbable cation exchange resin
Side effects	Nausea, vomiting, gastric irritation, and sodium retention
Dose	15–30 g in 50–100 ml NS, or 20% sorbitol PO every 3–4 hr, or 50 g in 200 ml 20% sorbitol of 20% dextrose in water PR by retention enema for 30–60 min.
Notes	20 mEq of Na^+ are exchanged for 20 mEq K^+ for each 15 g resin given PO. Mg^{2+} and Ca^{2+} may also be exchanged. Actual results are highly variable.

Spironolactone

Proprietary name(s)	Aldactone
Therapeutic class	Aldosterone antagonist and diuretic
Indications	Ascites, edema, hypertension, and hyperaldosteronism
Actions	Aldosterone antagonist
Metabolism	Hepatic (into many active metabolites)
Excretion	Renal > biliary
Side effects	Hyponatremia, gynecomastia, confusion, and headache
Dose	50–100 mg PO per day (may be divided into 4 doses per day as desired). Higher doses may be required in states of hyperaldosteronism.
Notes	Most effective in states of hyperaldosteronism; however, equipotent to thiazide diuretics in the treatment of hypertension.

Sucralfate

Proprietary name(s)	Carafate
Therapeutic class	Sulfated disaccharide
Indications	Peptic ulcer disease, prophylaxis, and treatment
Actions	Formation of an ulcer-adherent complex that acts as a barrier to damage from gastric acid, bile salts, and pepsin; minimal antacid properties
Excretion	Fecal, not absorbed
Side effects	Side effects are rare: constipation, nausea, gastric discomfort, pruritus, rash, dizziness, headache, insomnia, and vertigo
Dose	1 g PO 4 times per day.
Notes	May reduce the absorption and effects of many medications including cimetidine, ciprofloxacin, digoxin, ketoconazole, norfloxacin, phenytoin, ranitidine, tetracycline, and theophylline. Sucralfate binds and sequesters aluminum. Use with caution in renally impaired patients.

Sumatriptan succinate

Proprietary name(s)	Imitrex
Indications	Intermittent treatment of migraine

Actions	Selective 5-hydroxytryptamine-like receptor agonist Causes vasoconstriction, particularly of the dilated carotid circulation in migraine disorder
Side effects	May cause coronary artery spasm. Contraindicated in patients with coronary artery disease, concomitant use of ergot alkaloid medication, concomitant use of MAO inhibitors, uncontrolled hypertension, or hemiplegic migraine disorder. Flushing, dizziness, feelings of heat, pressure, malaise, fatigue, drowsiness, nausea, and vomiting
Dose	6 mg SC or 100 mg PO. If initial dose is partially or completely successful, may repeat doses with an additional 6 mg SC or 100 mg. Do not exceed a maximum daily PO dose of 300 mg. Do not repeat if initial dose has no effect.
Notes	Peak effect in 15 min with SC dose, in 0.5–5 hr with PO dose.

Tetracycline	**See antibiotic listing in Appendix E**

Thiamine (vitamin B₁)

Therapeutic class	Vitamin replacement
Indications	Thiamine deficiency and prophylaxis of Wernicke's encephalopathy
Actions	Water soluble vitamin B_1 replacement
Side effects	IV administration associated with hypotension or anaphylactic shock
Dose	100 mg PO/IM/IV every day × 3 days. If given IV, administer over 5 min.
Notes	Well absorbed orally. Consider the PO route, even in emergencies.

Tobramycin	**See antibiotic listing in Appendix E**

Vancomycin	**See antibiotic listing in Appendix E**

Verapamil

Proprietary name(s)	Isoptin and Calan
Therapeutic class	Calcium channel blocker
Indications	Angina pectoris, treatment of SVTs,

	hypertension, and left ventricular diastolic dysfunction
Actions	Calcium channel blockade and depresses AV conduction
Metabolism	Hepatic
Excretion	Renal (70%) and fecal
Side effects	CHF, bradycardia, hypotension, headache, dizziness, and constipation
Dose	For angina and hypertension, 80–120 mg PO 3 times per day. For SVT, 5–10 mg IV; IV administration should only occur in monitored patients.
Notes	Calcium gluconate 1–2 g IV may reverse the negative inotropic and hypotensive effects, but not the AV block.

Warfarin

Proprietary name(s)	Coumadin
Therapeutic class	Oral anticoagulant
Indications	Prophylaxis and treatment or DVT, pulmonary embolism, and embolic CVA
Actions	Inhibits vitamin K–dependent clotting factors
Metabolism	Hepatic and microsomal
Excretion	Renal
Side effects	Hemorrhage, nausea, vomiting, skin necrosis, fever, and rash
Dose	10 mg PO every day × 2 days, then estimate maintenance dose at 5–7.5 mg every day PO based on PT.
Notes	Dosage must be individualized to maintain PT in the desired range. Many medications interact to increase or decrease the effects of warfarin. Always look up the interactions with warfarin of any newly prescribed medication. Fresh frozen plasma is the treatment of choice to reverse warfarin-associated hemorrhage. Vitamin K is used if further warfarin therapy is not desired.

APPENDIX E

ANTIBIOTIC STANDARD DOSES AND SUSCEPTIBILITY GUIDELINES

Table E–1 □ ANTIBIOTIC STANDARD DOSES AND INDICATIONS FOR PATIENTS WITH NORMAL RENAL FUNCTION

Drug	Dosage Range (g/day) IV/IM*	Usual Dosage (g/dosing interval) IV/IM*	Special Comments and Usage
Amikacin	15 mg/kg	7.5 mg/kg every 12 hr	Good coverage for Gram-negative rods Useful for organisms resistant to gentamicin and tobramycin Consider use in patients with Gram-negative infections with contraindication to aminoglycoside use
Amoxicillin	1–6	0.5–1.0 every 8 hr	Good for group B streptococcus, Streptococcus viridans, S. pneumoniae, and staphylococcus
Ampicillin	2–12	1 every 6 hr	Drug of choice for enterococcus, group B streptococcus, Listeria, and actinomycete Useful for treatment of sepsis in combination with an aminoglycoside and either metronidazole or clindamycin
Aztreonam	1–8	0.5–2 every 8 hr	Good Gram-negative coverage Consider use in patients with Gram-negative infections with renal insufficiency or contraindication to aminoglycoside use

Table continued on following page

Table E–1 □ ANTIBIOTIC STANDARD DOSES AND INDICATIONS FOR PATIENTS WITH NORMAL RENAL FUNCTION *Continued*

Drug	Dosage Range (g/day) IV/IM*	Usual Dosage (g/dosing interval) IV/IM*	Special Comments and Usage
Cefazolin	3–6	1 every 8 hr	Most common preoperative antibiotic Good *Staphylococcus aureus* and *Staphylococcus epidermidis* coverage Moderate streptococcus groups A and B coverage Does not cover enterococcus
Cefotaxime	3–8	1–2 every 6–8 hr	Moderate coverage of streptococcus and staphylococcus, but does not cover enterococcus Useful in meningitis due to Gram-negative rods resistant to ampicillin
Cefoxitin	3–6	1–2 every 6–8 hr	Some staphylococcus and streptococcus coverage, and moderate anaerobic Gram-positive (*Clostridium*) and anaerobic Gram-negative coverage (*Bacteroides fragilis*) with a single agent
Ceftazidime	3–6	1 every 8 hr	Good *Pseudomonas* coverage Consider use when Gram-negative infection and aminoglycosides inappropriate
Ceftriaxone	1–4	1–2 every 12–24 hr	Longer half-life than other cephalosporins Moderate staphylococcus and streptococcus coverage Useful in meningitis due to Gram-negative rods resistant to ampicillin
Cefuroxime	2–4.5	0.5–1 every 8 hr	Mixed lung infections in penicillin-allergic patients *Haemophilus influenzae* resistant to ampicillin Good coverage for streptococcus and staphylococcus except MRSA and enterococcus
Ciprofloxacin	0.4–0.8	200–400 mg every 12 hr	Broad-spectrum agent for urinary tract infections and as adjunct for complicated skin infection; also, good bone penetration 500 mg PO every 12 hr has equal bioavailability as 400 mg IV every 12 hr
Clindamycin	0.6–2	0.6 every 8 hr	Good coverage for anaerobes "above the diaphragm" *B. fragilis* dosing

Drug	Dose*	Notes
Erythromycin	1–4	Drug of choice for *Legionella, Chlamydia, Mycoplasma*
	0.5 every 6 hr	Moderate *S. aureus* and streptococcus groups A and B coverage
		Does not cover *S. epidermidis* or enterococcus
Gentamicin	3–5 mg/kg	Serious aerobic Gram-negative rod infections
	1–1.5 mg/kg every 8 hr	Follow gentamicin levels and creatinine
Imipenem	1–2	Good staphylococcus coverage, except MRSA
	0.5 every 6 hr	Good anaerobic and aerobic enteric coverage
		Consider "big-gun agent"
Metronidazole	1–2	Good Gram-negative enteric coverage
	0.5 every 8 hr	Good for anaerobes "below the diaphragm"
		Well absorbed orally
		Good for pseudomembranous colitis caused by *Clostridium difficile*
Penicillin	2–20 mu	Drug of choice for streptococcal infections
	1–4 mu every 4–6 hr	Good for oral infections, human bites, and anaerobic infections "above the diaphragm"
Piperacillin	6–12	Use for *Pseudomonas* infections
	1.5–2 every 4 hr	Moderate Gram-negative enteric coverage
Tetracycline	1–2	Avoid use in children or pregnant patients, because bone and tooth development
	0.5 every 6 hr	are affected
Tobramycin	3–5 mg/kg	More effective than gentamicin for *Pseudomonas* infection
	1.5 mg/kg every 8 hr	
Vancomycin	1–2	Drug of choice for MRSA
	1 every 12 hr	Useful in multidrug-resistant Gram-positive infections

*Unless otherwise specified.
MRSA = methicillin-resistant *Staphylococcus aureus*; mu = million units.

Table E–2 □ ANTIBIOTIC SUSCEPTIBILITY GUIDELINES (SENSITIVITIES MUST BE CHECKED)

Drug	Aerobes								Anaerobes	
	Pneumococci	Staphylococcus aureus (penicillin resistant)	Haemophilus influenzae	H. influenzae, (ampicillin resistant)	Escherichia coli (community acquired)	Klebsiella	Pseudomonas	Coliforms	Above Diaphragm Excluding Bacillus fragilis	B. fragilis
Amikacin	−	?	−	−	+	+	+	+	−	−
Ampicillin/amoxicillin	+	−	+/+	−	+/+	−	−	±	+	−
Cefazolin	+	+	−	−	+	+	−	±	+	−
Cefotaxime	+	?	+	+	+	+	−	±	?	−
Cefoxitin	+	+	−	−	+	+	−	±	+	+
Ceftazidime	?	?	+	+	+	+	+	+	−	−
Ceftriaxone	+	?	+	+	+	+	−	±	?	−

Antibiotic								
Cefuroxime	+	++	+	+	+	±	+	—
Chloramphenicol	+	++	+	+	+	±	+	+
Ciprofloxacin	—	+	—	—	—	+±	—	+
Clindamycin	+	+±	—	—	—	—	+	+
Cloxacillin	+	+	—	—	—	—	—	—
Co-trimoxazole	+±	±	+	+	+	—	—	—
Erythromycin	+	+	?	?	?	—	—	?
Gentamicin	—	?	+	+	+	+	—	—
Imipenem	+	+	+	+	+	+	+	+
Metronidazole	±	—	—	—	—	—	+	+
Penicillin	+±	—	—	—	—	—	—	—
Piperacillin	+	—	+	+	+	+	++	++
Tetracycline	±	?	+	+	+	±	±	+
Tobramycin	—	+	—	—	—	+	—	+
Vancomycin	+	+	—	—	—	+	—	—

Courtesy of St. Paul's Formulary, St. Paul's Hospital, Vancouver, British Columbia, Canada.
+ + = drug of choice; + = effective; − = not effective; ± = depends on sensitivities; ? = clinical efficacy not proven.

APPENDIX F

PROPRIETARY NAMES OF COMMON MEDICATIONS

Adalat	nifedipine
Aldactone	spironolactone
ALternaGEL	aluminum hydroxide gel
Alupent	metaproterenol sulfate
Amicar	aminocaproic acid
Amphojel	aluminum hydroxide gel
Apresoline	hydralazine hydrochloride
AquaMEPHYTON	phytonadione (vitamin K_1)
Aquasol A	retinol (vitamin A)
Atarax	hydroxyzine hydrochloride
Ativan	lorazepam
Beclovent	beclomethasone dipropionate
Benadryl	diphenhydramine hydrochloride
Bumex	bumetanide
Calan	verapamil hydrochloride
Capoten	captopril
Carafate	sucralfate
Cardizem	diltiazem hydrochloride
Colace	docusate sodium
Compazine	prochlorperazine maleate
Coumadin	warfarin sodium
Cytotec	misoprostol
Demerol HCl	meperidine hydrochloride
Diabinese	chlorpropamide
Dialose	docusate
Diflucan	fluconazole
Dilacor	diltiazem hydrochloride
Dilantin XR	phenytoin sodium
Dulcolax	bisacodyl
Edecrin	ethacrynic acid
Esidrix	hydrochlorothiazide
Gelusil	aluminum hydroxide; magnesium hydroxide; simethicone
Haldol	haloperidol
HydroDIURIL	hydrochlorothiazide
Imitrex	sumatriptan succinate
Inderal	propranolol hydrochloride
Indocin	indomethacin
Isoptin	verapamil hydrochloride
Isordil	isosorbide dinitrate
Kay Ciel	potassium chloride
Kayexalate	sodium polystyrene sulfonate
Lanoxin	digoxin
Lasix	furosemide
Librium	chlordiazepoxide hydrochloride
Lopurin	allopurinol
Lotrimin	clotrimazole

Maalox	aluminum hydroxide; magnesium hydroxide
Metaprel	metaproterenol
Micro-K	potassium chloride
Motrin	ibuprofen
Mycelex	clotrimazole
Mycostatin	nystatin
Mylanta	aluminum hydroxide; magnesium hydroxide; simethicone
Naprosyn	naproxen
Narcan	naloxone hydrochloride
Nilstat	nystatin
Nizoral	ketoconazole
Noctec	chloral hydrate
Normodyne	labetalol hydrochloride
Osmitrol	mannitol
Pentam 300	pentamidine isoethionate
Pepcid	famotidine
Phenergan	promethazine hydrochloride
Phytonadione	vitamin K_1
Prilosec	omeprazole
Procan	procainamide hydrochloride
Procardia	nifedipine
Proventil	albuterol sulfate
Pyridium	phenazopyridine hydrochloride
Quinamm	quinine sulfate
Retinol	vitamin A
Romazicon	flumazenil
Serax	oxazepam
Sinemet	levodopa; carbidopa
Slow-K	potassium chloride
Sorbitrate	isosorbide dinitrate
Tagamet	cimetidine hydrochloride
Thiamine	vitamin B_1
Thorazine	chlorpromazine
Trandate	labetalol hydrochloride
Tylenol	acetaminophen
Valium	diazepam
Vanceril	beclomethasone dipropionate
Vasotec	enalapril maleate
Ventolin	albuterol sulfate
Versed	midazolam hydrochloride
Vistaril	hydroxyzine pamoate
Vitamin A	retinol
Vitamin B_1	thiamine hydrochloride
Vitamin K_1	phytonadione
Xylocaine	lidocaine
Zantac	ranitidine hydrochloride
Zaroxolyn	metolazone
Zyloprim	allopurinol

INDEX

Note: Page numbers in *italics* refer to illustrations; page numbers followed by t refer to tables.

489